KETO ONCOLOGY

A Comprehensive Guide

Jocelyn L. Tan, M.D.

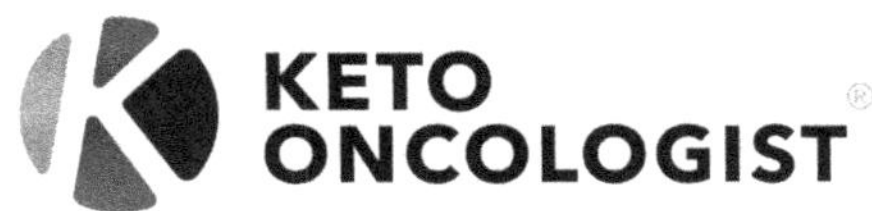

PITTSBURGH, PENNSYLVANIA

2024

Dr. Jocelyn Tan has written an important book that addresses many misconceptions about ketogenic diets and their use for cancer management. The information presented will help both cancer patients and their caregivers understand better the science of ketogenic metabolic therapy, which will eventually become a major therapeutic strategy for the non-toxic management of cancer.

— Thomas N. Seyfried, Ph.D.
AUTHOR OF CANCER AS A *METABOLIC DISEASE, ON THE ORIGIN, MANAGEMENT, AND PREVENTION OF CANCER*

[Keto Oncology] is a sweeping examination of metabolic oncology. Dr. Tan does a wonderful job summarizing the important points for patients interested in understanding this emerging field of cancer therapy.

— Travis Christofferson, MS
AUTHOR OF *CURABLE & TRIPPING OVER THE TRUTH,*
AND *KETONES, THE FOURTH FUEL*
FOUNDER OF THE FOUNDATION FOR METABOLIC CANCER THERAPIES

Dr. Tan shines a light on the predominant feature common to most cancers: a disruption in cellular metabolism. Her simple explanations of complex topics, such as cancer-promoting pathways, help break the science into manageable bits. She references her clinical experience as an integrative oncologist, lending authenticity to her support for repurposed drugs and supplements, metabolic treatments, and powerful nutritional strategies…

— Miriam Kalamian, EdM, MS, CNS
AUTHOR OF *KETO FOR CANCER* AND FOUNDER OF DIETARY THERAPIES LLC

[Keto Oncology] is one book you want to pick up to understand the real Keto Diet and filter out the monetized media hype-filled with misinformation. If you are interested in preventing cancer, getting healthy, or using the keto diet as an adjunct to chemotherapy/ immunotherapy/radiation, [Keto Oncology] is for you. This book is written in a way everyone can read and benefit from…

— Zorica Kurtesevic, RN
VETERAN AFFAIRS PITTSBURGH HEALTHCARE SYSTEM

First Edition was published in April 2024 under the title "The Keto Code."
Second Edition was published in August 2024 under the new title.

Keto Cancer Doctor
1151 Freeport Road #388
Pittsburgh, PA 15238

This book contains advice and information relating to health care. It should be used as a supplement rather than as a replacement for the advice of your doctor or another trained health professional. If you know or suspect you have a health problem, it is recommended that you seek your physician's advice before embarking on any medical program or treatment. All efforts have been made to assure the accuracy of this book's information and internet addresses as of the publication date. The author, entities, and non-entities associated with this work assume no responsibility for the topicality, correctness, completeness, or quality of the information provided. The author, entities, and non-entities associated with this work disclaim liability for any medical outcomes resulting from applying the methods mentioned in this book. This work was published by Jocelyn Tan of Wholesome Ideas LLC in her personal capacity. The opinions expressed in this article are the author's own and do not reflect the view of The United States Department of Veterans Affairs, or The United States government.

Imprint Logo and Cover Design by Sharif El Komi of Komi Studio
Pre-press & Editing by Thomas A. Kilian III of Kilian Enterprises LLC
Partially Edited by Author Connections, LLC
Diagrams used under CC BY-NC 4.0 from Kilian Enterprises LLC unless otherwise stated.

Library of Congress Cataloging-in-Publication Data:
Tan, Jocelyn L.
KETO ONCOLOGY: A Comprehensive Guide
p. cm.
Includes bibliographical references, index, and appendices
Identifiers: ISBN: 978-0-9815827-5-7
Subjects: Diet therapy | Nutrition for Cancer Prevention | Therapeutics | Oncology | Immunotherapy | Nutrition and Holistic Medicine | Pharmacology and Therapeutics | Wellness | Specific therapies and kinds of therapies
Classification: LCC: RM214-258 | DDC 615.8/54—dc23

Printed in the United States of America under the imprint of Keto Oncologist®, a division of Wholesome Ideas LLC • U.S.A. - ID 6972651

This book is dedicated to:

My parents

Contents

PART I: UNDERSTANDING THE SCIENCE BEHIND CANCER

PART II:
TAKING ACTION

Contributors

Author:

Jocelyn L. Tan, M.D.

UNIVERSITY OF PITTSBURGH, CLINICAL ASSOCIATE PROFESSOR OF MEDICINE, VETERAN AFFAIRS PITTSBURGH HEALTHCARE SYSTEM

Contributors:

Apurva K. Pandey, M.D.

OREGON HEALTH SCIENCE UNIVERSITY, ASSISTANT PROFESSOR OF MEDICINE

Arisha Patel, M.D., MBA

SANARE ONCOLOGY, pLLC
ONCOLOGY ASCLEPICIA, pLLC
ADJUNCT FACULTY, STANFORD UNIVERSITY

Christine A. Garcia, M.D., MPH

WEILL CORNELL MEDICINE—NEW YORK PRESBYTERIAN HOSPITAL, ASSISTANT PROFESSOR

Hema Rai, M.D.

UNIVERSITY OF PITTSBURGH, CLINICAL ASSISTANT PROFESSOR OF MEDICINE, VETERAN AFFAIRS PITTSBURGH HEALTHCARE SYSTEM

Mariam Shalaby, M.D.

MOUNT SINAI BETH ISRAEL MEDICAL CENTER

Chaoyuan Kuang, M.D., Ph.D.

MONTEFIORE MEDICAL CENTER, ALBERT EINSTEIN COLLEGE OF MEDICINE, DEPARTMENT OF ONCOLOGY AND MOLECULAR PHARMACOLOGY, ASSISTANT PROFESSOR

Jennifer Carrick, R.N., M.S.

PAREXEL, SENIOR CLINICAL RESEARCH ASSOCIATE

Manuscript Reviewers:

Brittaney-Belle Gordon, M.D.

UPMC HILLMAN CANCER CENTER, DIVISION OF HEMATOLOGY ONCOLOGY

Joseph Tan, M.D.

BON SECOURS MEMORIAL REGIONAL CENTER, MECHANICSVILLE, VA

Kevin A. Quann, M.D., Ph.D.

UPMC HILLMAN CANCER CENTER, DIVISION OF HEMATOLOGY ONCOLOGY, PITTSBURGH, PA

Mujahed Lateef, M.D.

UNITED HEALTHCARE, MEDICAL DIRECTOR, (PHYSIATRIST)

Nadia Shalaby, Ph.D.

AIN SHAMS UNIVERSITY, PROFESSOR, DEPARTMENT OF ENGLISH LANGUAGE AND LITERATURE, CAIRO, EGYPT

Sharif El Komi

KOMI STUDIO, CREATIVE DIRECTOR AND FOUNDER

Thomas Seyfried, Ph.D.

BOSTON COLLEGE, PROFESSOR OF BIOLOGY, GENETICS, AND BIOCHEMISTRY

Tomás Duraj, M.D., Ph.D.

BOSTON COLLEGE, BIOLOGY DEPARTMENT, POST DOCTORAL RESEARCHER

Zorica D. Kurtesevic, R.N.

VETERAN AFFAIRS PITTSBURGH HEALTHCARE SYSTEM

Introduction

Cancer is a scary word. I almost always sense a brief pause when I reveal my profession to new friends and colleagues. As I have continued my training through the years, the word *cancer* no longer instills fear in me but rather interest.

Know your enemy. Cancer has a way of interrupting our busy lives when we least expect it. Learning more about this intruder is the best way to deal with it. By flipping open this book, you have just taken the first step towards fighting cancer, the metabolic way.

Most of us have heard about traditional treatments—surgery, radiation, and chemotherapy.

Early-stage cancers can sometimes be cured by surgery alone. Radiation therapy is added to treatment plans when there is a high possibility of "leftover" cancer after surgery. If surgery is not possible, radiation may be a substitute as the first-line option. Chemotherapy is offered later to "mop up" any cancer cells that may be left floating around in the bloodstream or lymphatics.

For people with more advanced cancers, a cure is still possible for some, but more work is needed. Larger cancers need more extensive surgery. Therefore, chemotherapy is offered upfront to try to shrink a bulky tumor before surgery. This strategy accomplishes two things. A smaller cancer will be easier to operate on, making a cure more likely. Cancer patients will benefit from better outcomes with chemotherapy before operating since the intact blood vessels have not yet been disrupted by surgery, so they can efficiently carry the chemotherapy to the area of concern. Metastatic cancers (cancers that have moved on to other organs) are much more challenging to treat with surgery or radiation; therefore, chemotherapy becomes the first choice. Some metastatic patients can still be cured if the wayward tumors are small, few, and easy to remove. Once the original cancer and the metastases are removed, we add a few months of chemotherapy. For the rest, when a cure is not possible, symptom control and prolongation of life become the main goals.

As a medical oncologist, I spend most of my time treating patients with traditional methods. Many of my early-stage cancers, indeed, have not relapsed after treatment. About half of them, however, do relapse. Our usual rule that "five years in remission equals a cure" isn't always true. Some cancers not only return but also change into aggressive cancers that no longer respond to any chemotherapy.

On rare occasions, I have witnessed metastatic cases disappear entirely with chemotherapy alone. Over seven years later, these patients are still enjoying remission. Surely, there must be some underlying difference in the metabolism of these patients that defies the rules of curability. For these patients, *the reversal of a deeper underlying process* could have played a role.

You may have picked up this book because you or a loved one discovered cancer. You are wondering what the ketogenic diet can do for you. This book is not a recipe book, nor is it a textbook. It is written for the motivated layperson who has little or no medical knowledge yet is interested in learning more about the metabolic side of cancer.

New cancer patients often begin searching for information on alternative treatments. A lot of "complementary cancer therapies" are out there for sale to the public. Some are backed by scientific evidence, while others claim "evidence" but are not legitimate. Some have real benefits "tied in" with the metabolic pathways of cancer.

You will find the names of many metabolically related supplements and new compounds in the corresponding chapters in Part One. This information is for reference only. It is not intended as medical advice or to replace a doctor's care.

The past few years saw the ketogenic diet evolve into a popular weight loss program. It is sometimes advertised as a medical "cure-all." While this is certainly an overstatement, ketogenic diets do have benefits that deserve some serious attention.

The first half of this book explores the history of cancer, its hallmarks, and the basics behind the metabolic theory of cancer. We will dive into dense concepts. This will include Warburg's Hypothesis, cancer's dependence on glucose, glutamine, fatty acid synthesis, and other alternative energy pathways. While Part One in this book features, in the simplest possible terms, some dense, highly technical topic data, Part Two focuses on the ketogenic diet itself—what it involves and how to implement it effectively.

Health professionals wishing to learn more about the metabolic side of oncology might also find this book interesting and valuable. Although medical doctors know the basics about ketosis, most are unaware of the underlying mechanisms for its anti-cancer benefits. In many cases, practitioners confuse nutritional ketosis with *diabetic ketoacidosis* (DKA). These are two entirely separate and different clinical states.

One reason for writing this book is to clear many misconceptions about ketogenic diets (KDs). I want to help others understand more about its science and encourage future research. Near the book's end is valuable information on current ketogenic diet research.

For people without cancer, this book will hopefully help you learn more about metabolism so that you can live longer and healthier lives!

PART I:

Understanding the Science Behind the Cancer

Chapter 1

Cancer Basics

Thinking outside the box: What is the root of cancer?

To defeat cancer, we must first understand what makes it begin and what makes it grow.

Too many people develop cancers despite following what they believe is the ideal lifestyle. They exercise, eat mostly vegetables, avoid meat and fat, and get enough sleep. But they still get cancer. What are they missing?

Many patients receive treatment and then relapse. Why does cancer keep returning? Is there something still fueling its embers?

Just like a burning fire, it might return if you only extinguish the flame. You must also remove any fuel—dry leaves, twigs, or charcoal embers—to prevent it from igniting again. To effectively treat cancer, one must remove the cause of the sustaining energy that it feeds on.

Did you know that years ago, when lifespans were much shorter, cancer was rare?

Cancer cases only began to rise with the development of modern times (Wallis, 2018). According to the National Cancer Institute, 1,918.030 new cases in the United States and 609,360 cancer deaths were expected in the year 2022 (Siegel, *et al.*, 2022, pp. 7-33). Compare this to 2006, when we had 1,399,790 new cases and 564,830 expected deaths (Jemal, *et al.*, 2006).

38.4% of men and women living in the United States will develop cancer in their lifetime (Siegel, *et al.*, 2022, pp. 7-30). Understanding how and why cancers develop can help us pursue the most effective and durable therapies.

The words cancer and tumor:

For our purposes in this book, there are two words that mean the same thing and are used interchangeably: *tumor* and *cancer*. The word *tumor* is a Latin word that means "a swelling" or "lump," while *cancer* comes from the Greek word *karkínos,* which means "crab."

The current state of thinking:

Being a medical oncologist, I routinely offer chemotherapy treatments to my patients. After all, we know these are the 'standard of care,' with ample scientific evidence to back up their usefulness.

Chemotherapy drugs kill cancers by making cells die. They create unstable oxygen molecules called *reactive oxygen species* or ROS. When ROS rise, cells reach a fatal point. Unfortunately, nearby normal cells also suffer.

Patients dislike chemotherapy mainly because of the accompanying side effects. Nausea, fatigue, hair loss, and possibly secondary cancers arising years later are all valid concerns. However, I try to remind them to focus on the side effect that matters—the effect of killing tumors. For frail or elderly patients, we can minimize side effects by reducing doses or tweaking the schedules of chemotherapy cycles to allow longer breaks in between. When side effects are mild, treatments have a greater chance of continuing for many months. It is difficult but not impossible to reach complete remission with chemotherapy, even if one has Stage 4 cancer. I have a handful of patients with Stage 4 cancers who tolerated chemotherapy for at least two years, and they entered complete remissions! We declare someone to be in complete remission when there are no signs of cancer in the urine, blood, or imaging scans. Yet, despite these few successes, complete remission in Stage 4 cases is rare.

Over the past two decades, I've witnessed a boom in new cancer therapies, each seemingly more exciting than the previous. Cancer textbooks have gotten thicker each year. The Food and Drug Administration (FDA) has approved new therapies such as *biologics* and *immune therapy* at record speed. These new drugs initially promised better results with fewer side effects. Unlike traditional chemotherapy, the new drugs focus on blocking rather than poisoning cancer cells' growth signals.

Some *targeted therapies* work by blunting or cutting off specific biochemical signaling pathways that fuel cancers. Examples of these new drugs include *bevacizumab* and *sorafenib*. Both target and block the *vascular endothelial growth factor* (VEGF) pathway—the signals that make new blood vessels. *Vascular* refers to the blood vessels that supply the tumor. *Endothelial* refers to the inside lining of the blood vessels. By targeting VEGF pathways, we essentially shrink the blood vessels supplying the cancer and kill cancers by blocking their blood supply. Bonus benefit: We avoid harming normal cells.

Other *targeted therapies* aim to 'fix' the genetic defects that presumably cause cancers to develop. *Imatinib,* or *Gleevec*, is a drug that targets the *bcr-abl* gene defect of chronic myelogenous leukemia. It is so effective that most patients are expected to have complete remission and live normal lifespans.

We also have immune therapy. *Immunotherapy* trains the immune system to recognize cancers as foreign so that we can naturally destroy them. Immunotherapy attacks cancers without the usual side effects of hair loss, nausea, and vomiting.

When these cancer-directed therapies first appeared on the scene, we hoped to reach a new era of oncology—one that promises cure rather than palliation. Unfortunately, more than two decades later, the promise of a complete cure for all has not materialized. Additional immunotherapy and targeted therapies have improved outcomes, but cures are still rare.

How do environmental causes increase our risk of developing cancer?

Chronic cell stress and inflammation are well-recognized

triggers of cancer. The risk of cancer increases due to our environment—chemicals, radiation, bacterial and viral infections—that can cause cancer. These irritants slowly damage normal cells; while some cells die, the damaged ones repair themselves. Multiple exposures to *smoke, alcohol, chemicals, and/or viral infections* will cause repeated cell recovery followed by repair. At some point, the repair process may 'go bad,' and a cell transforms into a cancerous one. A weakened immune system caused by autoimmune disease, steroids, immunity-suppressing medications, and certain viruses can also increase our risk of cancer.

How do genetic or metabolic defects increase our cancer risk?

Do all cancers have an underlying genetic or metabolic defect? We can explain this phenomenon molecularly by explaining how cells function and get energy.

A normal cell is widely believed to have a 'brain' or 'control center,' officially called the *nucleus*. The nucleus is located near the center of the cell and contains our *deoxyribonucleic acid* (DNA), which holds our genetic information.

Next to the nucleus is the *mitochondrion* (plural—*mitochondria*), considered our cells 'powerhouse' or 'battery.' The process of *respiration* (converting food into energy) is performed inside the mitochondria. We think of cell respiration as breathing, but in biochemistry, mitochondrial respiration refers to the process by which food transforms into useful energy. Respiration keeps cells alive and functioning well. When cancers develop, the nucleus and the mitochondria may develop defects (Gaude, 2014).

The genetic theory:

With the nucleus as the control center or brain of the cell, Hanahan and Weinberg (2011) state that defects begin in the nuclear genes, which cause mitochondrial defects that disrupt energy production (pp. 646-74). Cells with poor energy production become cancer cells.

Warburg, however, believed the opposite. To create cancer, Warburg declared that the actual cancer-causing defect begins from mitochondrial defects and <u>not</u> from nuclear gene defects (Seyfried, *et al.*, 2014). This is also known as Warburg's hypothesis.

How do internal stressors cause metabolism to malfunction, and what does that mean for cancer risk?

Normal cells possess natural antioxidants to protect themselves from damaging ROS. Unfortunately, during the energy-creating process, new *damaging ions* are made. For example, some electrons escape and damage nearby mitochondria during the *electron transport chain* (ETC) process (see page 28). These ions come in *superoxide anions,* ROS, *and hydroxyl radicals.* Soon, these highly charged ions will overpower the antioxidants, leading to serious mitochondrial damage. Amid all this inflammation, the mitochondrial energy output drops drastically and loses its energy charge. Meanwhile, the mitochondria develop new DNA defects and create new cancers.

Despite the defective DNA and energy shutdown, these new cancers somehow survive because they can get their energy elsewhere—from *glycolysis*. Glycolysis is the process by which glucose (usually from food) breaks down and transforms into energy.

Inflammation ➡ Damaged Mitochondria ➡ Cancer

How do external stressors affect cell health and cancer risk?

Many cancers develop after normal cells experience some form of repetitive stress. This stress is typically in the form of repeated exposure to a deadly inflammation or toxic chemical irritant. As cells die, cells also renew. This cyclical repetition of cell death and renewal over time can lead to faulty renewal.

Like a smartphone sent multiple times to the manufacturer for repair, a 'refurbished' product is no longer as good as new. It is the same for us. Our refurbished cells aren't as good as new ones; over time, after multiple 'refurbishings,' cells can develop into cancers.

Smoking and regular alcohol drinking are linked to many cancers. The chemicals in smoke and alcohol can damage cells repeatedly with each use. Therefore, anti-cancer campaigns strongly discourage these two social habits.

What impact does psychologic stress have on the risk of cancer?

Modern society thrives in an atmosphere of stress. Excess

psychologic stress can cause *norepinephrine* (adrenaline hormone) to rise. Yes, psychologic stress can cause cancers, too.

Norepinephrine is a stress hormone produced when we get excited or aroused. It affects our sleep-wake cycle and changes the spleen's *macrophages* (special internal white blood cells). The spleen is the organ found under our left rib cage. Because the spleen is part of our immune system, this internal disruption can cause cancer.

This carcinogenic effect of psychologic stress was seen in experiments of mice that developed liver cancer after stressing them with physical restraints (Jiang, 2019).

Conclusion: Yes, psychologic stress can cause cancer cells to grow.

What are disrupted biologic clocks, and how can they affect cancer risk?

Melatonin is a hormone that helps regulate sleep. It also acts as a powerful antioxidant to protect us against cancer.

Our body has an internal clock. Sleep helps regulate this clock and gives us a refreshed feeling when we wake up. When the sleep cycle is disrupted, melatonin levels drop, and diseases, including cancer, can develop (Gery, 2010). Odd working hours, 'blue light' from electronics, and interrupted sleep are all ways our internal clocks may be disrupted. Night shift workers (e.g., nurses, flight attendants, telephone operators, security guards) have increased cancer risk (Brudnowska, 2011).

What do all cancers have in common?

The Hallmarks of Cancer lists several common cancer characteristics: persistent tumor signaling, evasion from growth suppressors, *angiogenesis* (new blood vessel formation), invasion and metastasis, immortality, and resistance to cell death (Hanahan & Weinberg, 2011, pp. 646-75).

Let's go over these hallmarks.

Hallmarks of Cancer:

A. Persistent tumor signaling

Tumor cells communicate and receive signals or chemical instructions from the surrounding cells. Some signals tell the cancer to grow, move, and invade other body parts. These signals are endless. So, the tumor keeps growing.

B. Evasion of growth suppressors

Normal cells reach maturity and stop growing because growth suppressors tell them so. Cancers have *oncogenes* or cancer-promoting genes inside them, telling them to ignore anti-growth signals from tumor suppressors.

C. Angiogenesis

Angio refers to blood vessels, while *genesis* means to generate or produce. Angio + genesis, therefore, means to make new blood vessels. Like newcomers to a neighborhood, cancers must find food and build their personalized blood vessel network to supply themselves with nutrition.

D. Invasion and metastasis

Cancers like metastasizing, which means moving away and intruding into other organs. The cancer cells accomplish this by riding in the blood or lymph vessels en route to their destination. Early-stage cancers can be silent. They exist in the body, dormant and suppressed by their surrounding microenvironment. Changes in the microenvironment will allow cancers to scavenge and recycle parts of old proteins, carbohydrates, and nucleic acids that fill the cancers with *adenosine triphosphate* (ATP) energy. Once fully charged with ATP energy, cancer cells overcome suppressive forces and leave their home microenvironment. They move (metastasize) to cancer-free areas, implanting new roots and multiply uncontrollably (Hanahan & Weinberg, 2011).

E. Resistance to cell death

Normal cells age and eventually *apoptose* (a form of programmed cell death) or die. Unlike normal cells, cancer cells forget how to die. They lose the pro-death signals that tell cells it's time to break down and make way for new ones. Cancers can also stay alive by escaping immune destruction.

When standard therapies fail to eradicate all cancer cells, any dormant remnants of cancer will eventually resurrect and use any of these special powers to survive.

Chapter Summary/Key Takeaways:

Cancer is a complex disease that has affected countless lives around the world. The incidence and number of deaths remain high despite the development of new therapies. Cancer has many causes, with cell damage and stress often involved. We know that cancer is a manipulative disease and uses multiple strategies to maintain its survival, growth, and multiplication.

End Notes

Brudnowska J, Pepłońska B. Praca zmianowa nocna a ryzyko choroby nowotworowej-przeglad literatury [Night shift work and cancer risk: a literature review]. *Med Pr.* 2011;62(3): pp. 323-38. Polish. PMID: 21870422.

Gaude E, Frezza C. Defects in mitochondrial metabolism and cancer. *Cancer Metab.* 2014 Jul 17;2: p.10. doi: 10.1186/2049-3002-2-10. PMID: 25057353; PMCID: PMC4108232.

Gery S, Koeffler HP. Circadian rhythms and cancer. *Cell Cycle.* 2010 Mar 15;9(6): pp. 1097-1103. doi: 10.4161/cc.9.6.11046. PMID: 20237421.

Hanahan D, Weinberg RA. Hallmarks of cancer: the next generation. *Cell.* 2011 Mar 4;144(5): pp. 646-74. doi: 10.1016/j.cell.2011.02.013. PMID: 21376230.

Jemal A, Siegel R, Ward E, Murray T, Xu J, Smigal C, Thun MJ. Cancer statistics, 2006. *CA Cancer J Clin.* 2006 Mar-Apr;56(2): pp. 106-30. doi: 10.3322/canjclin.56.2.106. PMID: 16514137.

Jiang W, Li Y, Li ZZ, Sun J, Li JW, Wei W, Li L, Zhang C, Huang C, Yang SY, Yang J, Kong GY, Li ZF. Chronic restraint stress promotes hepatocellular carcinoma growth by mobilizing splenic myeloid cells through activating β-adrenergic signaling. *Brain Behav Immun.* 2019 Aug;80: e825-838. doi: 10.1016/j.bbi.2019.05.031. Epub 2019 May 21. PMID: 31125710.

Seyfried TN, Flores RE, Poff AM, D'Agostino DP. Cancer as a metabolic disease: implications for novel therapeutics. *Carcinogenesis.* 2014 Mar;35(3): pp. 515-27. doi: 10.1093/carcin/bgt480. Epub 2013 Dec 16. PMID: 24343361; PMCID: PMC3941741.

Siegel, R. L., Miller, K. D., Fuchs, H. E., & Jemal, A. (2022). Cancer statistics, 2022. *CA: A Cancer Journal for Clinicians*, *72*(1), pp. 7-33. doi: 10.3322/caac.21708

Wallis, C. (2018, April). Coming down from opioids. *Scientific American Magazine*, 318(4), p. 24. doi: 10.1038/scientificamerican0418-24.

Chapter 2

Normal Metabolism

In this chapter, we will discuss normal cell metabolism and learn how disrupted glucose metabolism can contribute to the development and sustenance of cancers. You will also learn about preclinical studies that explain how the metabolic theory can dictate the eventual cancerous fate of a cell.

Before you begin this chapter, please know that this material is packed with details. If you are convinced that the ketogenic diet is for you and are not interested in knowing how and why it works, you may skip directly to your topic of interest in the Table of Contents.

For those of you who are hungry for deeper knowledge, all are welcome to proceed. This chapter features the basic information needed to understand the deeper chapters of this book.

Before I discuss the technical side of cancer metabolism, recall that all food must pass through digestion in the gut, and on the molecular level, it must transform from food into energy.

There are three general types of food:

1. *Carbohydrates:* Examples include starches, such as bread, pasta, potatoes, rice, and all sweets.
2. *Proteins:* Examples include meats, seafood, eggs, cheeses, milk proteins, and soy products.
3. *Fats:* Examples include oils, butter, lard, and cream.

Imagine these three food groups taking three separate highways to their destination—the energy-rich *Krebs cycle.* But they must convert into *acetyl-CoA* (acetyl-coenzyme A) before entering the roundabout, which is the Krebs cycle, as shown in Figure 1. For this chapter, we will discuss only the first highway, *glycolysis*.

Figure 1

Krebs Cycle

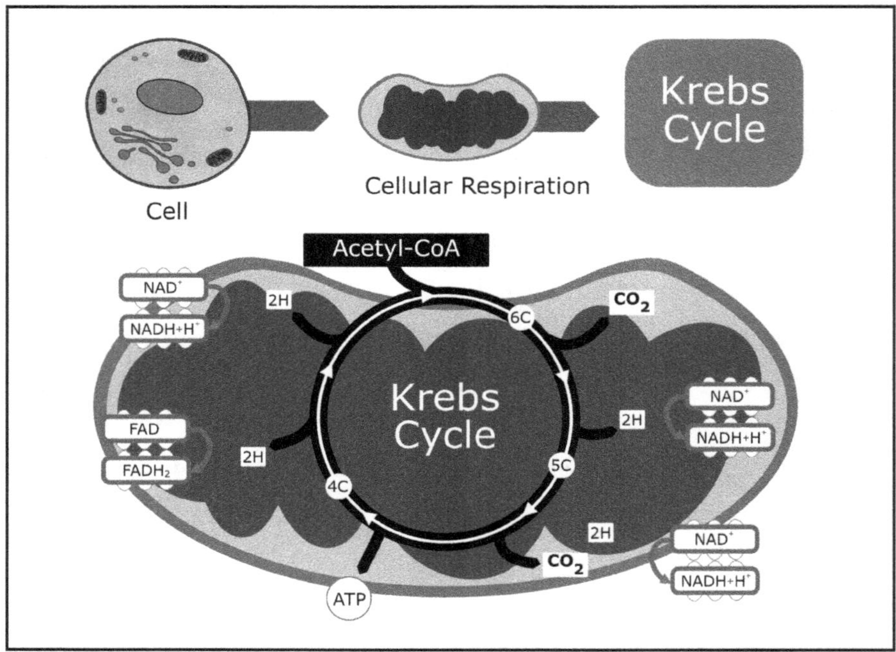

Glycolysis traces the path of carbohydrates or glucose as it transforms into *pyruvate* (simple acid), then acetyl-CoA, which can enter the Krebs cycle and become energy.

What is the role of glycolysis (glucose breakdown) in metabolism? It is a small energy maker.

Glycolysis is the process of breaking down *glucose*—a simple sugar—and turning it into energy. As you can see in Figure 2 (page 24), glucose is at the top of the pathway, and as it passes through the pathway, it changes its form and gets new names. Finally, you will see that it turns into pyruvate at the bottom of the path. Once glucose molecules become pyruvate, they must decide where to go. Pyruvate is an acid that comes from the breakdown of glucose. The pathway from glucose to pyruvate is a series of chemical chain reactions. When the reactions stop, we have pyruvate at the end of the chain. When there is plenty of oxygen, pyruvate will keep going into another set of reactions, as shown in the Krebs cycle (see Figure 1, page 20) and the ETC (see Figure 5, page 26), to make large amounts of energy. However, low oxygen will not make energy but lactic acid, as shown in Figure 6 (Chapter Three, page 42).

Figure 2

Steps of Glycolysis

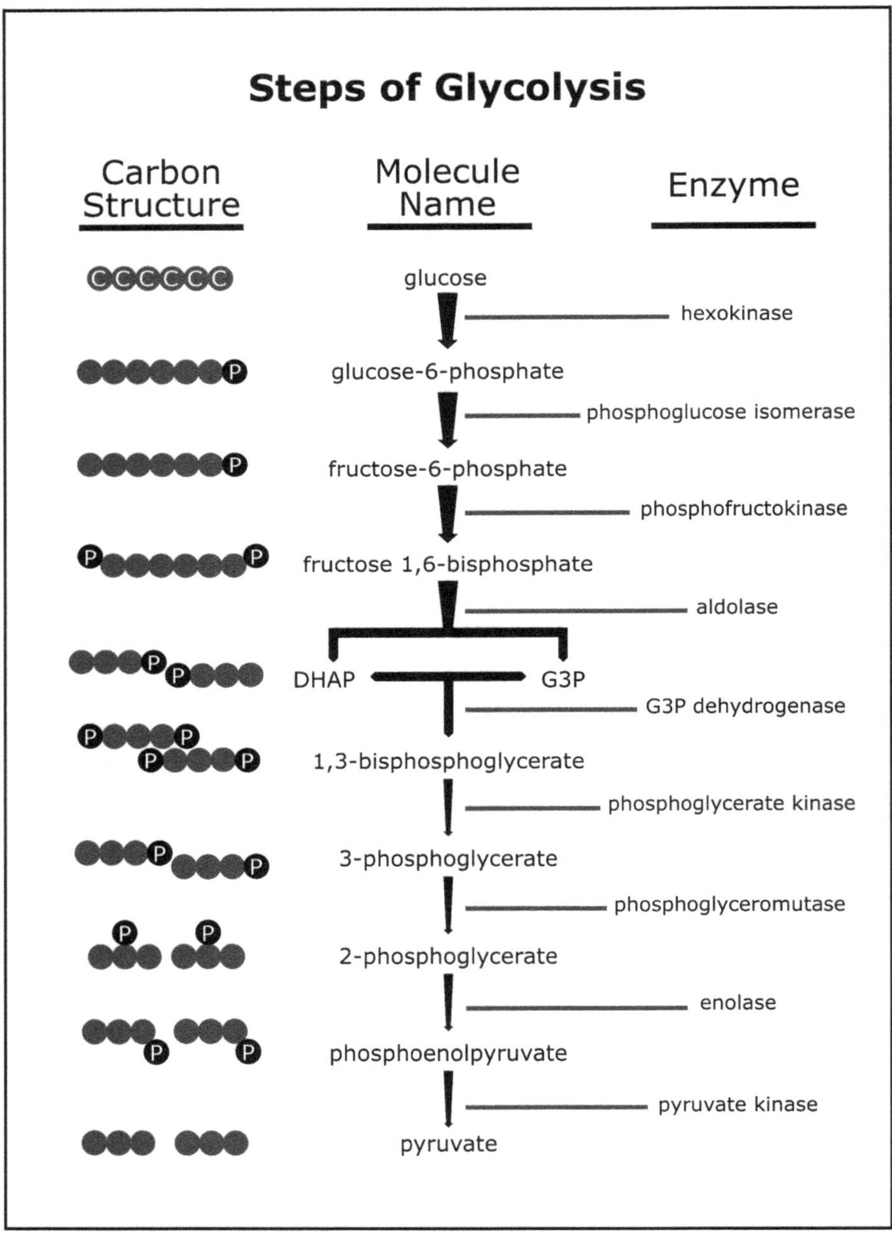
Steps of Glycolysis
Carbon Structure
Molecule Name
Enzyme
CCCCCC
glucose
hexokinase
P
glucose-6-phosphate
phosphoglucose isomerase
P
fructose-6-phosphate
phosphofructokinase
P P
fructose 1,6-bisphosphate
aldolase
P P
DHAP
G3P
G3P dehydrogenase
P P P P
1,3-bisphosphoglycerate
phosphoglycerate kinase
P P
3-phosphoglycerate
phosphoglyceromutase
P P
2-phosphoglycerate
enolase
P P
phosphoenolpyruvate
pyruvate kinase
pyruvate

How do mitochondria function as large energy makers?

Suspended in the *cytoplasm* is the mitochondrion (plural—mitochondria). Mitochondria serve as the cell's 'powerhouses' or 'batteries.'

If you recall, although we typically think of respiration as the act of breathing; however, in biochemistry, mitochondrial respiration refers to the process by which food transforms into useful energy. Our body's biochemical reactions transform food into energy-rich ATP.

When mitochondria are damaged, respiration suffers, and the cell loses much of its energy. Cancers have defective mitochondria, presumed to be the cause of their existence, yet they manage very well (Seyfried, 2014).

Think of mitochondrion as an energy factory. Let's explore the inside to understand how it makes energy. Inside mitochondria, we can find two large 'machines.' One is the wheel-shaped Krebs cycle displayed in Figure 1 (page 20) (the Krebs cycle's main job is to make energy for the living cell). The second machine is a short 'train' called the electron transport chain, ETC, as shown in Figure 5 (page 26) (its job is to connect energy to the Krebs cycle).

Figure 3

Parts of the Mitochondrion

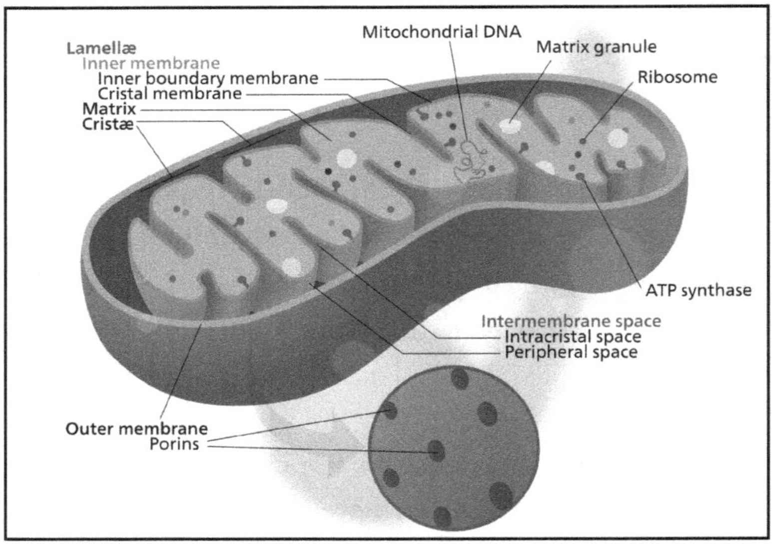

"*File:Mitochondrion structure.svg*," from Wikimedia Commons, CC BY-SA 3.0, (www.creativecommons.org/licenses/by-sa/3.0/). Access for free at https://en.wikipedia.org/wiki/File:Mitochondrion_structure.svg

Figure 4

Citric Acid Cycle

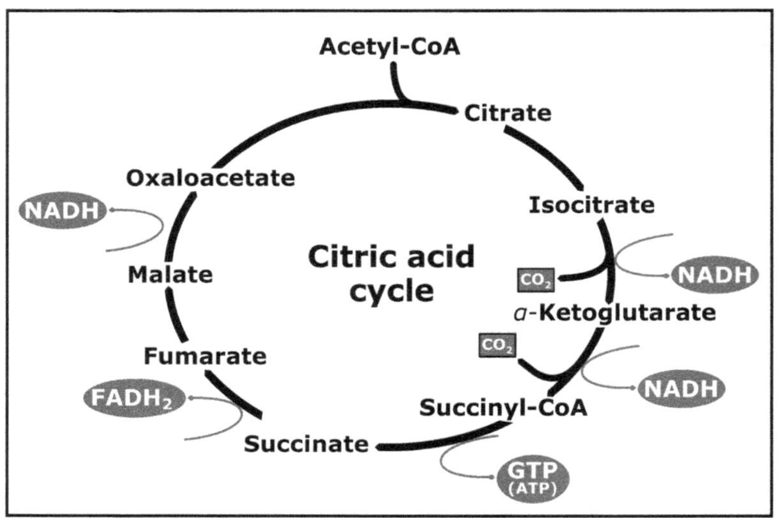

How does the Krebs or citric acid cycle in the mitochondrion produce energy for cells?

Another name for the Krebs cycle is the *tricarboxylic acid cycle* (TCA) because *citrate* is the first step upon entering this process. The Krebs cycle or the citric acid cycle, as displayed in Figure 4 (page 24), is found in the mitochondrial "matrix" (innermost chamber), found in Figure 3 (page 24), of every living cell that uses oxygen to make energy. A set of enzymatic reactions runs the cycle.

Enzymes are proteins that help 'grease' the machines, maintaining and protecting the lines that connect each acid. The cycle is made up of several acids. You know they are acids because their names end with 'ate.' Citrate or citric acid, *Isocitrate,* or isocitric acid, you get the picture.

Beginning with citrate, several reactions happen one after the other in a clockwise fashion, as shown in Figure 4 (page 24). Finally, we make the final acid, *oxaloacetate,* and return to the first citrate step.

Try to picture a ferris-wheel-like structure with many passenger chairs. The 'chairs' represent special molecules—*citrate, iso-citrate, alpha-ketoglutarate, succinate, succinyl-CoA, fumarate, malate*, and *oxaloacetate*. There is no need to remember all these names right now except for *citrate,* which is the first member of this machine, and *alpha-ketoglutarate* or AKG.

Acetyl-CoA is the first, very important molecule entering the Krebs cycle. Think of acetyl-CoA as raw material for energy-making machines. Acetyl-CoA comes from glucose and other food sources (fat, protein, etc.). With every turn of the cycle, our food (carbohydrates, fats, and proteins) will turn into acetyl-CoA, entering this Krebs cycle to produce energy, as Figure 4 (page 24) shows.

Electron transport chain (ETC) + ATP synthase or *OXPHOS*

The ETC is the other high-energy maker. It 'sits' on the inner membrane of the mitochondrion, as shown in Figure 5. The Krebs cycle sends *electrons* to the ETC to make another set of energy 'units'—roughly 30 to 34 units.

Figure 5
Electron Transport Chain

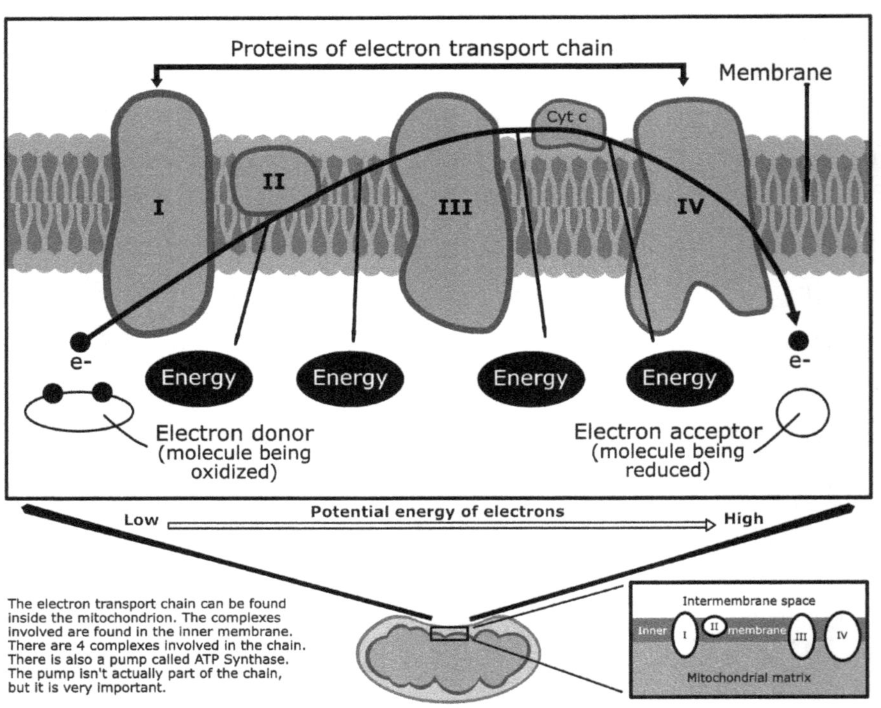
Proteins of electron transport chain
Membrane
Cyt c
I
II
III
IV
e-
e-
Energy
Energy
Energy
Energy
Electron donor
(molecule being
oxidized)
Electron acceptor
(molecule being
reduced)
Low
Potential energy of electrons
High
The electron transport chain can be found inside the mitochondrion. The complexes involved are found in the inner membrane. There are 4 complexes involved in the chain. There is also a pump called ATP Synthase. The pump isn't actually part of the chain, but it is very important.
Intermembrane space
Inner
membrane
Mitochondrial matrix

We need electrons as raw material to feed the ETC. Electrons pass along a string of proteins (*cytochromes*) pulled along an imaginary string. At the end of this string is oxygen. During this passage, the ETC spits out positively charged hydrogen molecules (protons), which pass through the inner membrane, as shown in Figure 5 (page 26). Protons leave the inner matrix chamber and enter the other side, the space sandwiched between the inner and outer membranes.

Think of the mitochondrion like two rubber balloons, one inside the other. The protons are leaving the center of the inner balloon and entering the space between the two balloons. As hydrogen molecules accumulate, this will build pressure in the space sandwiched between the inner and outer mitochondrial membranes.

Soon, the pressure is too much and needs relief, so the mitochondria allow the hydrogen protons to exit through a 'valve' called ATP *synthase*. As hydrogen ions squeeze through the ATP synthase, they propel hydrogen back into the mitochondria's center (matrix), as shown in Figure 5 (page 26). This makes lots of ATP! The process, the ETC plus the energy pressure buildup and hydrogen movement to make ATP, is called *oxidative phosphorylation* (OXPHOS). Scientists discovered that in many cancers, there are defects in the ATP synthase 'valve,' causing a dysfunctional OXPHOS process (Gaude & Frezza, 2014; Viale, *et al.*, 2015).

Looking again at Figure 1 (page 20), as the Krebs cycle turns, it releases 'sparks' of NADH and FADH2—high-energy molecules 'carrying' negatively charged electrons.

This makes a total of 36 (Krebs) units of ATP energy. Let's call this energy pathway the 'roundabout' or OXPHOS to make it easy to remember. If you imagine a road map with glucose traveling on a straight road until it reaches pyruvate and then acetyl-CoA, the acetyl-CoA will enter a roundabout—the Krebs cycle found in Figure 4 (page 24).

Everything explained so far is what goes on in a normal cell. This is very important to know because, as you will soon see, when parts of this fancy metabolic machinery are damaged, cancers may develop.

Chapter Summary/Key Takeaways:

I gave a quick overview of the normal energy-making processes in the cell. This will be very helpful in understanding how cancers develop. Inflammation can create defects in the mitochondria and disrupt our energy-making metabolism. Cancers will follow. The next chapter will reveal the defects in metabolism and how cancers develop because of these defects.

End Notes

Seyfried TN, Flores RE, Poff AM, D'Agostino DP. Cancer as a metabolic disease: implications for novel therapeutics. *Carcinogenesis.* 2014 Mar;35(3): pp. 515-27. doi: 10.1093/carcin/bgt480. Epub 2013 Dec 16. PMID: 24343361; PMCID: PMC3941741.

Gaude E, Frezza C. Defects in mitochondrial metabolism and cancer. *Cancer Metab.* 2014 Jul 17;2: p. 10. doi: 10.1186/2049-3002-2-10. PMID: 25057353; PMCID: PMC4108232.

Viale A, Corti D, Draetta GF. Tumors and mitochondrial respiration: a neglected connection. *Cancer Res.* 2015 Sep 15;75(18): pp. 3685-6. doi: 10.1158/0008-5472.CAN-15-0491. PMID: 26374463.

Chapter 3

Abnormal Glucose Metabolism

For purposes of this chapter, we will discuss glucose metabolism and what goes wrong before cancers develop.

Before we do, here is a quick refresher on what normal metabolism looks like.

We learned that the normal cell makes energy. There is the process of glycolysis, which breaks down glucose (simple sugar) to make energy. Inside the mitochondria is the bigger energy maker, the Krebs cycle, which is connected to the ETC and makes enormous amounts of energy.

Feed the Krebs cycle with raw material (acetyl-CoA), and after several passes through the machinery, our molecules will reach the electron transport chain, where even more energy is made. At the very end, we will have the final product, which contains as much as 36 units of ATP. Compare this to the 2ATP made with glycolysis.

While glycolysis is an energy producer, it uses glucose as raw material to produce less energy.

What goes on during abnormal cancer metabolism?

Before we discuss what's abnormal, be aware that there are at least <u>four</u> different areas of cancer metabolism:

A. Glucose metabolism

B. Glutamine metabolism

C. Fat metabolism (*de novo* fatty acid synthesis)

D. Ketone metabolism

Mess up any of these, and the risk of cancer goes up.

For purposes of this chapter, we will discuss glucose metabolism and what goes wrong before cancers develop.

What is glucose metabolism, and how is it linked to cancers?

Glucose (simple sugar) is a cancer's favorite food. Cancers use glucose for energy. Cancers need many enzymes to do this.

Glycolytic enzymes have many roles in cancer:

1. They 'grease' the glycolysis pathway to make pyruvate.

2. They make energy: 2ATP units.

3. They make lactic acid to surround cancers and help them move.

4. They maintain cell death pathways. Cancers forget how to die.

Let's look at glucose and how it changes within cancer metabolism. Glucose breaks down into pyruvate (simple acid from glucose) through a straightforward pathway. At the end of this pathway, pyruvate has two possible destinations, which are chosen depending on the oxygen levels.

When there is enough oxygen, pyruvate chooses the path toward acetyl-CoA to enter the Krebs cycle and make ATP energy. When oxygen is low, pyruvate chooses the lactic acid path.

Warburg-type cancers, however, do not follow the rules of oxygen. They love low oxygen conditions and keep the lactate going. The pyruvate-to-lactate pathway remains active with the help of oncogenes (pro-cancer genes) like C-MYC and RAS.

This is the ripe scenario: low oxygen, oncogenes, defective OXPHOS, and now, hyperactive glycolysis enzymes.

Glycolysis pathways, active as they are, will only reward cancer with two 'units' of energy, compared to the 34-36 units that come out of the other, more complicated route—acetyl-CoA followed by the Krebs cycle followed by ETC and ATP synthase. (Let's call the Krebs cycle the roundabout.) Since we believe that cancers all have mitochondrial defects, we don't expect them to use the Krebs cycle efficiently. Therefore, they need to use glycolysis. Because glycolysis only gives us two units of energy, cancers must rely on this pathway more frequently to compensate for the lower energy yield. At the end of glycolysis, we will find lactate (lactic acid).

Lactate is more than just an acid. It makes cancers aggressive and mobile. Aggressive, metastatic cancers often have high blood levels of *lactate dehydrogenase* (LDH). We will discuss lactate more in Chapter Four.

What we call "glucose hunger" seems to be a universal feature of cancer (Seyfried, *et al.*, 2014; Martinez-Outschoorn, *et al.*, 2014).

Stop. Did I lose you there? Let me go over the key facts again but in an easier way.

We need food to survive. We change food into energy once we take it inside our bodies. All metabolic pathways that involve food will ultimately connect to the Krebs cycle and the electron transport chain. When we eat carbohydrates, protein, and fat, we must process these foods through these biochemical processes to create energy and building blocks.

Examining the 'road map' version of the metabolism:

The first map represents a normal cell; the highways are green, meaning traffic flows well.

The second map represents cancer. In it, you will find areas of traffic and roadblocks.

At the northern position, you will find the house of sweets, or, in other words, glucose (simple sugar), on the north side of the map.

Imagine a car made of glucose leaving the house of sweets and heading south on the glucose highway. This highway is where we process and break down glucose.

At the end of the road, the vehicle reaches a point where it must either turn east towards Acid City (lactic acid) or try to enter the ramp that leads into the circular highway or Route 36 (Krebs cycle).

If the car follows the straight path down, it will find a rest station, the letter *P*, where a farmer sells pies. Pay attention because this is where Pyruvate is, the last stop on the glucose highway (glycolysis). After this rest stop, the car that visited Pyruvate must make a couple more turns before entering the ramp that leads into the roundabout (Krebs cycle). Every time it travels one revolution around Route 36's roundabout (Krebs cycle), a moderate amount of energy for fuel. However, only tiny amounts of energy will be picked up each time the car rides through Warburg Avenue.

The Warburg side street is pointed to the east. This side street or pathway will eventually end at Acid City (lactic acid). Not all 'sugar cars' will enter the roundabout because some will decide to detour to the Home of Acids (Intersection A [see page 39].

Meanwhile, you will see another busy green street called Protein Alley at the four o'clock position. If the car follows this green street or pathway, it will end up at the meat packer's home. It will be glutamine there. Glutamine is part of a protein. The car will then discover the *pyruvate dehydrogenase kinase* (PDK) enzyme at point *X*.

The roads in red are traffic-congested pathways. When cancer strikes, the entryway into the roundabout (the Krebs cycle) becomes inactive with traffic. Cancers can no longer make energy, so they turn east into Warburg Avenue and head toward Acid City. While traveling through Warburg Avenue, cancers can pick up some 'small change'—tiny packets of energy. They need a lot of energy; therefore, cancers take the glucose highway—Warburg Avenue path—often.

P = Pyruvate

X = Pyruvate kinase enzyme

A = Entry ramp into the Krebs cycle

Remember, Warburg Avenue leads to Acid City, where there is a lot of lactic acid or lactate. Lactate helps make cancers more mobile and prone to metastases.

At the two o'clock position, a small side street, Slippery Road, leads to the Land of Fats—the *fatty acid synthesis* (FAS) or fat-making pathway. Slippery Road becomes very active when cancer reprograms the energy machines to increase traffic in this direction.

Cancers use this Slippery Road to make new fats (yes, cancers can make fats, but not eat them) to make building material for more cancer cells. Sometimes, glutamine enters the roundabout at the four o'clock ramp and goes up to reach Slippery Road.

This map does not include the Mega Energy Warehouse (the ETC), where we make most of our cellular energy. It is nowhere on the map because we don't have a functional road to get there. Unfortunately, these roads are blocked off by cancer. Oil is needed to run the car, but now it will use enzymes instead of oil to make the travel smooth through the roadmap.

If you understand this simple lay explanation, you can dive into the next section.

How do we know if our cancer is glucose-hungry?

Cancer's hunger for glucose is often visible on a *positron emission tomography* (PET) CT scan. This scan uses glucose tagged to a radioactive tracer. Both slow and fast-growing cancers are visible based on their ability to attract glucose. Cancers that rapidly eat glucose will appear very bright in the final images, while slower-growing tumors will appear less intense (color intensity like background tissue) (Travaini, *et al.*, 2007).

Patients must fast for at least six hours before a PET scan because when blood glucose is high, the heart and skeletal muscles absorb some of that glucose, and the tumor image quality will suffer. Therefore, fasting improves images (Travaini, *et al.*, 2007).

The enzyme that changes pyruvate into lactic acid is called *lactate dehydrogenase* or LDH. When glucose breakdown is very active, the LDH is high. There is a blood test that your doctor can order (serum LDH), which, if high, may mean your cancer is very actively using up glucose.

Overactive glycolytic enzymes

Okay, we now know there are overactive glycolytic enzymes (enzymes that make cancers break down glucose). What else is involved?

Warburg believes cancers have faulty mitochondria. When mitochondria get damaged, we cannot go through 'Route 36' in the Krebs cycle, which eventually leads to ETC or OXPHOS.

Because defective mitochondria cannot benefit from OXPHOS energy, they must look elsewhere for energy to survive. They develop new but abnormal genes—oncogenes. Oncogenes are pro-cancer genes. Famous examples are C-MYC and RAS. These oncogenes over-activate the enzymes of glycolysis so that glucose can make 100 times more lactate and energy than usual.

Three enzymes are worth mentioning:

A. Hexokinase (HK)

B. Phosphofructokinase (PFK)

C. Lactate dehydrogenase (LDH)

Aggressive cancers often have excessive amounts of these enzymes (Justus & Sanderlin, 2015).

Special mention goes to *hexokinase* (HK) because it has a special mission: deactivating the BAK, BAD, and BAX cell death pathways (see page 50), thereby allowing cancers to almost live forever.

The fourth overactive enzyme in glucose metabolism is the PDK.

This part is getting technical, but please bear with me. It's important. To understand how PDK helps cancers, you need to know pyruvate.

What do we need to know about pyruvate? Pyruvate is a step near the end of the glycolysis (the glucose breakdown) pathway, located right before glucose turns into acetyl-CoA, heading into the Krebs cycle and then OXPHOS. Pyruvate sits with the PDK enzyme.

Remember the road map? Pyruvate is the rest station located at the end of the glucose highway but before the ramp to enter the roundabout (Krebs cycle). OXPHOS (regular energy making) and glycolysis (smaller amount of energy from the breakdown of glucose) make the crossroads. Once your food turns into pyruvate, it has a fate's choice. Either enter the pathway towards acetyl-CoA, then go into the roundabout (Krebs cycle) and then to the crossroads (OXPHOS) to make energy (Route 36). Or turn towards glycolysis to break down glucose into lactate (Route 2) headed to Acid City, or even *gluconeogenesis* (GNG) to make more glucose.

The part where the glucose car reaches the entrance ramp but instead turns east towards Acid City to make lactic acid? Cancers like to go 'down south' through the glucose highway, then follow the pathway going East (Warburg Avenue) towards lactate because lactate provides energy and helps cancers invade and spread to other places (metastasize).

Two more enzymes are involved to allow cancers this freedom of choice between lactate or OXPHOS. The first is *Pyruvate dehydrogenase* (PDH), known as the 'gate.' I call it the 'helper.' PDH helps pyruvate become acetyl-CoA and enter OXPHOS. PDH turns pyruvate into acetyl-CoA to keep the good energy flowing. Cancers don't want a good energy flow because they would rather use the energy that comes from sugar. Therefore, cancers rely on the second enzyme, PDK, to block or 'kill' the PDH (helper of OXPHOS). With PDH gone, cancers can no longer use pyruvate to make acetyl-CoA.

As you can see, these two enzymes—PDH and PDK—work together. They act as a control valve to maintain traffic. We want some level of glycolysis and OXPHOS, but not too much. Cancers, however, want to sabotage this traffic control and divert traffic to lactate.

Overactive PDK enzymes

The gatekeeper, PDH, controls whether pyruvate makes lactate with the glycolysis pathway or enters OXPHOS to make lots of energy.

Cancers with high PDK can block PDH and, therefore, the traffic into OXPHOS, too. Pyruvate must make a detour towards glycolysis and lactate. PDK makes defective death pathways to allow cancers to live. Aggressive cancers bear a lot of PDK enzymes.

Dichloroacetate (DCA) is an experimental drug that can fight cancer by attacking the PDK enzyme. Pyruvate no longer must be forced into glycolysis, and PDK reopens the pathway to OXPHOS. The glycolytic-loving cancer will revert to normal OXPHOS metabolism (Lian, *et al.*, 2015).

Why do cancers hate oxygen?

As cancer cells multiply and crowd each other, oxygen becomes scarce, and HIF-1 proteins come alive. The letters HIF stand for *hypoxia-inducible factor.* Hypoxia is a state of low oxygen. We know that low oxygen triggers cancer growth signals. Therefore, HIF-1 is considered a "switch" that turns on cancers, as shown in Figure 6 (page 42).

We currently have no FDA-approved drugs targeting HK, PFK, or LDH. However, becoming familiar with these enzyme names is still a good idea if you search for clinical trials.

We want to try to avoid activating the HIF-1 protein. Smoking causes low oxygen conditions or hypoxia. Hypoxia triggers HIF-1, which promotes cancer signals. Avoid smoking to avoid hypoxia!

Figure 6
HIF1a

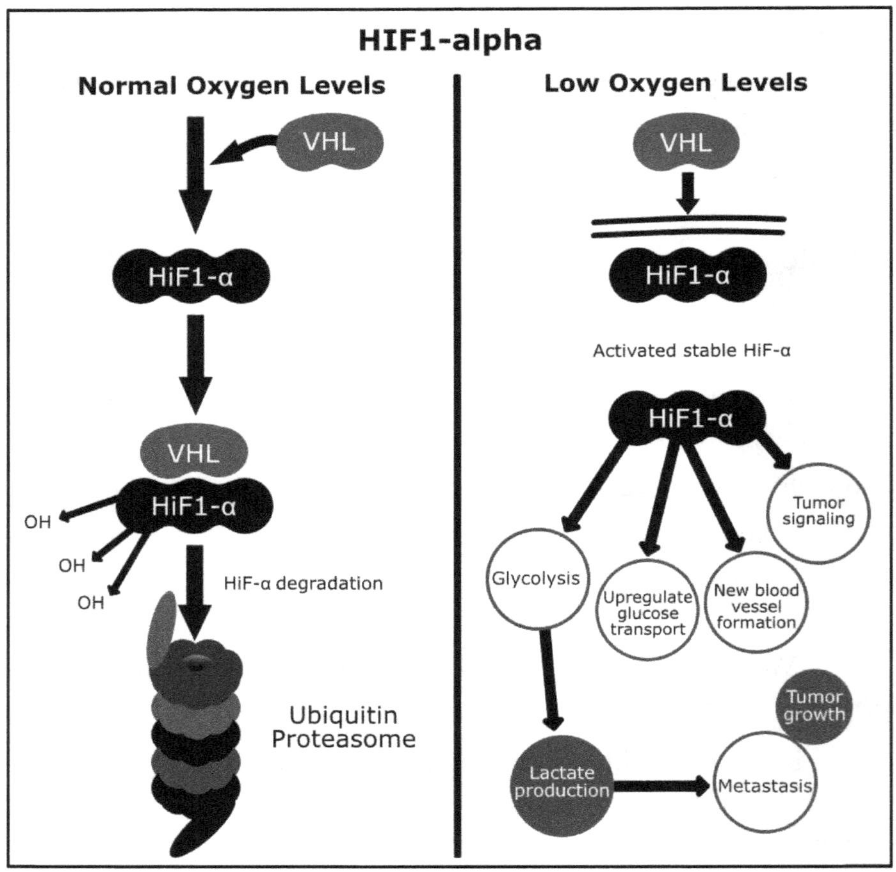

Potential metabolic therapies:

Below are some drugs and supplements that help fight cancer by targeting these defective metabolic areas.

A. 2-deoxy-D-glucose (2DG)

2DG is a glucose look alike. It is also known as a HK inhibitor. HK is the first enzyme in the glycolysis pathway. 2DG can block this by acting as a 'dummy' instead of the real glucose molecules. Since 2DG is not glucose, it cannot be metabolized in the same way as glucose. If present, 2DG can seriously slow down the rest of the glycolytic pathways, making it highly effective in limiting glucose to cancers. Still, at high doses, 2DG can be very toxic to the brain (Zhang, *et al.*, 2014). It isn't commercially available to the public.

B. 3-bromo-pyruvate (3-BrPA)

3-BrPA also targets the glycolysis pathway. 3-BrPA looks very similar to two of the acidic members of the glycolysis pathway. These two are *pyruvic acid* (pyruvate) and lactic acid (lactate). Just like 2DG, 3-BrPA is very effective in blocking the HK enzyme. How does 3-BrPA do this? 3-BrPA looks for the glycolysis controller enzyme protein called *glyceraldehyde 3-phosphate dehydrogenase* or GAPDH. GAPDH is one of the main enzymes that grease the glycolysis pathway. Once located, 3BPA can 'squeeze itself into and bind to' (i.e., alkylate) the active protein of the GAPDH and disable it. With GAPDH down, we block the HK enzymes and stop glycolysis, so cancers lose access to ATP energy and die (Konstantakou, *et al.*, 2015).

For cancer, this is a major crisis. ATP energy shutdown will also mess up several pro-cancer signals: Akt/ FOXO, mTOR, AMPK, MAPK, ERK, and BCL2JNK (to name just a few). 3-BrPA is so effective that it helps stop cancers with mutated BRAFV600 and KRAS cancer proteins (Konstantakou, *et al.*, 2015)!

As a bonus, 3-BrPA also blocks the cancer-loving fat-making pathway called *de novo fatty acid synthase*. Glucose pathways link to the fat pathway by using the molecule acetyl-CoA. 3-BrPA directly foils acetyl-CoA production by acting as a great impersonator of pyruvate. The real pyruvate can become acetyl-CoA, but not 3-BrPA. Acetyl-CoA is important because it sits at the main intersection of our glucose, fat, and protein metabolic pathways. In summary, 3-BrPA prevents us from having a good supply of acetyl-CoA. Because this central loss leads to a work stoppage of the multiple processes that fuel cancer (glycolysis, fatty acid synthesis, and even glutaminolysis), cancers will die. So far, 3BPA is very effective in killing cancer because it can make tons of damaging oxidants; however, it is also highly toxic to normal cells and, therefore, not available for medical use, at least not yet (Byrne, *et al.*, 2014).

C. Koningic acid (KA) or heptelidic acid

KA is a natural antibiotic/antiparasite that acts like

3-BrPA. KA inhibits glycolysis and HK by targeting GAPDH. It is effective against thyroid, colorectal, lung cancers, and leukemias (blood cancers). In thyroid cancers, KA has stopped cancer growth by blocking BCL2 without toxicity to the liver or kidneys (Jing, *et al., 2022*).

D. MicroRNA-199a-5p

MicroRNA-199a-5p is another HK inhibitor that can attack the noncoding areas of HK and limit cancer growth. Unfortunately, scientists are having trouble making this into a drug for public consumption (Guo, *et al.*, 2015).

E. Metformin

Metformin is a popular antidiabetic drug, has anti-hexokinase effects, and controls cell death pathways. It is active in lung, ovarian, liver, and other cancers. However, its clinical potency against cancers appears to be mild. Clinical trials are using high-dose metformin in combination with other treatments to help improve outcomes (Rio, *et al.*, 2013; Simcikova, *et al.*, 2021; Mathupala, *et al.*, 2006).

F. Benitrobenrazide (BNBZ)

BNBZ was studied in mouse models carrying human pancreatic adenocarcinoma cells. It appears to stop cancers by binding to HK. BNBZ has also shown high potency with very little toxicity (Zheng, *et al.*, 2020).

G. Euxanthone

Euxanthone, an ingredient found in the Chinese medicinal plant *Polygala caudata*, showed anti-cancer effects in mice models of epithelial ovarian cancer with few side effects noted. Euxanthone appeared to cause mitochondrial destruction and stopped glycolysis through HK inhibition (Zou & Wang, 2018). In liver cancer (hepatocellular carcinoma), blood caspase levels are usually low. We need caspase to fight inflammation. Euxanthone has anti-cancer properties through the help of antioxidant caspase enzyme activity and promotes cell death through the process of pyroptosis (Chen, *et al.*, 2018).

H. Dichloroacetate (DCA)

DCA is a PDK blocker. As mentioned earlier, DCA is a drug that can stop glycolysis. There is a lot of talk on social media regarding the drug. DCA stops the PDK enzyme by killing or blocking the PDK. With PDK gone, PDH (the helper) can help pyruvate change into acetyl-CoA and enter OXPHOS instead of glycolysis.

What happens next? Glycolysis stops, and lactate levels drop. This starves cancer. Pro-death factors (apoptotic factors) and hyperactive oxygen molecules rise. This makes conditions toxic for cancer, to kill them faster (Tataranni & Piccoli, 2019).

Bottom line: DCA tries to make cancer cells 'return to a normal lifestyle' and stop using sugar by allowing OXPHOS to run again, shutting down the path to glycolysis.

Another benefit of DCA is how lactate production will slow down. We know cancers use lactate for metastasis, and some feel it is also a fuel. By using DCA to force the mitochondria's metabolism to change from glycolysis into OXPHOS, we also reactivate the death pathways (i.e., BAK, BAD, and BAX [see page 49]), hopefully killing the cancer.

DCA is also a drug used to treat mitochondrial diseases that make too much lactic acid and is a byproduct of chlorine. Yes, we can find traces of DCA in our drinking water! In the past, it was used to treat diabetes. It is still considered a hazardous chemical and used only in the laboratory. Despite its anti-cancer activity in prostate, non-small cell lung cancers, glioblastoma, and breast cancer, DCA is not FDA-approved for cancer therapy. It also has activity against cancer stem cells but presents no side effects for normal cells. It is available for lab use, but to be effective for cancer, we need high doses. Unfortunately, in higher doses, DCA is too toxic (i.e., causes nervous system damage and death) to be used in clinical practice. There is also concern that DCA can be carcinogenic and may cause solid tumors such as liver cancer (Sutendra, *et al.*, 2013).

Interest in this pathway, however, is still alive. There are currently over a dozen potential PDK inhibitors under clinical study.

I. Ketogenic diets (KDs)

KDs fight cancers by lowering blood glucose and *insulin growth factor-1* (IGF-1), signaling and limiting *glucose transporter proteins* (GLUTs) numbers (Groleau, *et al.*, 2014). KDs also lessen the damaging effect of inflammation on mitochondrial respiration.

Where do cancers get energy if their mitochondria are defective?

Substrate-level phosphorylation (SLP) is mentioned in many scientific articles on cancer metabolism. SLP is very active in cancers as it means making ATP outside of OXPHOS or 'Route 36.'

Remember, OXPHOS is in mitochondria. SLP involves adding one phosphate group to two phosphate groups—*adenosine diphosphate* (ADP)—to make three *adenosine-triple-phosphate* (ATP). Instead of going through the Krebs cycle, using the ETC/OXPHOS energy pathway or 'Route 36', we are using other materials and making ATP energy through the 'backroads.' This is displayed in Figures 7 and 8 (page 55).

Many cancer cells have limited access to ATP energy and cannot make ATP via the Krebs cycle and OXPHOS (Route 36). Cancers use glucose and SLP to survive. One example of SLP is using glycolysis. Another example of SLP is using glutamine through the *glutamine glutamate alpha-ketoglutarate pathway (*α-Ketoglutaramate or AKG). Both are forms of SLP. One uses glucose, while the other pathway uses glutamine to make ATP outside of the Krebs cycle.

How do defective death pathway proteins keep cancers immortal?

Normal aging cells eventually die and are replaced by new ones. Cancers, however, know how to escape death. The glycolytic enzymes have one more contribution to cancer: they can deactivate anti-cell death (apoptosis) pathways. This is a case of a deactivator deactivating another deactivator.

We all have inbuilt programs that send instructions to our cells as we age. One of these programs includes the apoptosis or 'pro-death pathways.'

Old, defective cells reach a point when the pro-death pathways kick in, and the aging cell naturally dies, allowing new cells to replace them.

Cancers don't follow the rules. They multiply almost endlessly because they developed gene mutations that inactivated their ability to die. In chronic myelogenous leukemia, the BCR-ABL oncogene is one known cause of apoptosis.

HK is the first glycolytic pathway enzyme and is plentiful in cancers. HK can dampen the death pathways and allow cancers to live. This is another good reason to avoid sugar!

Alert: Technical material ahead.

BAD, BAX, and BAK proteins control the death pathways. An easy way to remember these proteins is by the ominous way they are each named:

- BAD = Bcl-2-Associated *Death* protein
- BAX = Bcl-2-Associated *X* protein
- BAK = Bcl-2-Associated *Killer* protein

These proteins keep cancers alive, mobile, and productive (Kim & Dang, 2005).

HK works closely with a *serine/threonine-protein kinase* (AKT) (another enzyme protein). HK uses AKT to 'relocate' itself from the *cytosol*, traveling to the *mitochondria*, where it connects to a special 'channel' on the outer mitochondrial membrane called the *voltage-dependent anion channel* or VDAC.

The VDAC controls the opening and closing of the pore (opening) through which the BAD, BAX, and BAK anti-cell death proteins pass (Cytochrome C).

This peculiar marriage between HK and VDAC will deactivate the apoptosis or 'death pathways.' Without an active death pathway, cancers can become immortal, losing the ability to die.

AKT can cause further damage by activating the mTOR signaling pathway, which feeds cancer and prevents programmed cell death or *autophagy*. This could be a target for a new anticancer drug. However, drug discovery programs are still working hard on this topic.

Potential metabolic therapies:

1. *MK-2206* is a drug that blocks the AKT protein (death pore protein) and has activity against stomach and ovarian cancer cells in the lab (Nitulescu, *et al.*, 2018).

2. *Epigallocatechin-3-gallate* (EGCG), an anticancer extract found in green tea, appears to block both HK and *phosphofructokinase* (PFK), the second glycolytic enzyme. It also deactivates the death pathway by meeting the BAD (Bcl-2-Associated Death) protein. EGCG in green tea might block PFK and HK and push cancers into the death pathway (Li, *et al.*, 2016).

3. *Sinomenine acutum*, an extract from a Chinese medicinal plant, has anti-hexokinase activity. In laboratory cell cultures of non-small cell lung cancer, *sinomenine* effectively slowed cancer growth (Liu, *et al.*, 2020).

What are lesser-known side streets that supply building blocks to cancers?

A. The pentose phosphate side pathway (PPP)

Glucose-loving cancer cells grow fast and multiply. They need lots of energy, and aside from getting energy from the glycolysis pathway, they also use another 'side pathway.'

This side pathway, PPP, branches out early from glycolysis (glucose breakdown) and produces two important products. One is NADPH, and the other is a sugar called *ribose 5-P* or *pentose.* Both are used to make fats, which cancers need as building blocks to grow. The PPP also helps build nucleotides, building blocks for more DNA. We cover this in detail in Chapter Five.

B. Insulin-related pathways

When blood glucose rises, the pancreas produces the hormone *insulin*. Think of insulin as the butler of your body (house). When sugar arrives at your door, the insulin butler helps lead your sugar to where it is needed.

Another hormone similar to insulin is *insulin growth factor-1* (IGF-1), which resembles insulin. Think of IGF-1 as your second butler. Because it is a growth factor, IGF-1 encourages cancers to grow and multiply. IGF can also control cell death so cancers will not die. Many cancers of the prostate, lung, and colon have high levels of IGF-1.

Finally, on the surface of cells, there is a protein called the IGF-1 receptor. IGF-1 needs to 'dock' with this receptor before it can do any work. Once the IGF-1 'locks' into place with its 'docking station,' the receptor, the cell stops growing and goes into a slower phase, called the *S phase*. The *S phase* is when the cell cycle pauses to allow duplication of genetic DNA material (Grimberg, 2000; Giovannucci & Cohen, 1999).

Cancers don't always grow and multiply. The *S* phase is necessary for cancers because they get a chance to make copies of their genes before the cell splits into two.

IGF-1-rich cancers often have abundant IGF-1 receptors, and as a result, there is accelerated cell growth and turnover.

How can we stop IGF-1?

A drug that targets the IGF-1 receptor would be nice. Ketogenic diets (KDs) can lower insulin growth factor levels and GLUTs (Groleau, *et al.*, 2014).

C. Excess GLUTs, Genes, and Signaling Pathways

Glucose enters cells with the help of GLUTs, which are found on cell membranes and allow glucose to enter the cell. GLUTs are the glucose gateways on the cell. Cancers want lots of glucose. They use pro-cancer oncogenes to help increase the number of gates. Oncogenes send signals via signaling pathways to increase the number of GLUTs (Kuo, *et al.*, 2019). MYC is probably the most popular and well-known oncogene to many cancer doctors. It earns itself a badge as a GLUT1 promoter (Nagarajan, *et al.*, 2016).

MYC uses the *phosphoinositide 3-kinase* (PI3K/Akt)—a protein kinase—signaling pathway. PI3K/Akt (extracellular signal-regulated kinase and phosphatidylinositol-3-kinase) stimulates glucose transporters GLUT 1, 2, 3, and 4.

Look for clinical trials that target PI3K/Akt pathways. Currently, we have some already approved for clinical use in certain cancers. *Alpelisib*, or *Piqray*, is a PI3K inhibitor, FDA-approved for breast cancers and some *B-cell* blood cancers.

We also have genes that block GLUTs. The opposite of oncogenes is tumor suppressor genes such as TP53 (tumor protein 53), which help protect us against cancers. Tumor suppressors will stop or limit GLUTs. However, many people with defective tumor suppressors, such as TP53-mutated genes, lose the tumor suppressor protection and are at higher risk of developing more aggressive cancers that fail to respond to therapy (Sano, *et al.*, 2011).

Another pro-cancer pathway, called the *IkappaB kinase complex* (IKK) and *nuclear factor kappa B* (NF-κB) pathway, likes to boost the GLUT numbers.

The TP53 gene can normally help us by stopping the IKK NF-κB pathway. However, many cancers have defective or mutated TP53s, allowing IKK NF-κB to favor the GLUT transporters, helping glucose enter easily. NF-κB adds more damage by protecting cancer cells from the toxic effects of chemotherapy.

Why am I showing you all these little pathways? It is important to see how complex the pathways are. It isn't simply glucose heading straight to feed cancers. There are many players, like in a football game with twists and turns.

What are the possible 'future drugs'? Here are some potential therapies in Research & Development. To be clear, research in this field doesn't excite me yet. In case you are

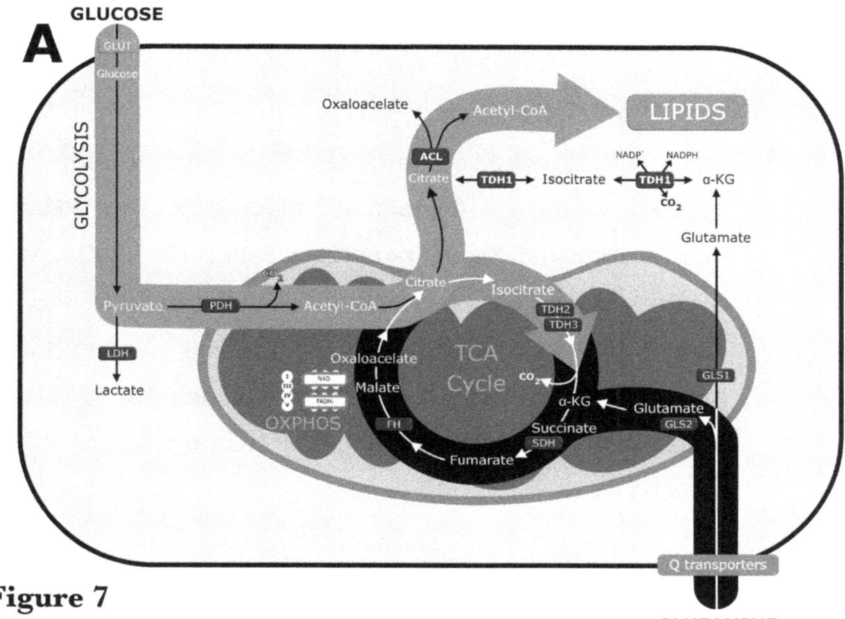

Figure 7

Normal Metabolic Pathways

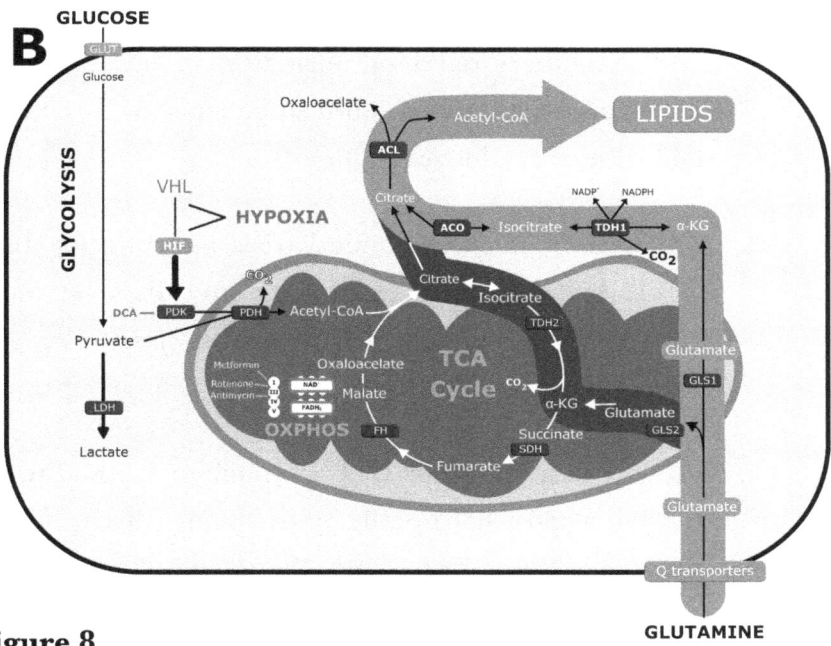

Figure 8

Abnormal Pathways Seen In Cancer—glycolysis, lipid pathway and glutamine pathways (SLP)

searching for clinical trials, I include these only for your information.

1. *AMG 479 (ganitumab)* (anti-IGF-1) is an antibody that appears to have some activity against neuroendocrine, neuroectodermal, and pancreatic cancers. Trials were begun by Amgen in pancreatic cancer, in addition to gemcitabine chemotherapy. There was a trend for improved six months beyond survival, but the trial was unfortunately abandoned in 2012 (Kindler, *et al.*, 2012, e2834-42).

2. *Figitumumab* (an anti-IGF-1) is another example that was studied pre-clinically. It is an antibody that targets the insulin-like growth factor receptor. Unfortunately, a few years ago, figitumumab research stopped after a non-small cell lung cancer trial showed poor results (Arcaro, 2013). Another trial used this drug in adrenocortical cancer, and eight out of fourteen patients (57%) enjoyed stable disease (Haluska, *et al.*, 2010).

3. *IKK inhibitors.* Look for clinical trials targeting the IKK NF-κB pathways. An example is the IKK inhibitor *PS1145*, which has some activity against nasopharyngeal cancer (Lung, *et al.*, 2019).

4. *BAY-876* is a synthetic GLUT1 inhibitor shown to be effective against hepatocellular carcinoma (liver cancer). When injected directly into the bloodstream, serious brain and muscular toxicities were expected because these

organs, like the liver, also have high levels of GLUT1. However, when injected directly into liver cancers of mice, BAY-876 spread slowly outside of the tissue and had few side effects. This drug could be a future option for liver cancers treated with chemotherapy applied directly to the cancer (*transarterial chemoembolization* or TAC) (Yang, *et al.*, 2021; Schwartzenberg-Bar-Yoseph, *et al.*, 2004; Ma, *et al.*, 2018).

5. *Resveratrol*, a substance found in red grape skins and statin drugs (anti-cholesterol), can help starve cancer by blocking GLUT 1, 3, and 4 (Ako, *et al.*, 2021).

D. Glycogen related pathways

Glycogen is a storage form of glucose. Excess glucose is packaged into glycogen and stored in our liver and muscles for future use. When we need glucose, we can get some of this stored glycogen and release glucose for energy. Interestingly, certain aggressive cancers, such as clear-cell kidney cancer, clear-cell breast, osteosarcoma, and cancers with peritoneal metastases, are linked to accelerated glycogen breakdown. Glycogen itself is a fuel that facilitates the metastatic spread of cancers. Therefore, targeting these glycogen-related pathways might be a novel way to fight these aggressive cancers (Khan, *et al.,* 2020). See Figure 9 (page 58).

Figure 9

Glycogen

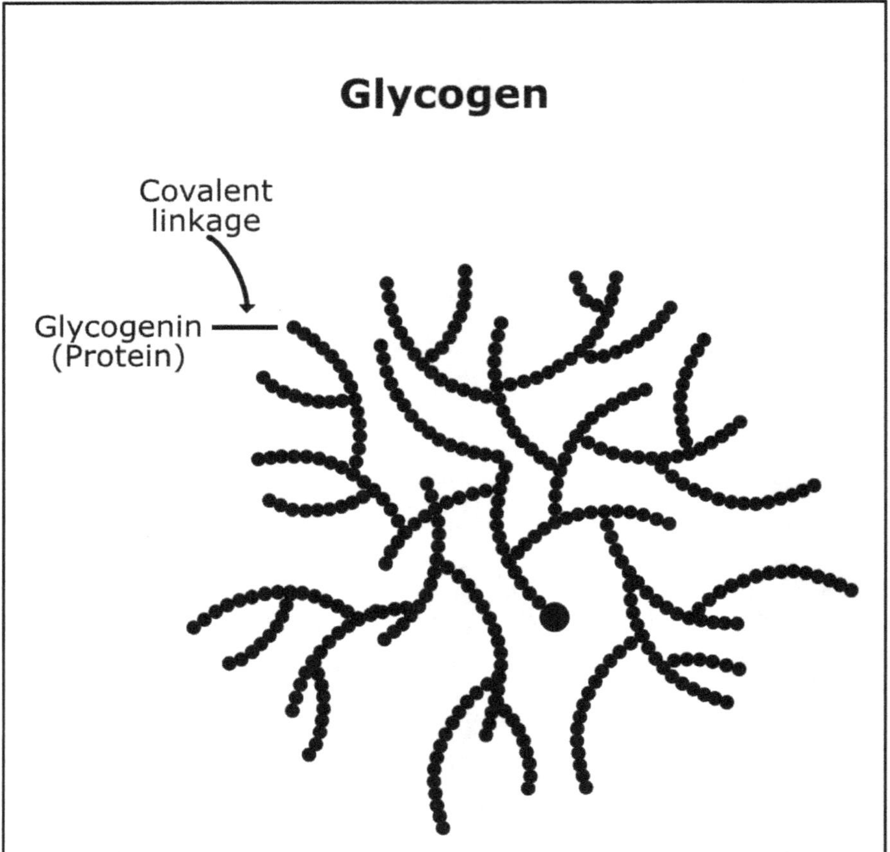

Chapter Summary/Key Takeaways:

You have now completed the densest chapter in this book. Cancers are complex, just as our metabolism is. There are many signals and pathways involved. Some go in a straight line (like glucose to lactic acid), while other pathways intersect, take detours, and have gates and receptors. Enzymes of many types are involved; some are overactive, and some are dampened. Like our highways, our metabolism, too, has tolls, gates, and checkpoints. You will recognize some of these pathways because many of our newer chemotherapy drugs are poised to target them.

Glucose appears to be a central ingredient that drives most of these pathways. Glycolysis makes lactate, which contributes to cancer growth and cancer cell survival. There is also the HIF-1 protein, which we believe is the metabolic switch that turns on cancers. This switch is activated by glucose, low oxygen, and acidity.

FAQs

From the Facebook group "Keto For Cancer"

QUESTION 01:

Any disadvantages or advantages to fasting during my chemotherapy? How long should I fast?

ANSWER 01:

Mouse studies show decreased levels of a hormone called IGF-1 (Insulin Growth Factor) after 72 hours (about 3 days) of fasting. IGF-1 promotes cell growth, but during fasting, lowered levels of IGF-1 can protect normal cells from chemotherapy-induced DNA damage while cancer cells remain unprotected.

QUESTION 02:

As a cancer patient, does fasting cause cancer to feed from apoptosis instead of ketones? Also, what are your thoughts on autophagy-fed cancers?

ANSWER 02:

Apoptosis is the process of cells dying. Both cancer and normal cells do that, but normal cells are better at this because cancer cells often lose the ability to die. The death pathways of cancer cells are messed up. Therefore, we try to fight cancer by triggering the death pathways that lead to apoptosis. By poisoning them with chemo or by starving them by diet, cancers go into apoptosis and die. It is a win when cells die, but the cell nucleus can extrude (spits out) a protein, activating another cancer-promoting pathway. It is what we call the "downstream phenomena." In other words, it is cancer's way of fighting back. Does this mean you avoid fasting or refuse chemo? Not really. We must figure out another way to fight the downstream effects.

Autophagy is a double-edged sword. Autophagy's primary role is to protect us against cancer by mopping up old cell debris that could cause irritation and inflammation. However, it can also boost cancers by stimulating downstream effects. I would be careful about taking hydroxychloroquine (HCQ) without a doctor's supervision or if you do not have an autoimmune disease. Too many patients have come to me with the most horrific cancers, and they were all previously on HCQ or some other immune-modifying drug. They can alter the immune system to a cancer's advantage and, in turn, allow new cancers to flourish and multiply. HCQ should be reserved for people with an autoimmune disease requiring treatment.

End Notes

Ako Bahrami, Esmail Ayen, Mazdak Razi, Mehdi Behfar, Effects of atorvastatin and resveratrol against the experimental endometriosis; evidence for glucose and monocarboxylate transporters, neoangiogenesis, *Life Sciences*, Volume 272, 2021, e119230, ISSN 0024-3205 https://doi.org/10.1016/j.lfs.2021.1192

Arcaro A. Targeting the insulin-like growth factor-1 receptor in human cancer. *Front Pharmacol.* 2013 Mar 22;4: p. 30. doi: 10.3389/fphar.2013.00030. PMID: 23525758; PMCID: PMC3605519.

Giovannucci E. Insulin-like growth factor-I and binding protein-3 and risk of cancer. *Horm Res*. 1999;51 Suppl 3: pp. 34-41. doi: 10.1159/000053160. PMID: 10592442.

Gottlob K, Majewski N, Kennedy S, Kandel E, Robey RB, Hay N. Inhibition of early apoptotic events by Akt/PKB is dependent on the first committed step of glycolysis and mitochondrial hexokinase. *Genes Dev.* 2001 Jun 1;15(11): e1406-18. doi: 10.1101/gad.889901. PMID: 11390360; PMCID: PMC312709.

Frances L. Byrne, Ivan K.H. Poon, Susan C. Modesitt, Jose L. Tomsig, Jenny D.Y. Chow, Marin E. Healy, William D. Baker, Kristen A. Atkins, Johnathan M. Lancaster, Douglas C. Marchion, Kelle H. Moley, Kodi S. Ravichandran, Jill K. Slack-Davis, Kyle L. Hoehn; Metabolic Vulnerabilities in Endometrial Cancer. *Cancer Res.* 15 October 2014; 74 (20): e5832–45.

Grimberg A, Cohen P. Role of insulin-like growth factors and their binding proteins in growth control and carcinogenesis. *J Cell Physiol.* 2000 Apr;183(1): pp. 1-9. doi: 10.1002/(SICI)1097-4652(200004)183:1<1:AID-JCP1>3.0.CO;2-J. PMID: 10699960; PMCID: PMC4144680.

Groleau V, Schall JI, Stallings VA, Bergqvist CA. Long-term impact of the ketogenic diet on growth and resting energy expenditure in children with intractable epilepsy. *Dev Med Child Neurol.* 2014 Sep;56(9): e898-904. doi: 10.1111/dmcn.12462. Epub 2014 Apr 20. PMID: 24749520; PMCID: PMC4133288.

Guo W, Qiu Z, Wang Z, Wang Q, Tan N, Chen T, Chen Z, Huang S, Gu J, Li J, Yao M, Zhao Y, He X. MiR-199a-5p is negatively associated with malignancies and regulates glycolysis and lactate production by targeting hexokinase 2 in liver cancer. *Hepatology*. 2015 Oct;62(4): e1132-44. doi: 10.1002/hep.27929. Epub 2015 Jul 4. PMID: 26054020.

Haluska P, Worden F, Olmos D, Yin D, Schteingart D, Batzel GN, Paccagnella ML, de Bono JS, Gualberto A, Hammer GD. Safety, tolerability, and pharmacokinetics of the anti-IGF-1R monoclonal antibody figitumumab in patients with refractory adrenocortical carcinoma. *Cancer Chemother Pharmacol.* 2010 Mar;65(4): e765-73. doi: 10.1007/s00280-009-1083-9. Epub 2009 Aug 2. PMID: 19649631; PMCID: PMC2875253.

Jing, C., Li, Y., Gao, Z., *et al.* Antitumor activity of Koningic acid in thyroid cancer by inhibiting cellular glycolysis. *Endocrine* 75, pp. 169–77 (2022). https://doi.org/10.1007/s12020-021-02822-x

Justus CR, Sanderlin EJ, Yang LV. Molecular Connections between Cancer Cell Metabolism and the Tumor Microenvironment. *Int J Mol Sci.* 2015 May 15;16(5): e11055-86. doi: 10.3390/ijms160511055. PMID: 25988385; PMCID: PMC4463690.

Khan T, Sullivan MA, Gunter JH, Kryza T, Lyons N, He Y, Hooper JD. Revisiting Glycogen in Cancer: A Conspicuous and Targetable Enabler of Malignant Transformation. Front Oncol. 2020 Oct 30;10: e592455. doi: 10.3389/fonc.2020.592455. PMID: 33224887; PMCID: PMC7667517.

Kim JW, Dang CV. Multifaceted roles of glycolytic enzymes. *Trends Biochem Sci.* 2005 Mar;30(3): pp. 142-50. doi: 10.1016/j.tibs.2005.01.005. PMID: 15752986.

Kindler HL, Richards DA, Garbo LE, Garon EB, Stephenson JJ Jr, Rocha-Lima CM, Safran H, Chan D, Kocs DM, Galimi F, McGreivy J, Bray SL, Hei Y, Feigal EG, Loh E, Fuchs CS. A randomized, placebo-controlled phase 2 study of ganitumab (AMG 479) or conatumumab (AMG 655) in combination with gemcitabine in patients with metastatic pancreatic cancer. *Ann Oncol.* 2012 Nov;23(11): e2834-42. doi: 10.1093/annonc/mds142. Epub 2012 Jun 13. PMID: 22700995.

Konstantakou, E.G., Voutsinas, G.E., Velentzas, A.D. et al. 3-BrPA eliminates human bladder cancer cells with highly oncogenic signatures via engagement of specific death programs and perturbation of multiple signaling and metabolic determinants. *Mol Cancer.* 14, p. 135 (2015). https://doi.org/10.1186/s12943-015-0399-9

Kuo CC, Ling HH, Chiang MC, Chung CH, Lee WY, Chu CY, Wu YC, Chen CH, Lai YW, Tsai IL, Cheng CH, Lin CW. Metastatic Colorectal Cancer Rewrites Metabolic Program Through a Glut3-YAP-dependent Signaling Circuit. *Theranostics.* 2019 Apr 13;9(9): e2526-40. doi: 10.7150/thno.32915. PMID: 31131051; PMCID: PMC6525983.

Lian S, Shao Y, Liu H, He J, Lu W, Zhang Y, Jiang Y, Zhu J. PDK1 induces JunB, EMT, cell migration and invasion in human gallbladder cancer. *Oncotarget.* 2015 Oct 6;6(30): e29076-86. doi: 10.18632/oncotarget.4931. PMID: 26318166; PMCID: PMC4745712.

Li, Li, S., Wu, L., Feng, J. *et al. In vitro* and *in vivo* study of epigallocatechin-3-gallate-induced apoptosis in aerobic glycolytic hepatocellular carcinoma cells involving inhibition of phosphofructokinase activity. *Sci Rep* 6, e28479 (2016). https://doi.org/10.1038/srep28479

Liu W, Yu X, Zhou L, Li J, Li M, Li W, Gao F. Sinomenine Inhibits Non-Small Cell Lung Cancer via Downregulation of Hexokinases II-Mediated Aerobic Glycolysis. *Onco Targets Ther.* 2020 Apr 16;13: e3209-21. doi: 10.2147/OTT.S243212. PMID: 32368080; PMCID: PMC7176511.

Lung, H.L., Kan, R., Chau, W.Y. *et al.* The anti-tumor function of the IKK inhibitor PS1145 and high levels of p65 and KLF4 are associated with the drug resistance in nasopharyngeal carcinoma cells. *Sci Rep* 9, e12064 (2019). https://doi.org/10.1038/s41598-019-48590-7

Ma Y, Wang W, Idowu MO, Oh U, Wang XY, Temkin SM, Fang X. Ovarian Cancer Relies on Glucose Transporter 1 to Fuel Glycolysis and Growth: Anti-Tumor Activity of BAY-876. *Cancers (Basel).* 2018 Dec 31;11(1): p. 33. doi: 10.3390/cancers11010033. PMID: 30602670; PMCID: PMC6356953.

Mathupala, S., Ko, Y. & Pedersen, P. Hexokinase II: Cancer's double-edged sword acting as both facilitator and gatekeeper of malignancy when bound to mitochondria. *Oncogene* 25, e4777–86 (2006). https://doi.org/10.1038/sj.onc.1209603

Martinez-Outschoorn, U., F. Sotgia, and M.P. Lisanti, Tumor microenvironment and metabolic synergy in breast cancers: critical importance of mitochondrial fuels and function. *Semin Oncol*, 2014. 41(2): pp. 195-216.

Nitulescu, G. M., Van De Venter, M., Nitulescu, G., Ungurianu, A., Juzenas, P., Peng, Q., Olaru, O. T., Grădinaru, D., Tsatsakis, A., Tsoukalas, D., Spandidos, D. A., Margina, D."The Akt pathway in oncology therapy and beyond (Review)." *International Journal of Oncology* 53.6 (2018): e2319-31

Nagarajan A, Malvi P, Wajapeyee N. Oncogene-directed alterations in cancer cell metabolism. *Trends Cancer.* 2016 Jul;2(7): pp. 365-77. doi: 10.1016/j.trecan.2016.06.002. Epub 2016 Jun 27. PMID: 27822561; PMCID: PMC5096652.

Salani, B., Marini, C., Rio, A. et al. Metformin Impairs Glucose Consumption and Survival in Calu-1 Cells by Direct Inhibition of Hexokinase-II. *Sci Rep* 3, e2070 (2013). https://doi.org/10.1038/srep02070

Sano D, Xie TX, Ow TJ, Zhao M, Pickering CR, Zhou G, Sandulache VC, Wheeler DA, Gibbs RA, Caulin C, Myers JN. Disruptive TP53 mutation is associated with aggressive disease characteristics in an orthotopic murine model of oral tongue cancer. *Clin Cancer Res.* 2011 Nov 1;17(21): e6658-70. doi: 10.1158/1078-0432.CCR-11-0046. Epub 2011 Sep 8. PMID: 21903770; PMCID: PMC3207013.

Schwartzenberg-Bar-Yoseph F, Armoni M, Karnieli E. The tumor suppressor p53 down-regulates glucose transporters GLUT1 and GLUT4 gene expression. *Cancer Res.* 2004 Apr 1;64(7): e2627-33. doi: 10.1158/0008-5472.can-03-0846. PMID: 15059920.

Seyfried TN, Flores RE, Poff AM, D'Agostino DP. Cancer as a metabolic disease: implications for novel therapeutics. *Carcinogenesis*. 2014 Mar;35(3): pp. 515-27. doi: 10.1093/carcin/bgt480. Epub 2013 Dec 16. PMID: 24343361; PMCID: PMC3941741.

Šimčíková, D., Gardáš, D., Hložková, K. *et al.* Loss of hexokinase 1 sensitizes ovarian cancer to high-dose metformin. *Cancer Metab* 9, p. 41 (2021). https://doi.org/10.1186/s40170-021-00277-2

Sutendra Gopinath, Michelakis Evangelos, Pyruvate dehydrogenase kinase as a novel therapeutic target in oncology, Frontiers in Oncology, Vol. 3, 2013, Sutendra G, Michelakis ED. Pyruvate dehydrogenase kinase as a novel therapeutic target in oncology. Front Oncol. 2013 Mar 7;3:38. doi: 10.3389/fonc.2013.00038. PMID: 23471124; PMCID: PMC3590642.

Tataranni T, Piccoli C. Dichloroacetate (DCA) and Cancer: An Overview towards Clinical Applications. *Oxid Med Cell Longev.* 2019 Nov 14;2019: e8201079. doi: 10.1155/2019/8201079. PMID: 31827705; PMCID: PMC6885244.

Travaini L, Trifiro G, Paganelli G. [18F] FDG uptake: pay attention to candies. *Ecancermedicalscience.* 2007;1: p. 48. doi: 10.3332/ecms.2007.48. Epub 2007 Aug 15. PMID: 22275952; PMCID: PMC3223976.

Yang Hua, Zhang Mu-Zi-he, Sun Hui-wei, Chai Yan-tao, Li Xiaojuan, Jiang Qiyu, Hou Jun; A Novel Microcrystalline BAY-876 Formulation Achieves Long-Acting Antitumor Activity Against Aerobic Glycolysis and Proliferation of Hepatocellular Carcinoma; *Frontiers in Oncology*. Vol.11. 2021. URL=https://www.frontiersin.org/articles/10.3389/fonc.2021.783194

Y.-F. Chen, H.-Y. Qi, F.-L. Wu; Euxanthone exhibits anti-proliferative and anti-invasive activities in hepatocellular carcinoma by inducing pyroptosis: preliminary results; *Eur Rev Med Pharmacol Sci*. Year: 2018 Vol. 22 - N. 23. e8186-96. doi: 10.26355/eurrev_201812_16511

Zheng M, Wu C, Yang K, Yang Y, Liu Y, Gao S, Wang Q, Li C, Chen L, Li H. Novel selective hexokinase 2 inhibitor Benitrobenrazide blocks cancer cells growth by targeting glycolysis. *Pharmacol Res*. 2021 Feb;164: e105367. doi: 10.1016/j.phrs.2020.105367. Epub 2020 Dec 8. PMID: 33307221.

Zhang D, Li J, Wang F, Hu J, Wang S, Sun Y. 2-Deoxy-D-glucose targeting of glucose metabolism in cancer cells as a potential therapy. *Cancer Lett*. 2014 Dec 28;355(2): pp. 176-83. doi: 10.1016/j.canlet.2014.09.003. Epub 2014 Sep 10. PMID: 25218591.

Zou J., Wang H. Euxanthone inhibits glycolysis and triggers mitochondria-mediated apoptosis by targeting hexokinase 2 in epithelial ovarian cancer. *Cell Biochem Funct*. 2018 Aug;36(6): pp. 303-11. doi: 10.1002/cbf.3349. Epub 2018 Jul 8. Retraction in: *Cell Biochem Funct*. 2021 Mar;39(2):344. PMID: 29984416.

Chapter 4

Lactate

Excess lactate sets the stage for cancer growth.

We know that lactate comes after fermenting glucose. Our body normally controls this process to avoid excess lactate formation. When there is a lot of oxygen or ATP energy, normal cells receive instructions to stop fermentation (de la Cruz-Lopez, *et al.*, 2019).

Cancer cells, however, will ignore oxygen. Even when oxygen is high, cancers will continue to make lactate despite the negative signals coming from oxygen. Aside from oxygen, the other negative feedback signal is ATP, but the cancer cells do not see that either because lactate returns to the liver to convert to glucose and does not enter the Krebs cycle to make ATP. Therefore, with no ATP made, there will be no signal to stop glycolysis (Koukourakis, *et al.*, 2005, 2006; Lin, *et al.*, 2017; Kolev, *et al.*, 2008; Ullah, *et al.*, 2006).

Lactate allows cancers to metastasize.

Cancers use glucose to produce much lactic acid waste. We know this happens when *lactate dehydrogenase* (LDH) levels are high. Colorectal cancers are filled with *oxidative stress,* which causes membranes to leak LDH into the blood circulation. LDH will raise *matrix metalloproteinases* (MMP) enzymes. MMPs are special proteins that break down barriers keeping cancers separate from normal cells. MMPs increase the likelihood of cancer invasion and metastases (Gopcevic, *et al.*, 2017).

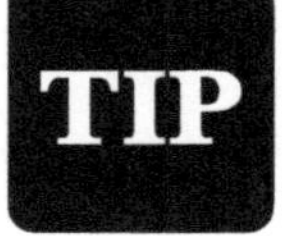

There is a blood test your doctors can order—the LDH test. LDH enzymes grease the last reaction of glycolysis, where glucose converts into lactate. High LDH levels are common in aggressive cancers.

Lactate will activate tumor-signaling pathways.

In addition to high lactate, low oxygen levels (hypoxia) will encourage glucose breakdown into lactate, which we know uses the enzyme LDH. Aside from making lactate, LDH can also stabilize and activate the pro-cancer HIF-1α:

Acidity ➡ Low oxygen ➡➡ LDH ➡➡ Active HIF-1α ➡➡➡ Signals

Epigallocatechin gallate (green tea) contains *catechins* (a type of antioxidant), which might help block the LDH activity in cancers (Han, *et al.*, 2021).

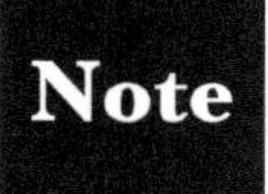

A drug that blocks LDH sounds like a great idea! Unfortunately, drug companies are not doing a very good job of making this type of drug come to reality (Di Stefano, *et al.*, 2016).

Lactate protects cancers from oxidative stress.

Lactate helps cancers. It protects cancers by reducing their exposure to ROS levels and tames stress. ROS are highly reactive oxygen molecules that damage cells and change them into cancers. By removing stress, cancers survive.

Chapter Summary/Key Takeaways:

There are many effects of lactate, including evasion of negative feedback, boosted signaling pathways, protection against chemotherapy, new blood vessel formation, and easier spreading to other organs. All these can give cancers an advantage. The next chapter will explore the pentose phosphate pathway, another pathway to cancer growth.

End Notes

de la Cruz-López KG, Castro-Muñoz LJ, Reyes-Hernández DO, García-Carrancá A, Manzo-Merino J. Lactate in the Regulation of Tumor Microenvironment and Therapeutic Approaches. *Front Oncol.* 2019 Nov 1;9: e1143. doi: 10.3389/fonc.2019.01143. PMID: 31737570; PMCID: PMC6839026.

Di Stefano G, Manerba M, Di Ianni L, Fiume L. Lactate dehydrogenase inhibition: exploring possible applications beyond cancer treatment. *Future Med Chem.* 2016 Apr;8(6): e713-25. doi: 10.4155/fmc.16.10. Epub 2016 Apr 7. PMID: 27054686.

Gopcevic K, Rovcanin B, Kekic D, Krivokapic Z, Dragutinovic V. Matrix Metalloproteinase-2 and -9, Lactate, and Malate Dehydrogenase and Lipid Peroxides in Sera of Patients with Colorectal Carcinoma. *Folia Biol (Praha).* 2017;63(5-6): pp. 190-96. PMID: 29687772.

Han JH, Kim M, Kim HJ, Jang SB, Bae SJ, Lee IK, Ryu D, Ha KT. Targeting Lactate Dehydrogenase A with Catechin Resensitizes SNU620/5FU Gastric Cancer Cells to 5-Fluorouracil. *Int J Mol Sci.* 2021 May 20;22(10): e5406. doi: 10.3390/ijms22105406. PMID: 34065602; PMCID: PMC8161398.

Kolev, Y., *et al.*, Lactate dehydrogenase-5 (LDH-5) expression in human gastric cancer: association with hypoxia-inducible factor (HIF-1alpha) pathway, angiogenic factors production and poor prognosis. *Ann Surg Oncol*, 2008. 15(8): e2336-44.

Koukourakis, M.I., *et al.*, Lactate dehydrogenase 5 expression in operable colorectal cancer: strong association with survival and activated vascular endothelial growth factor pathway—a report of the Tumour Angiogenesis Research Group. *J Clin Oncol*, 2006. 24(26): e4301-8.

Koukourakis, M.I., *et al.*, Lactate dehydrogenase 5 (LDH5) relates to up-regulated hypoxia inducible factor pathway and metastasis in colorectal cancer. *Clin Exp Metastasis*, 2005. 22(1): pp. 25-30.

Lin, S., *et al.*, Lactate-activated macrophages induced aerobic glycolysis and epithelial mesenchymal transition in breast cancer by regulation of CCL5-CCR5 axis: a positive metabolic feedback loop. *Oncotarget*, 2017. 8(66): e110426-43.

Ullah, M.S., A.J. Davies, and A.P. Halestrap, The plasma membrane lactate transporter MCT4, but not MCT1, is up-regulated by hypoxia through a HIF-1alpha-dependent mechanism. *J Biol Chem*, 2006. 281(14): e9030-7.

Chapter 5

The Pentose Phosphate Pathway (PPP)

An overactive side street: the PPP

Cancer cells grow rapidly and need plenty of glucose. Glucose makes energy through glycolysis but also enters the very active *pentose phosphate pathway* (PPP), which is important for fighting inflammation and making DNA.

The PPPs branch out early from glycolysis (glucose breakdown) and produce two important products. One is NADPH, and the other is a sugar called *ribose-5-phosphate.*

Let's focus on the first product, NADPH, which is very important for cancer to thrive in our body. A sufficient supply of NADPH protects cancers from oxidative stress (Fernandez-Marcos & Nóbrega-Pereira, 2016). NADPH inside red blood cells ensures that we have enough antioxidant *glutathione* to clean up any damaging

ROS. This may not be the ideal scenario, especially when one is trying to fight cancer with chemotherapy! Chemotherapy hopes to kill cancer cells via increased oxidative stress, and if the PPP is overactive, NADPH might protect cancers from the toxicity of chemotherapy. NADPH is also involved in 'building activities' that involve glucose and/or fat. Many cancers have the PPP actively involved in fatty acid synthesis (FAS) and glycolysis.

The second product of the PPP is *ribose-5-phosphate*, a building block for DNA. Because DNA construction is very important to cancers, the PPPs, like glycolysis, are highly important for normal and cancerous cell growth.

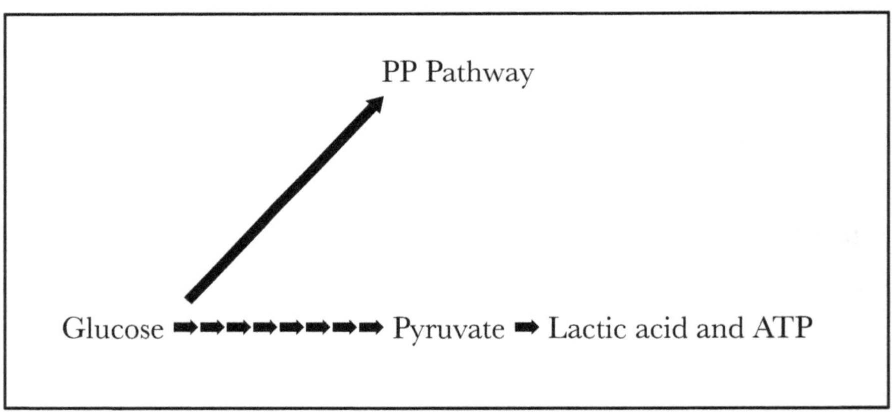

The PPP detour is seen branching off early from the glucose pathway, way before glucose gets close to becoming lactic acid.

How do we limit the PPP to slow down cancer?

G6PD (glucose-6-phosphatase dehydrogenase) is inside almost all cells and keeps carbohydrate metabolism working. Excess

G6PD, however, will keep cancers happy, protected, and growing endlessly! Many aggressive cancers, including cancers of the breast, prostate, stomach; lung, ovarian, brain; leukemias, and gut cancers, have elevated G6PD. G6PD is almost everywhere, and the PPP is overactive in most cancers (Patra & Hay, 2014).

TP53 is our security guard against cancer. As a functioning tumor suppressor gene, TP53 keeps G6PD under control to protect us from developing cancer from an overactive PPP. A defective TP53 will fail to deactivate G6PD, allowing the PPP to run unchecked and giving cancers easy access to building material for growth. Cancers have been observed adjusting the PPP to their advantage (Patra & Hay, 2014; Kather, *et al.*, 1972).

Possible anti-PPP therapies as anti-cancer tools:

The PPP is controlled by many players: tumor suppressors, oncoproteins, enzymes, and metabolites. The following are ways to fight cancer by targeting the PPP:

A. Diet

High glucose conditions make G6PD overactive; therefore, a low glucose diet may help tame G6PD activity and limit cancer (Wagle, *et al.*, 1998; Ge, *et al.*, 2020).

B. Dehydroepiandrosterone (DHEA)

The hormone DHEA targets the PPP by blocking G6PD. Currently, it is available as an over-the-counter health supplement but is not FDA-approved to treat any disease. Its effectiveness is still not well established. In laboratory studies, DHEA blocked G6PD and delayed the growth of hormone-positive and hormone-negative breast cancer cells. Unfortunately, DHEA is quickly inactivated in the body, so its true effectiveness is questionable. Other than DHEA, I know of no other commercially available G6PD inhibitor for use in oncology.

C. Glucose-6-Dehydrogenase Inhibitor 1 (G6PDi-1)

The small molecule named G6PD is an inhibitor with actions similar to DHEA. It is used mostly in the lab and unavailable to the public (Di Monaco, *et al.*, 1997; Mele, *et al.*, 2018; Ghergurovich, *et al.*, 2020; Luo, *et al.*, 2021).

D. Polydatin

Polydatin is a potent liver antioxidant G6PD inhibitor that comes from an extract of the roots of *Polygonum cuspidatum.* It is native to Asia but also found in Europe and America. In laboratory studies, polydatin had anticancer effects on head, neck, and breast cancer. There was no evidence of toxicity in a Phase 2 clinical trial of oral cancer patients. Cisplatin and Afatinib chemotherapy were more effective when combined with polydatin. Benefits were believed to be due to polydatin's ability to directly inhibit the PPP, decrease NADPH, and bring antioxidant and anti-inflammatory properties. This natural substance is popular in clinical research (Mele, *et al.*, 2018; Zhang, *et al.*, 2012).

E. Resveratrol

Resveratrol is a natural substance in grape skin and seeds that blocks IGF-1. Because the PPP also controls insulin secretion, resveratrol dampens many pro-cancer signaling pathways, such as Ras/Raf/Mek/Erk and PI3K/AKT/ mTOR. Advanced human colon cancers have elevated PPP activity in the lab and might benefit from resveratrol (Vanamala, *et al.*, 2011).

F. Wedelolactone

Wedelolactone, extracted from the medicinal herb *Eclipta prostrata*, is used in Brazil to treat hepatitis caused by snake venom. Anti-breast, head, and neck cancer effects were seen in the lab (Chen, *et al.*, 2013; Song, *et al.*, 2022; Sayanta, *et al.*, 2021; Zou, *et al.*, 2022).

G. Zoledronic acid

Zoledronic acid is a treatment for osteoporosis and metastatic bone disease, often offered to prostate cancer patients with bone metastases. It does more than just strengthen bones; it also blocks the PPP. In bladder cancer cell lines, zoledronic acid can slow growth and block the PPP by targeting the G6PD enzyme), which, you recall, is PPP's major step (Wang, *et al.*, 2015).

H. Metformin

Thanks to its ability to inhibit the complex 1 protein of the mitochondria, Metformin has anticancer properties, thus stopping mTOR tumor signaling pathways. However, its anticancer activity was weak when solo; when metformin was added to a G6PDH inhibitor—*6-amino nicotinamide* (6-AN), the combo increased levels of the antioxidant glutathione in a lab model of melanoma (Arbe, *et al.*, 2020).

Chapter Summary/Key Takeaways:

We learned how the pentose phosphate pathway branches out from glycolysis. We saw how the pentose phosphate pathway enables cancer cells to survive oxidative stress and use the elements from glucose breakdown to supply cell-building material. We reviewed some strategies to help fight these pro-cancer effects.

In the next chapter, we will discover cancer stem cells, learn why they are dangerous, and find new ways of preventing their pro-cancer effects.

End Notes

Arbe MF, Agnetti L, Breininger E, Glikin GC, Finocchiaro LME, Villaverde MS. Glucose 6-phosphate dehydrogenase inhibition sensitizes melanoma cells to metformin treatment. *Transl Oncol.* 2020 Nov;13(11): e100842. doi: 10.1016/j.tranon.2020.100842. Epub 2020 Aug 8. PMID: 32781368; PMCID: PMC7417947.

Chen Z, Sun X, Shen S, Zhang H, Ma X, Liu J, Kuang S, Yu Q. Wedelolactone, a naturally occurring coumestan, enhances interferon-γ signaling through inhibiting STAT1 protein dephosphorylation. *J Biol Chem.* 2013 May 17;288(20): e14417-27. doi: 10.1074/jbc.M112.442970. Epub 2013 Apr 11. PMID: 23580655; PMCID: PMC3656297.

Di Monaco, M., Pizzini, A., Gatto, V. *et al.* Role of glucose-6-phosphate dehydrogenase inhibition in the antiproliferative effects of dehydroepiandrosterone on human breast cancer cells. *Br J Cancer* 75, pp. 589–92 (1997). https://doi.org/10.1038/bjc.1997.102.

Fernandez-Marcos PJ, Nóbrega-Pereira S. NADPH: new oxygen for the ROS theory of aging. *Oncotarget.* 2016 Aug 9;7(32): e50814-15. doi: 10.18632/oncotarget.10744. PMID: 27449104; PMCID: PMC5239434.

Ge T, Yang J, Zhou S, Wang Y, Li Y, Tong X. The Role of the Pentose Phosphate Pathway in Diabetes and Cancer. *Front Endocrinol* (Lausanne). 2020 Jun 9;11: p. 365. doi: 10.3389/fendo.2020.00365. PMID: 32582032; PMCID: PMC7296058.

Ghergurovich JM, García-Cañaveras JC, Wang J, Schmidt E, Zhang Z, TeSlaa T, Patel H, Chen L, Britt EC, Piqueras-Nebot M, Gomez-Cabrera MC, Lahoz A, Fan J, Beier UH, Kim H, Rabinowitz JD. A small molecule G6PD inhibitor reveals immune dependence on pentose phosphate pathway. *Nat Chem Biol.* 2020 Jul;16(7): e731-39. doi: 10.1038/s41589-020-0533-x. Epub 2020 May 11. PMID: 32393898; PMCID: PMC7311271.

Kather, H., M. Rivera, and K. Brand, Interrelationship and control of glucose metabolism and lipogenesis in isolated fat-cells. Effect of the amount of glucose uptake on the rates of the pentose phosphate cycle and of fatty acid synthesis. *Biochem J*, 1972. 128(5): e1089-96.

Liu CL, Hsu YC, Lee JJ, Chen MJ, Lin CH, Huang SY, Cheng SP. Targeting the pentose phosphate pathway increases reactive oxygen species and induces apoptosis in thyroid cancer cells. *Mol Cell Endocrinol.* 2020 Jan 1;499: e110595. doi: 10.1016/j.mce.2019.110595. Epub 2019 Sep 26. PMID: 31563469.

Luo Z, Du D, Liu Y, Lu T, Liu L, Jiang H, Chen K, Shan C, Luo C. Discovery and characterization of a novel glucose-6-phosphate dehydrogenase (G6PD) inhibitor via high-throughput screening. *Bioorg Med Chem Lett.* 2021 May 15;40: e127905. doi: 10.1016/j.bmcl.2021.127905. Epub 2021 Mar 6. PMID: 33689874.

Mele, L., Paino, F., Papaccio, F. et al. A new inhibitor of glucose-6-phosphate dehydrogenase blocks pentose phosphate pathway and suppresses malignant proliferation and metastasis in vivo. *Cell Death Dis.* 9, p. 572 (2018). https://doi.org/10.1038/s41419-018-0635-5.

Patra KC, Hay N. The pentose phosphate pathway and cancer. *Trends Biochem Sci.* 2014 Aug;39(8): pp. 347-54. doi: 10.1016/j.tibs.2014.06.005. Epub 2014 Jul 15. PMID: 25037503; PMCID: PMC4329227.

Sayanta Dutta, Sushweta Mahalanobish, Parames C. Sil, Chapter 8 - Phytoestrogens as Novel Therapeutic Molecules Against Breast Cancer, In Natural Product Drug Discovery, Discovery and Development of Anti-Breast Cancer Agents from Natural Products, *Elsevier,* 2021, pp. 197-229, https://doi.org/10.1016/B978-0-12-821277-6.00008-8.

Song J, Sun H, Zhang S, Shan C. The Multiple Roles of Glucose-6-Pchosphate Dehydrogenase in Tumorigenesis and Cancer Chemoresistance. *Life (Basel).* 2022 Feb 12;12(2): p. 271. doi: 10.3390/life12020271. PMID: 35207558; PMCID: PMC8875868.

Vanamala J, Radhakrishnan S, Reddivari L, Bhat VB, Ptitsyn A. Resveratrol suppresses human colon cancer cell proliferation and induces apoptosis via targeting the pentose phosphate and the talin-FAK signaling pathways-A proteomic approach. *Proteome Sci.* 2011 Aug 17;9(1): p. 49. doi: 10.1186/1477-5956-9-49. PMID: 21849056; PMCID: PMC3175442.

Wagle A, Jivraj S, Garlock GL, Stapleton SR. Insulin regulation of glucose-6-phosphate dehydrogenase gene expression is rapamycin-sensitive and requires phosphatidylinositol 3-kinase. *J Biol Chem.* 1998 Jun 12;273(24): e14968-74. doi: 10.1074/jbc.273.24.14968. PMID: 9614103.

Wang X, Wu G, Cao G, Yang L, Xu H, Huang J, Hou J. Zoledronic acid inhibits the pentose phosphate pathway through attenuating the Ras-TAp73-G6PD axis in bladder cancer cells. *Mol Med Rep.* 2015 Sep;12(3): e4620-25. doi: 10.3892/mmr.2015.3995. Epub 2015 Jun 24. PMID: 26126921.

Zhang H, Yu CH, Jiang YP, Peng C, He K, Tang JY, Xin HL. Protective effects of polydatin from Polygonum cuspidatum against carbon tetrachloride-induced liver injury in mice. *PLoS One.* 2012;7(9): e46574. doi: 10.1371/journal.pone.0046574. Epub 2012 Sep 28. PMID: 23029551; PMCID: PMC3461010.

Zou YX, Mu ZQ, Wang J, Tian S, Li Y, Liu Y. Wedelolactone, a component from Eclipta prostrata (L.) L., inhibits the proliferation and migration of head and neck squamous cancer cells through the AhR pathway. *Curr Pharm Biotechnol.* 2022 Mar 7. doi: 10.2174/1389201023666220307110554. Epub ahead of print. PMID: 35255785.

Chapter Six

The Reverse Warburg Effect and Other Controversial Topics

This is probably the most controversial and highly debated topic in cancer metabolism. Despite ample emerging literature, authorities continue to debate *for* or *against* the Warburg effect. I will showcase the evidence for the reverse Warburg effect.

Interest in cancer metabolism is rising. At present, Warburg's teachings remain very popular. Warburg and many others after him believed that glucose-loving cancer cells have non-functioning mitochondria (contains the defective Krebs and ETC-ATPase) and OXPHOS failure. Remember the pathway that I called Route 36? Warburg-type cancers don't use this; instead, they use the low energy-yielding Route 2. Because the energy harvested from this route is so tiny, cancers must run through it multiple times to get enough energy from glucose to supply its massive needs. Cancers become hungry for glucose, and this small but busy energy-making route is the main reason behind the Warburg effect.

Conflicting versions of the Warburg effect

Recently, conflicting versions of the Warburg effect began to appear. Some researchers claimed that certain cancers have some functioning OXPHOS, which uses lactate and ketones.

In 2009, a group of investigators came up with a new idea that Warburg-type cancers have not only one but two compartments. There is the cancer itself, which doesn't use glucose, and the *stroma* (the surrounding connective tissue) around it, which does. Their theory still preserves some parts of Warburg's theory. For example, the new version believes that hypoxia (low oxygen) is still the reason behind glucose addiction.

Lisanti and Locasale's 2016 paper proposes that to keep cancers happy and active, one compartment will have cancer cells with low sugar appetites and intact OXPHOS, while the second compartment, the stroma, is where glucose is processed to make lactate (pp. 577-8). The lactate will then pass back to the cancer side and feed it.

The cancer cells in the first compartment will begin transforming into the reverse Warburg variety. The cancers will send some hydrogen peroxide (a very irritating compound) to 'infect' the stroma's fibroblasts (cells that build connective tissue) and change them into glucose-loving cells (Martinez-Outschoorn, *et al.*, 2011; Liberti & Locasale, 2016; Sotgia, *et al.*, 2012). Once that transformation happens, the stroma will use glucose to make lactate.

Here is the step that triggers cancer. As fibroblasts begin loving glucose, they lose *Caveolin-1 proteins* (Cav-1), the oncogenic membrane protein that helps cell membranes maintain shape. As the tissues around cancer cells lose Cav-1, oxygen levels appear low (just like a deflated balloon) and will activate the HIF-1α (hypoxia-inducible factor) protein (see Figure 6, page 41).

HIF-1α is a mighty switch that turns on pre-cancer signals. Glucose breaks down, and acidity rises due to accumulating lactate. Excess lactate must leave, so it 'rides' the special lactate transporter (monocarboxylate transporter 4 [MCT4]) to enter and feed the low-sugar cancers found on the other side (Boscher & Nabi, 2012).

Indeed, some aggressive breast cancers have low Cav-1 levels, which partly supports this theory (Pavlides, *et al.*, 2009).

The 'two-compartment setup' sounds like an efficient way to energize cancers. The Warburg effect is still functioning, with the bulk of glycolysis appearing in the fibroblasts (second compartment), not in the tumor itself. Lactate also activates metalloproteinase enzymes, which break cancer barriers and help them metastasize to other organs (Liberti & Locasale, 2016; Sotgia, *et al.*, 2012).

Turning the focus back to the first compartment, where the cancers appear to have little appetite for sugar, they apparently have functioning mitochondria—contrary to Warburg, who claimed all cancers have defective mitochondria.

What are current ways to treat 'reverse Warburg' (RW) cancers?

Assuming the RW cancers do exist, how can we fight them? They are indeed a different creature. Sugar-loving while at the same time making lots of lactate and ketones, then feeding these into a functioning OXPHOS.

One way is to target lactate by blocking the MCT lactate transporters responsible for transferring lactate from the fibroblast compartment into the cancer.

We can also target glycolytic enzymes. Others have thought of targeting *succinyl-CoA:3-ketoacid CoA transferase* or SCOT, the enzyme that breaks down ketones, and another way is to target glutamine. More on this in Chapter Eleven.

How about targeting OXPHOS itself?

Before reading about possible treatments, let's briefly review the inside of the mitochondrion. After the Krebs cycle, we meet OXPHOS. This energy-making machinery has two synchronized steps:

1. *The electron transport chain (ETC)*—electrons get passed along a string/chain of proteins. One of these proteins is CoQ10. We know the CoQ10 is an over-the-counter supplement. It is an antioxidant and fights inflammation. CoQ10 helps us in the energy-making process in the ETC by helping pass the electrons along the chain, as displayed in Figure 5 (page 26).

2. *A shift of pressure* from one compartment to another—space *A* to space *B*—results in ATP energy production.

(See: Gaude & Frezza, 2014; Viale, *et al.*, 2015.)

Which experimental drugs can fight abnormal OXPHOS?

I am not entirely convinced of the existence of reverse Warburg tumors. But I included the following for completion. We still need more evidence that the reverse Warburg effect exists. Hence, the drugs mentioned below are still highly experimental and best used under clinical trial supervision. These experimental therapies are meant to attack cancers that still have some form of functioning OXPHOS.

A. Metformin

Metformin is an antidiabetic drug with two anti-cancer effects. Metformin blocks insulin and targets OXPHOS, effectively reducing ATP energy levels in cancers (Thakur, *et al.*, 2018).

B. Atovaquone

Atovaquone is a commercially available antimalarial treatment. It was first available in 2000 and currently treats Pneumocystis carinii pneumonia. Atovaquone inhibits Cytochrome *B*, one of the ETC proteins. It fights cancer by attacking OXPHOS to kill stem cells (Fiorillo, *et al.*, 2016).

C. IACS-010759

IACS-010759 is another investigational OXPHOS blocker. If you were hoping this would be a potent anti-cancer drug, think again. This drug is highly toxic. A Phase 1 clinical trial studied this drug in patients with relapsed/ refractory acute myeloid leukemia. The researchers saw toxic side effects such as increased acidity from lactate and significant nerve damage or neuropathy!

D. Cyanides

Cyanides are highly fatal to cells because they inhibit cellular respiration in the mitochondria, hit the ETC's *Cytochrome C oxidase protein*, and block electrons transferring to oxygen. The result is blocked ATP production, so energy escapes as heat. Because OXPHOS is down, the cell metabolism switches to glycolysis, and lactate accumulates. In its natural form, small amounts of cyanide can safely be found in food such as almonds and lima beans. Cyanide toxicity can cause immediate death (Graham & Traylor, 2022).

E. Atorvastatin

Atorvastatin (an anti-cholesterol drug) is being studied as a potential cancer treatment. Statins can reduce CoQ10—an electron passer, mentioned on page 90—and enzyme levels and stop the abnormal OXPHOS. Strangely, the pravastatin version did not have the same effects (Urbano, *et al.*, 2017).

What are the implications of cancers feeding on fats and ketones?

"How can fats feed cancers?" This sentence is not entirely accurate. Cancers don't use fats for food. Instead, cancers need a lot of fat to use as a building material for more cancer cells. Since cancers must build quickly, they reprogram and make their fats.

The Krebs cycle develops defective parts (mutated intermediates) and begins to make lots of citrate (acid at the end of the Krebs cycle). Citrate accumulates, so to eliminate the excess, some citrate must leave the mitochondria and travel to the fat-making pathway (fatty acid synthesis). How convenient!

Cancers need lots of fat to build membranes and cell structures, etc.; therefore, an active fat acid synthesis pathway is required. As citrate heads towards fatty acid synthesis (FAS), it produces *malonyl-CoA*, which (although unfortunate for us but good for cancers) stops fats from *beta-oxidizing* (breaking down) into acetyl-CoA.

How can ketones feed cancers?

This is another thought-provoking topic: Do we have cancers feeding on ketones? Here is the technical explanation. The glycolysis pathway can get blocked at the pyruvate step, so that path cannot make acetyl-CoA. If both glycolysis and fatty acid β-oxidation cannot make acetyl-CoA, the cancer might turn to ketones and begin breaking them down. In this special situation, the *ketolytic* enzyme SCOT begins breaking down (using up) ketones to make acetyl-CoA (Liberti & Locasale, 2016; Israel & Schwartz, 2020).

In another scenario, some cancers have mutations in the Krebs cycle at the *succinate dehydrogenase* (SDH) step. As a result, the Krebs cycle ends up making too much *succinyl-CoA*. The rewired cancer uses SCOT enzymes and takes succinyl-CoA and ketone acetoacetate to make more acetyl-CoA and run its OXPHOS. Of course, this 'keto-adaptation' assumes that the cancer cell has some functional OXPHOS. This response to Krebs cycle defects is an elegant explanation of how ketones can fuel cancer. However, Israël and Schwartz (2020) mentioned that there is "still no direct evidence of this because there were no actual measurements" (e1755-7).

What are the arguments against the reverse Warburg and ketone-loving cancer theories?

We just reviewed the reverse Warburg effect. We also reviewed some research on cancers loving ketones and some of the investigational drugs that could fight these non-Warburg cancers.

I had the opportunity to discuss these thought-provoking issues with Dr. Thomas Seyfried, Professor of Biochemistry at Boston College, who stands firmly by Warburg's original hypothesis. Dr. Seyfried (2014) feels that the statement that "cancers have functioning mitochondria" is wrong (pp. 515-27). The function is vague here and needs to be defined. What do the authors mean when they reference 'functional mitochondria'? They use oxygen consumption as evidence of intact respiration (getting energy from food). Oxygen consumption might appear normal in some cancer cells, but this does not mean cancer cells can produce enough ATP. Cancer cells can use oxygen, but uncoupling disrupts ATP production. (More on uncoupling in Chapter Seventeen.) Moreover, mitochondrial SLP can produce ATP through a non-oxidative process, giving the appearance of normal function.

Therefore, we cannot prove the presence of normal respiration (OXPHOS) based on the Krebs cycle or *tricarboxylic acid cycle* (TCA) activity.

In addition, the studies that showed tumors had "normal" respiration had improper assignment of controls. Furthermore, culture media setups in the laboratory cannot truly represent what goes on in the human body. On further examination of their research setups, flaws were present. The experiments allowed some amount of glucose, glutamine, other sugars, uridine, etc., to invade the experimental design (Seyfried, *et al.*, 2014).

These experiments show that OXPHOS is present but cannot entirely compensate for SLP. All the experiments here appear to have SLP fuels present. The researchers can prove "utilization" (additive) of these substrates (ketones, lactate, fat) in addition to, but not substitution for, the absence of SLP.

My lay explanation: We can't use oxygen consumption alone as evidence against the Warburg effect. Just because you see smoke doesn't mean there is a fire. Just because you see cancers using oxygen does not mean functional mitochondria exist. Cancers use up oxygen to make ROS. The fact that we have some operational ETC does not necessarily prove that there is ATP production. Cancers may get their ATP energy from the Krebs cycle (the main power supply) and glycolysis (glucose breakdown) or via the SLP of glutamine (Seyfried, *et al.*, 2014). (Note: SLP is the alternate but also powerful energy-making pathway.)

Cancer cells can also develop an 'uncoupling' of their *oxidative phosphorylation*, making it possible to appear that the ETC is functional, yet it is not (Seyfried, *et al.*, 2014). Many cancers do uncouple (see Chapter Seventeen).

Other evidence for faulty mitochondria points to abnormal cancer respiration based on abnormal lipid (fat) membranes. Glucose-loving, lactic acid-producing cancers all had defects in the inner mitochondrial membrane's *cardiolipin* (special membrane fat) lipid layers. The result? ETC deficits and poor ATP production (Kosaki, *et al.*, 1958; Merchant, *et al.*, 1991).

Evidence from mitochondrial transfer experiments further supports the Warburg effect. The cytoplasm controls whether cancer develops and not the nucleus (Minocherhomji, *et al.*, 2012; Israel & Schaeffer, 1988).

Should I worry about ketones worsening melanomas?

A mouse model of BRAF-V600E-positive melanomas showed tumor growth after exposure to the acetoacetate ketone, presumably boosting BRAF-V600E-dependent MEK1 signaling pathways (Weber, *et al.*, 2020; Xia, *et al.*, 2017). This research study brought some concern regarding using the ketogenic diet (KD) in patients positive for this mutation.

Surprisingly, a human male with BRAF-V600E-positive melanoma from the US Veterans ketogenic diet pilot trial consumed a KD for over two years and did exceptionally well. He remains in complete remission, more than nine years past his initial diagnosis. We need more human research before jumping to conclusions based on a single mouse study.

Chapter Summary/Key Takeaways:

Most cancers need glucose desperately. Sugar hunger is the central feature common to almost all cancers. Others disagree and talk about cancers that "do not love glucose" and instead depend on lactate and ketones using a two-compartment strategy. These investigators believe some cancers can feed on ketones and fat. They also believe that the cancers have functioning OXPHOS/ mitochondria. Warburg's camp and Seyfried both disagreed. They both believed that all cancers have defective mitochondria. Seyfried also pointed out the flaws in the lactate-ketone-loving cancer studies. Despite the lab experiments suggesting that cancers can feed on fats and ketones, scientists still cannot explain why cancer patients are doing well on ketogenic diets and fasting ketones. The ketogenic paradox highlights the benefits of ketones on real-life patients despite negative results in lab studies (Abolhassani, *et al.*, 2022). The debate will continue, but more quality research is still needed.

In the next chapter, we will glance at the progress of the ketogenic diet over the years.

End Notes

Abolhassani, Mohammad & E, Berg & G, Tenenbaum & Israël, Maurice. (2022). Inhibition of SCOT and Ketolysis Decreases Tumor Growth and Inflammation in the Lewis Cancer Model. *JOCR*. 3. p. 104. 10.17303/jocr.2022.3.104.

Bonuccelli G, Tsirigos A, Whitaker-Menezes D, Pavlides S, Pestell RG, Chiavarina B, Frank PG, Flomenberg N, Howell A, Martinez-Outschoorn UE, Sotgia F, Lisanti MP. Ketones and lactate "fuel" tumor growth and metastasis: Evidence that epithelial cancer cells use oxidative mitochondrial metabolism. *Cell Cycle.* 2010 Sep 1;9(17): e3506-14. doi: 10.4161/cc.9.17.12731. Epub 2010 Sep 21. PMID: 20818174; PMCID: PMC3047616.

Bonuccelli G, Whitaker-Menezes D, Castello-Cros R, Pavlides S, Pestell RG, Fatatis A, Witkiewicz AK, Vander Heiden MG, Migneco G, Chiavarina B, Frank PG, Capozza F, Flomenberg N, Martinez-Outschoorn UE, Sotgia F, Lisanti MP. The reverse Warburg effect: glycolysis inhibitors prevent the tumor promoting effects of caveolin-1 deficient cancer associated fibroblasts. *Cell Cycle.* 2010 May 15;9(10): e1960-71. doi: 10.4161/cc.9.10.11601. Epub 2010 May 15. PMID: 20495363.

Boscher C, Nabi IR. Caveolin-1: role in cell signaling. *Adv Exp Med Biol.* 2012;729: pp. 29-50. doi: 10.1007/978-1-4614-1222-9_3. PMID: 22411312.

Daniela D. Weber, Sepideh Aminzadeh-Gohari, Julia Tulipan, Luca Catalano, René G. Feichtinger, Barbara Kofler, Ketogenic diet in the treatment of cancer—Where do we stand?. *Molecular Metabolism*, Volume 33,2020, pp. 102-21, ISSN 2212-8778, https://doi.org/10.1016/j.molmet.2019.06.026.

Ertel, A., Tsirigos, A., Whitaker-Menezes, D., Birbe, R. C., Pavlides, S., Martinez-Outschoorn, U. E., Pestell, R. G., Howell, A., Sotgia, F., & Lisanti, M. P. (2012). Is cancer a metabolic rebellion against host aging?: In the quest for immortality, tumor cells try to save themselves by boosting mitochondrial metabolism. *Cell Cycle*, *11*(2), pp. 253-263. https://doi.org/10.4161/cc.11.2.19006.

Fiorillo M, Lamb R, Tanowitz HB, Mutti L, Krstic-Demonacos M, Cappello AR, Martinez-Outschoorn UE, Sotgia F, Lisanti MP. Repurposing atovaquone: targeting mitochondrial complex III and OXPHOS to eradicate cancer stem cells. *Oncotarget.* 2016 Jun 7;7(23): e34084-99. doi: 10.18632/oncotarget.9122. PMID: 27136895; PMCID: PMC5085139.

Gaude E, Frezza C. Defects in mitochondrial metabolism and cancer. *Cancer Metab.* 2014 Jul 17;2: p. 10. doi:10.1186/2049-3002-2-10. PMID: 25057353; PMCID: PMC4108232.

Graham J, Traylor J. Cyanide Toxicity. [Updated 2022 Feb 17]. In: *StatPearls* [Internet]. Treasure Island (FL): StatPearls Publishing; 2022 Jan-. Available from: https://www.ncbi.nlm.nih.gov/books/NBK507796/.

Israel BA, Schaeffer WI. Cytoplasmic mediation of malignancy. *In Vitro Cell Dev Biol.* 1988 May;24(5): pp. 487-90. doi: 10.1007/BF02628504. PMID: 3372452.

Israël, M, Schwartz, L. Inhibition of the ketolytic acetyl CoA supply to tumors could be their "Achilles heel." *Int. J. Cancer*, 2020, 147: e1755-57. https://doi.org/10.1002/ijc.32979.

Kosaki T, Ikoda T, Kotanti Y, Nakagawa S, Saka T. A new phospholipid, malignolipin, in human malignant tumors. *Science.* 1958 May 16;127(3307): e1176-7. doi: 10.1126/science.127.3307.1176. PMID: 13555861.

Liberti MV, Locasale JW. Metabolism: A new layer of glycolysis. *Nat Chem Biol.* 2016 Jul 19;12(8): pp. 577-8. doi: 10.1038/nchembio.2133. PMID: 27434766.

Martinez-Outschoorn U, Sotgia F, Lisanti MP. Tumor microenvironment and metabolic synergy in breast cancers: critical importance of mitochondrial fuels and function. *Semin Oncol.* 2014 Apr;41(2): pp. 195-216. doi: 10.1053/j.seminoncol.2014.03.002. Epub 2014 Mar 5. PMID: 24787293.

Martinez-Outschoorn UE, Lin Z, Trimmer C, Flomenberg N, Wang C, Pavlides S, Pestell RG, Howell A, Sotgia F, Lisanti MP. Cancer cells metabolically "fertilize" the tumor microenvironment with hydrogen peroxide, driving the Warburg effect: implications for PET imaging of human tumors. *Cell Cycle.* 2011 Aug 1;10(15): e2504-20. doi: 10.4161/cc.10.15.16585. Epub 2011 Aug 1. PMID: 21778829; PMCID: PMC3180189.

Merchant TE, Kasimos JN, de Graaf PW, Minsky BD, Gierke LW, Glonek T. Phospholipid profiles of human colon cancer using 31P magnetic resonance spectroscopy. *Int J Colorectal Dis.* 1991 May;6(2): pp. 121-6. doi: 10.1007/BF00300208. PMID: 1875121.

Minocherhomji S, Tollefsbol TO, Singh KK. Mitochondrial regulation of epigenetics and its role in human diseases. *Epigenetics*. 2012 Apr;7(4): pp. 326-34. doi: 10.4161/epi.19547. Epub 2012 Apr 1. PMID: 22419065; PMCID: PMC3368816.

Pavlides S, Whitaker-Menezes D, Castello-Cros R, Flomenberg N, Witkiewicz AK, Frank PG, Casimiro MC, Wang C, Fortina P, Addya S, Pestell RG, Martinez-Outschoorn UE, Sotgia F, Lisanti MP. The reverse Warburg effect: aerobic glycolysis in cancer associated fibroblasts and the tumor stroma. *Cell Cycle*. 2009 Dec;8(23): e3984-4001. doi: 10.4161/cc.8.23.10238. Epub 2009 Dec 5. PMID: 19923890.

Seyfried TN, Flores RE, Poff AM, D'Agostino DP. Cancer as a metabolic disease: implications for novel therapeutics. *Carcinogenesis*. 2014 Mar;35(3): pp. 515-27. doi: 10.1093/carcin/bgt480. Epub 2013 Dec 16. PMID: 24343361; PMCID: PMC3941741.

Sotgia F, Whitaker-Menezes D, Martinez-Outschoorn UE, Flomenberg N, Birbe RC, Witkiewicz AK, Howell A, Philp NJ, Pestell RG, Lisanti MP. Mitochondrial metabolism in cancer metastasis: visualizing tumor cell mitochondria and the "reverse Warburg effect" in positive lymph node tissue. *Cell Cycle*. 2012 Apr 1;11(7): e1445-54. doi: 10.4161/cc.19841. Epub 2012 Apr 1. PMID: 22395432; PMCID: PMC3350881.

Sotgia F, Whitaker-Menezes D, Martinez-Outschoorn UE, Salem AF, Tsirigos A, Lamb R, Sneddon S, Hulit J, Howell A, Lisanti MP. Mitochondria "fuel" breast cancer metabolism: fifteen markers of mitochondrial biogenesis abel epithelial cancer cells, but are excluded from adjacent stromal cells. *Cell Cycle*. 2012 Dec 1;11(23): e4390-401. doi: 10.4161/cc.22777. Epub 2012 Nov 21. PMID: 23172368; PMCID: PMC3552922.

Thakur S, Daley B, Gaskins K, Vasko VV, Boufraqech M, Patel D, Sourbier C, Reece J, Cheng SY, Kebebew E, Agarwal S, Klubo-Gwiezdzinska J. Metformin Targets Mitochondrial Glycerophosphate Dehydrogenase to Control Rate of Oxidative Phosphorylation and Growth of Thyroid Cancer In Vitro and In Vivo. *Clin Cancer Res.* 2018 Aug 15;24(16): e4030-43. doi:10.1158/1078-0432.CCR-17-3167. Epub 2018 Apr 24. PMID: 29691295; PMCID: PMC6095745.

Urbano, F., Bugliani, M., Filippello, A. et al. Atorvastatin but Not Pravastatin Impairs Mitochondrial Function in Human Pancreatic Islets and Rat β-Cells. Direct Effect of Oxidative Stress. *Sci Rep* 7, e11863 (2017). https://doi.org/10.1038/s41598-017-11070-x.

Viale A, Corti D, Draetta GF. Tumors and mitochondrial respiration: a neglected connection. *Cancer Res.* 2015 Sep 15;75(18): e3685-6. doi: 10.1158/0008-5472.CAN-15-0491. PMID: 26374463.

Xia S, Lin R, Jin L, Zhao L, Kang HB, Pan Y, Liu S, Qian G, Qian Z, Konstantakou E, Zhang B, Dong JT, Chung YR, Abdel-Wahab O, Merghoub T, Zhou L, Kudchadkar RR, Lawson DH, Khoury HJ, Khuri FR, Boise LH, Lonial S, Lee BH, Pollack BP, Arbiser JL, Fan J, Lei QY, Chen J. Prevention of Dietary-Fat-Fueled Ketogenesis Attenuates BRAF V600E Tumor Growth. *Cell Metab.* 2017 Feb 7;25(2): pp. 358-373. doi: 10.1016/j.cmet.2016.12.010. Epub 2017 Jan 12. PMID: 28089569; PMCID: PMC5299059.

Chapter Seven

Changing Opinions Over the Years

Many scientists did not take long to criticize Warburg for his simplistic theory. By the 1950s and 60s, his hypothesis on the metabolic basis of cancer was already less popular. Warburg was blamed for failing to link the cause of cancers with the prevailing gene mutation theory.

Warburg was also criticized because his theory failed to explain the reason behind the many "hallmarks" of cancers.

In 1956, Sidney Weinhouse insisted that Warburg was wrong and that cancer cells do not have faulty respiration (e8927-30). In that year's August issue of *Science*, Weinhouse (1956) publicly disputed Warburg's theory and pointed out that despite the high levels of glycolysis in cancer cells, tumors use oxygen the same way as normal cells (e8927-30). He stated that since cancers use oxygen, cancers must have normal respiration. Weinhouse (1956) also pointed out that the concept of aerobic glycolysis was not new nor unique to cancer (e8927-30). In fact, normal brain, kidney, retina, and intestines also had aerobic glycolysis despite near-normal rates of complete glucose and *fatty acid oxidation* (FAO) (Weinhouse, 1956).

Because of Weinhouse's statements, the Warburg theory lost credibility. For many years, little was published on tumor metabolism. Attention focused on the genetic theory of cancer and remained that way for decades. Tumor suppressor genes and tumor oncogenes took center stage.

In 1970, renewed interest in the metabolic basis of cancer began when the Atkins diet became popular. 1994 was the year when the Charlie Foundation for Ketogenic Therapies began to increase awareness about diet therapies for people with neurological disorders, seizures, and cancers. After that, many others supported the premise behind the ketogenic diet's beneficial effects on medical conditions. Today, the ketogenic diet is gaining popularity and credibility in the medical field.

Chapter Summary/Key Takeaways:

We are a long way from actually using the ketogenic diet in clinical practice. However, the research could expand faster. When we conducted a trial of the modified Atkins diet in advanced cancers in 2013, the ketogenic diet was still largely unknown. Indeed, the last decade has seen a phenomenal rise in interest regarding the ketogenic diet and its potential benefits.

The next chapter will showcase several interesting cases that benefitted from early metabolic therapies.

End Notes

Kim JW, Dang CV. Cancer's molecular sweet tooth and the Warburg effect. *Cancer Res.* 2006 Sep 15;66(18): e8927-30. doi: 10.1158/0008-5472.CAN-06-1501. PMID: 16982728.

Weinhouse S., On respiratory impairment in cancer cells. *Science.* 1956 Aug 10;124(3215): pp. 267-9. doi: 10.1126/science.124.3215.267. PMID: 13351638.

Chapter Eight

Two Interesting Case Studies

There are very few published reports of cancers treated with metabolic therapy. The metabolic-focused publications that exist are few and are usually case reports. Below are two worth mentioning.

In 1956, the New York State Department of Mental Hygiene reported two cases of biopsy-proven metastatic cancers (melanoma and cervical cancer) successfully treated with insulin (Koroljow, 1956, pp. 261-70). The insulin brought down their blood sugars and put the patients into a coma. The doctors prescribed a series of daily, half-hour to one-and-a-half-hour sessions of medically induced *hypoglycemia* (low blood glucose). The two patients not only cured their depression, but their gross tumors completely disappeared (Koroljow, 1962).

Chapter Summary/Key Takeaways:

These two cases had astounding results, even though the disappearance of their tumors was unanticipated.

Since then, there have been many other case reports and reviews of cancer patients treated with dietary plus standard-of-care therapies. However, these were limited to case series and feasibility studies. We need larger-scale, randomized control studies covering cancers in humans. (See this chapter's End Notes for further sources of more case reports and reviews.)

In the next chapter, we will study glutamine, the other major cancer fuel, and how it can reprogram the cell into a cancer-sustaining machine.

End Notes

Abdelwahab, M.G., *et al.*, The ketogenic diet is an effective adjuvant to radiation therapy for the treatment of malignant glioma. *PLoS One*, 2012. 7(5): e36197.

Iyikesici, M.S., *et al.*, Efficacy of Metabolically Supported Chemotherapy Combined with Ketogenic Diet, Hyperthermia, and Hyperbaric Oxygen Therapy for Stage IV Triple-Negative Breast Cancer. *Cureus*, 2017. 9(7): e1445.

Koroljow, S., Two cases of malignant tumors with metastases apparently treated successfully with hypoglycemic coma. *Psychiatr Q*,. 1962. 36: pp. 261-70.

Koroljow, S.A., An investigation of the role played by oxygen and by cellular respiration in hypoglycemic coma. *Psychiatr Q*,. 1956. 30(1): pp. 123-40.

Maroon, J., *et al.*, Restricted calorie ketogenic diet for the treatment of glioblastoma multiforme. *J Child Neurol*, 2013. 28(8): e1002-8.

Nebeling, L.C. and E. Lerner, Implementing a ketogenic diet based on medium-chain triglyceride oil in pediatric patients with cancer. *J Am Diet Assoc*, 1995. 95(6): pp. 693-7.

Perez, A., *et al.*, Comment on: Ketogenic diet treatment in recurrent diffuse intrinsic pontine glioma in children: A safety and feasibility study. *Pediatr Blood Cancer*, 2019. 66(7): e27664.

Schwartz, K., *et al.*, Treatment of glioma patients with ketogenic diets: report of two cases treated with an IRB-approved energy-restricted ketogenic diet protocol and review of the literature. *Cancer Metab*, 2015. 3: p. 3.

van der Louw, E., *et al.*, Ketogenic diet treatment in recurrent diffuse intrinsic pontine glioma in children: A safety and feasibility study. Pediatr Blood Cancer, 2019. 66(3): e27561.

Winter, S.F., F. Loebel, and J. Dietrich, Role of ketogenic metabolic therapy in malignant glioma: A systematic review. *Crit Rev Oncol Hematol*, 2017. 112: pp. 41-58.

Zuccoli, G., *et al.*, Metabolic management of glioblastoma multiforme using standard therapy together with a restricted ketogenic diet: Case Report. *Nutr Metab (Lond)*, 2010. 7: p. 33.

Chapter Nine

Glutamine Basics

Glutamine (Gln) is an amino acid receiving more attention than usual. Surfacing news shows that glutamine may be feeding some cancers. This chapter is essential because most of us have a profound lack of information regarding how glutamine 'feeds' cancer.

A complete overview of glutamine metabolism is beyond the scope of this book. However, here is some basic information to help you follow news about potential metabolic therapies as they become available.

Amino Acids:

Protein is found in chicken, beef, cheese, eggs, nuts, lentils, seafood, and soy. These proteins found in animal products are also found in many plant-based foods. When we digest, the stomach secretes acids to help deconstruct protein into a simpler form—small units called amino acids. Once we digest proteins into small amino acids, they are absorbed into the bloodstream as they pass through intestinal surface cells. Most amino acids arrive at the liver to be broken down further, then sent back to the blood towards their final destinations. Depending on the amino acid, they might have different destinations.

Breaking down amino acids results in excess nitrogen and a carbon skeleton. The carbon skeleton is vital to new cancer survival. It supplies the scaffolding needed to create new cellular building material while the excess nitrogen becomes ammonia, which is toxic and therefore excreted as urea in the urine.

While some amino acids come from the diet, others are produced naturally inside the body and are 'non-essential.' We have twenty amino acids in the body, each breaking down to glutamate (Glu), the acidic version of glutamine (Gln).

Introduction to Glutamine:

The most abundant amino acid found in our blood is glutamine. Glutamine is a building block used to make other amino acids. We even use glutamine to make glucose, protein, and *glutathione,* an antioxidant. Antioxidants can, therefore, protect us from cancer.

Glutamine shuttles out excess ammonia from the body. We store it in our muscles and our lungs. Our gut lining depends on it to stay intact and healthy. Cancer patients lose a lot of glutamine when their muscles shrink, and use it to protect against infection, heal surgical wounds, and lessen the side effects of chemotherapy (Miller, 1999).

What are some sources of glutamine?

Glutamine is a non-essential amino acid. We don't need to find glutamine in the diet because we make it ourselves. But how?

Glutamine from glucose! Some carbon atoms can be retrieved and used to build glutamine by breaking down glucose through glycolysis. The glycolytic intermediates (aka, the middlemen steps) include glucose-6 phosphate, pyruvate, 3-phosphoglycerate, and *phosphoenolpyruvate* (PEP), any of which can be recycled to create glutamine in a '*de novo*' fashion.

What are the benefits of glutamine?

Many are aware that glutamine can feed cancers. It may also help some rewired cancers to grow, so it may surprise you that glutamine is also important for our health and is the most abundant amino acid in the bloodstream (Zhao, *et al.*, 2019; Piva & McEvoy-Bowe, 1998).

The benefits of glutamine deserve some mention.

Gut Health:

Glutamine is anti-inflammatory. Celiac and irritable bowel syndrome (IBS) patients often suffer from gut inflammation. During inflammation, the body activates several lines of defense—NF-κB protein, *interleukin-6* (IL-6), and *tumor necrosis factor-alpha* (TNF-α)—to kill the gut lining cells. Glutamine can blunt this inflammatory attack by activating its counterattack with *heat shock proteins* (HSP) to reduce the cell death enzyme (caspase) and keep cells alive (Wischmeyer,

2002). Glutamine supplements can also heal the gut lining by maintaining a 'tight junction' between the cells that line the gut (Li, *et al.*, 2004).

Healing From Surgery:

Glutamine supplements might help recovery after surgery and give additional antioxidant protection thanks to its byproduct, *glutathione*. This is important because intact guts guard against sepsis and infection (Li, *et al.*, 2004; Wischmeyer, *et al.*, 2014). However, a study of ten rectal cancer patients who underwent chemo-radiotherapy and received glutamine to help speed up gut healing failed to show improvement compared to those who received a placebo. Samples of both their healthy and cancerous tissue were examined by expert pathologists for signs of radiation-related damage. Unfortunately, they failed to prove that glutamine protected the rectal tissue from damage (Vidal-Casariego, 2015).

What are some of the anti-cancer benefits of glutamine?

Glutamine is feared to cause cancer, but so many do not know that glutamine can also protect us from cancer. Healthy cells need to stick together. We already mentioned that glutamine maintains tight cell junctions. These junctions stay tight to prevent cell leakage of water and electrolytes. Healthy cells use intact cell junctions to send communication signals to each other. Healthy junctions prevent metastasis by preserving cell-to-cell contacts (Li, *et al.*, 2004). Cancer cells begin to move when these contacts are broken.

Glutamine can also preserve the *epithelial-mesenchymal transition* (EMT) zone between surface cells and the underlying tissue. When the EMT is damaged, cancer cells are free to leave their origin and travel to distant organs like the liver, bone, or brain. When tumors use glutamine, eventually, their core gets depleted of glutamine. Glutamine depletion within the tumor weakens the EMT barrier, allowing cancers to move and metastasize. (Recouvreux, *et al.*, 2020).

Daily Benefits of Glutamine:

Glutamine helps our immune system:

The white blood cells (i.e., lymphocytes) that comprise our immune system depend on glutamine. The liver, gut, skeletal muscles, and kidneys all use glutamine. Without glutamine, we risk infections, wounds heal poorly, and our liver and kidneys may fail (Calder & Yaqoob, 1999).

Glutamine helps bodybuilding and recovery:

Excess glucose is stored as glycogen (as shown in Figure 9, page 57) in both the liver and muscles. Glutamine's carbons become part of the glycogen structure. During times of stress and inflammation, the liver and muscles release glutamine. Some examples of stressful times are when we undergo surgery, extensive physical exercise, or severe infections. Glutamine supplements can speed up recovery in surgical and critically ill patients (Li, *et al.*, 2004)

Glutamine as antioxidant protection:

Glutamine can also become glutathione, providing antioxidant protection against ROS damage (Li, *et al.*, 2004; Wischmeyer, *et al.,* 2014).

Building our genetic structure:

Our genetic material, DNA, is made up of nitrogen coming from glutamine. DNA is a structure that looks like a spiral staircase, with each step comprising two types of building blocks, called nucleic acid. Some of glutamine's nitrogen becomes part of nucleic acids (Coster, *et al.,* 2004).

Glutamine maintains the balance of cell energy forces.

Glutamine contributes to cell structures and ATP energy production. Part of the cell structure comprises protein, fats, steroids, and cholesterol, all of which receive energy from glutamine (Cruzat, *et al.*, 2018; Mansour, *et al.*, 2015).

Glutamine as a housekeeper:

Glutamine provides us with housekeeping as well as detoxification benefits. Its ability to transport nitrogen helps us keep our body clean by neutralizing excess toxic ammonia, which leaves our body through our liver as urea and through our kidneys as ammonia. Glutamine is vital for health.

Important glutamine enzymes:

Normal cells can control glutamine metabolism and slow production to avoid excess.

The process of glutamine metabolism will ultimately transform glutamine into *alpha-ketoglutarate* (AKG). Glutamine-sourced AKG is identical to the AKG from citrate in the Krebs cycle, but its goal is to use the Krebs cycle for a short segment and then head over to the fat-making pathway.

Cancers have very active glutamine enzymes.

Two important enzymes and two steps are needed in this transformation to AKG. The first enzyme is glutaminase (GLS), which changes glutamine into an acid called glutamate (Glu). The second enzyme is *glutamine dehydrogenase* (GDH). GDH helps glutamate (Glu) transform into AKG, the fourth Krebs cycle step. This is where glutamine (Gln) enters the Krebs cycle. But unlike the AKG that comes from citrate, this AKG arrives from glutamine (Gln) with a different purpose: joining the FAS pathway to make energy, membranes, and structural building blocks for AKG.

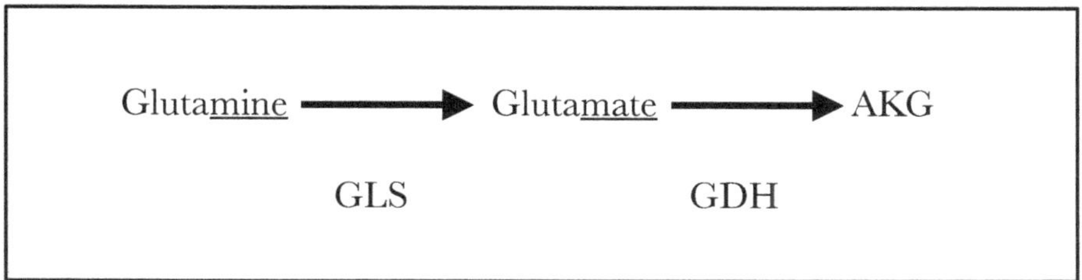

Alpha-ketoglutarate (AKG):

AKG is just another form of glutamine. It is currently sold as an over-the-counter nutritional supplement with possible anti-aging benefits. AKG from the Krebs cycle is a healthy thing to have.

If you examine the Krebs cycle closely, you will see that AKG is the fourth step. It is important for keeping metabolic machinery healthy and running well.

Aside from efficiency, AKG has many jobs. It controls gene expression, balances oxygen status in the cell, fights inflammation by reducing oxidative stress, removes waste, and helps make new building blocks for protein (amino acids).

Resistance exercise can increase AKG in the blood and muscle. Exercising with weights can make AKG stimulate the adrenal gland to produce adrenaline, which builds muscle mass and helps with fat loss (Yexian, *et al.*, 2020).

Oral AKG, in supplement form or the diet, appears to delay aging in mice, worms, fruit flies, and yeast cells. Its benefits may depend on AKG's ability to act as an antioxidant, mimic calorie restriction, and build DNA. AKG does have some bad effects, too, such as causing inflammation. The benefits of AKG, however, seem to outweigh its detriments (Bayliak & Lushchak, 2021).

Glutamine and Fat: How are they related?

We know glucose can work alongside glutamine to produce energy. Sometimes, glutamine pathways take an 'extra turn,' and the cancer begins to make its own fat (*de novo* fatty acid synthesis).

When does glutamine turn into fat? The 'Go' signal comes when oxygen is extremely low. Soon, a domino effect of reactions happens. HIF1-α protein becomes stable and active. Glutamine (Gln) turns into glutamate (Glu) (acid) and AKG (a form of glutamine). AKG enters the Krebs cycle, but instead of moving in the cycle to make energy, AKG becomes citric acid, which will now be used to make fat, which cancers use for construction purposes. This fat-making occurs in the *de novo* fatty acid synthesis pathway. Aggressive cancers often have cells that have overactive FAS.

We now know that glutamine plays a role in making fat synthesis overactive. Another enzyme involved is fatty acid synthase (FASN). You will see its name in many scientific articles on fat and cancer.

In addition, the AKG from glutamine will activate mTOR signaling pathways, another cancer growth promoter (Yoo, *et al.*, 2020).

TAKE AWAY POINT:

When cancers grow and crowd, oxygen levels drop. When oxygen is low, both glutamine and fat pathways become very active. We also know that behind all this, glucose breakdown pathways (glycolysis) are overactive, keeping oxygen levels low (Sun & Denko, 2014). The AKG coming from glutamine is not a friendly player here.

In tumors with *both* the fat and glutamine pathways active, blocking both pathways might be necessary.

Potential therapies:

A. Smoking cessation

Since low oxygen activates the HIF-1 protein to wake up many pro-cancer signals, could improving low oxygen conditions be useful? Smoking can worsen oxygen conditions, so it should be stopped.

B. Green tea

We know that glutamine (Gln) changes to AKG in two steps: 1) from glutamine (Gln) to glutamate (Glu) and 2) from glutamate (Glu) to AKG. The enzyme responsible for the second step (glutamate Glu to AKG) is GDH, which can be neutralized by EGCG, the active ingredient in green tea (Hensley, *et al.*, 2013). (Review page 119 for a visual timeline.)

C. Nutrition and healthy epigenetics

Nutrition plays a significant role in keeping us epigenetically sound. Proper nutrition and vitamins (B6, B12, and folate) help maintain our healthy genes by keeping our *epigenetic layer* healthy. Protein can also help. Proteins comprise amino acids, which can help us maintain advantageous epigenetics, improve our gene expression, and keep us healthy (Ji, *et al.*, 2016).

Chapter Summary/Key Takeaways:

You have just completed a basic introduction to glutamine, how it is useful for normal cells, and why we simply cannot live without it.

I've introduced you to some key enzymes that control glutamine metabolism. They will be useful as we advance to the next chapter, examining how and why glutamine can also benefit cancers.

End Notes

Bayliak MM, Lushchak VI. Pleiotropic effects of alpha-ketoglutarate as a potential anti-aging agent. *Ageing Res Rev.* 2021 Mar;66: e101237. doi: 10.1016/j.arr.2020.101237. Epub 2020 Dec 16. PMID: 33340716.

Calder PC, Yaqoob P. Glutamine and the immune system. *Amino Acids.* 1999;17(3): pp. 227-41. doi: 10.1007/BF01366922. PMID: 10582122.

Coster J, McCauley R, Hall J. Glutamine: metabolism and application in nutrition support. *Asia Pac J Clin Nutr.* 2004;13(1): pp. 25-31. PMID: 15003911.

Cruzat V, Macedo Rogero M, Noel Keane K, Curi R, Newsholme P. Glutamine: Metabolism and Immune Function, Supplementation and Clinical Translation. *Nutrients.* 2018 Oct 23;10(11): e1564. doi: 10.3390/nu10111564. PMID: 30360490; PMCID: PMC6266414.

Hensley CT, Wasti AT, DeBerardinis RJ. Glutamine and cancer: cell biology, physiology, and clinical opportunities. *J Clin Invest.* 2013 Sep;123(9): e3678-84. doi: 10.1172/JCI69600. Epub 2013 Sep 3. PMID: 23999442; PMCID: PMC3754270.

Ji Yun, Wu Z, Dai Z, Sun K, Wang J, Wu G. Nutritional epigenetics with a focus on amino acids: implications for the development and treatment of metabolic syndrome. *J Nutr Biochem*. 2016 Jan;27: pp. 1-8. doi: 10.1016/j.jnutbio.2015.08.003. Epub 2015 Aug 10. PMID: 26427799.

Li N, Lewis P, Samuelson D, Liboni K, Neu J. Glutamine regulates Caco-2 cell tight junction proteins. *Am J Physiol Gastrointest Liver Physiol.* 2004 Sep;287(3): G726-33. doi: 10.1152/ajpgi.00012.2004. Epub 2004 May 6. PMID: 15130874.

Mansour A, Mohajeri-Tehrani MR, Qorbani M, Heshmat R, Larijani B, Hosseini S. Effect of glutamine supplementation on cardiovascular risk factors in patients with type 2 diabetes. *Nutrition*. 2015 Jan;31(1): pp. 119-26. doi: 10.1016/j.nut.2014.05.014. Epub 2014 Jun 23. PMID: 25466655.

Miller AL. Therapeutic considerations of L-glutamine: a review of the literature. *Altern Med Rev.* 1999 Aug;4(4): pp. 239-48. PMID: 10468648.

Piva TJ, McEvoy-Bowe E. Oxidation of glutamine in HeLa cells: role and control of truncated TCA cycles in tumour mitochondria. *J Cell Biochem.* 1998 Feb 1;68(2): pp. 213-25. doi: 10.1002/(sici)1097-4644(19980201)68:2<213::aid-jcb8>3.0.co;2-y. PMID: 9443077.

Recouvreux, M. V., Moldenhauer, M. R., Galenkamp, K. M. O., Jung, M., James, B., Zhang, Y., Lowy, A., Bagchi, A., & Commisso, C. (2020). Glutamine depletion regulates slug to promote EMT and metastasis in pancreatic cancer. *Journal of Experimental Medicine*, 217(9), e20200388. https://doi.org/10.1084/jem.20200388.

Sun RC, Denko NC. Hypoxic regulation of glutamine metabolism through HIF1 and SIAH2 supports lipid synthesis that is necessary for tumor growth. *Cell Metab*. 2014 Feb 4;19(2): pp. 285-92. doi: 10.1016/j.cmet.2013.11.022. PMID: 24506869; PMCID: PMC3920584

Vidal-Casariego A, Hernando-Martín M, Calleja-Fernández A, Cano-Rodríguez I, Cordido F, Ballesteros-Pomar MD. Tissue effects of glutamine in rectal cancer patients treated with preoperative chemoradiotherapy. *Nutr Hosp*. 2015 Apr 1;31(4): e1689-92. doi: 10.3305/nh.2015.31.4.8521. PMID: 25795959.

Wischmeyer PE. Glutamine and heat shock protein expression. *Nutrition*. 2002 Mar;18(3): pp. 225-8. doi: 10.1016/s0899-9007(01)00796-1. PMID: 11882394.

Wischmeyer PE, Dhaliwal R, McCall M, Ziegler TR, Heyland DK. Parenteral glutamine supplementation in critical illness: a systematic review. *Crit Care*. 2014 Apr 18;18(2): R76. doi: 10.1186/cc13836. PMID: 24745648; PMCID: PMC4056606.

Yexian Yuan, Pingwen Xu, Qingyan Jiang, Xingcai Cai, Tao Wang, Wentong Peng, Jiajie Sun, Canjun Zhu, Cha Zhang, Dong Yue, Zhihui He, Jinping Yang, Yuxian Zeng, Man Du, Fenglin Zhang, Lucas Ibrahimi, Sarah Schaul, Yuwei Jiang, Jiqiu Wang, Jia Sun, Qiaoping Wang, Liming Liu, Songbo Wang, Lina Wang, Xiaotong Zhu, Ping Gao, Qianyun Xi, Cong Yin, Fan Li, Guli Xu, Yongliang Zhang, Gang Shu (2020, February 27). Exercise-induced α-ketoglutaric acid stimulates muscle hypertrophy and fat loss through OXGR1-dependent adrenal activation. *The EMBO Journal*. https://www.embopress.org/doi/full/10.15252/embj.2019103304. https://doi.org/10.15252/embj.2019103304.

Yoo, H.C., Yu, Y.C., Sung, Y. et al. Glutamine reliance in cell metabolism. *Exp Mol Med.* 52, e1496–1516 (2020). https://doi.org/10.1038/s12276-020-00504-8

Zhao, Y., Zhao, X., Chen, V. *et al.* Colorectal cancers utilize glutamine as an anaplerotic substrate of the TCA cycle in vivo. *Sci Rep.* 9, e19180 (2019). https://doi.org/10.1038/s41598-019-55718-2

Chapter Ten

Glutamine and Cancer

There is indeed proof that our friend glutamine can suddenly turn into a traitor and begin to feed and enable cancer. According to Warburg, cancers use up a lot of glucose, but most of that glucose will turn into lactic acid (lactate). These cancers prefer lactate and try to avoid making acetyl-CoA, the molecule that sits near the intersection of the glucose, amino acid, and fat pathways.

Once we reach the acetyl-CoA step, for normal cells, the next stop is the Krebs cycle. Warburg-type cancers normally avoid this step and prefer to stay in glycolysis to make lots of lactic acids.

However, some rewired cancers will turn some glucose into acetyl-CoA, which feeds into the Krebs cycle. Shortly after entering the cycle, citric acid (citrate), the first step of the circular chain reaction, will leave the mitochondria and head toward the fat-making (synthesis) pathway to make fat. Typically, we see this 'fat detour' when the body has a significant excess of glucose. This detour is also seen in rewired cancers, which also use fat to make structural supports for themselves. We now have a glucose <u>and</u> fat-loving cancer. This is similar to the detour glutamine takes while en route to the fat-making pathways.

When glucose sends acetyl-CoA to enter the Krebs cycle, it moves (rotates) a little, hoping to make energy. Still, the cycle does not continue because citrate leaves the cycle early and heads outside the mitochondria, landing in the jelly-filled cytosol to join the fat-making pathway.

Meanwhile, the cancers keep growing and crowding. Soon, the lack of oxygen will also trigger glutamine metabolism.

What happens when glutamine-related enzymes are overactive?

Let's take a moment to highlight the glutamine-related enzymes. Cancers have very active versions of these enzymes. Glutamine (Gln) can jumpstart the Krebs cycle by entering as AKG. However, glutamine (Gln) must undergo a few changes before turning into AKG. The glutaminase (GLS) enzyme changes glutamine (Gln) into glutamate (Glu); another enzyme, the glutamine dehydrogenase (GDH), turns it into AKG. Both enzymes (GLS and GDH) are very active in cancers. AKG can now enter the Krebs cycle and rotate it 'in reverse.' The reverse Krebs cycle goes backward towards citrate. It will make lots of citric acid, leaving the cycle and the mitochondria to head toward the fatty acid synthesis (FAS) pathway to build more fat (Nguyen & Durán, 2018).

In addition to the fat synthesis pathway, the mTORC pathway can sense the presence of glutamine (Gln). When GLS (the first enzyme) changes glutamine (Gln) to glutamate (Glu), the mTORC1 cancer-signaling pathway plus several other cancer pathways (such as PTEN, AMPK, and IGF-1/PI3K/Akt) become active (Durán, *et al.*, 2012).

GDH (the second enzyme) makes enough AKG to supply the fat needs of cancers and to balance antioxidant glutathione levels in cancers (Jin, *et al.*, 2015). Targeting these enzymes (GLS and GDH) is a way to control cancer growth metabolically.

AKG, aging, and cancer:

AKG is a form of glutamine that seems to be important for maintaining youth. Between ages 40 and 80, AKG drops significantly (Harrison & Pierzynowski, 2008). When aging mice received AKG supplements, it suppressed inflammation and prolonged their lifespans (Asadi Shahmirzadi, *et al.*, 2020).

When our glutamine metabolism becomes active, the cancers themselves become glutamine-depleted. Since AKG comes from glutamine, loss of glutamine means that AKG will also drop. Low AKG disturbs DNA strands, creating a new gene pattern that favors more cancer (Tran, *et al.*, 2020).

Another important enzyme, the *isocitrate dehydrogenase* (IDH), helps the Krebs cycle rotate and make energy. If you take another look at the cycle (Figure 8, page 55), you see that IDH normally becomes AKG. Some cancers have defective IDH enzymes. An example is IDH1. Acute myelogenous leukemia (blood cancer) and cholangiocarcinoma (bile duct cancer) are examples.

Dr. Thomas Seyfried mentioned that the "IDH1 mutation in glioblastoma is like winning the lottery". He was referring to the increased tumor killing seen when IDH1 mutated glioma cells were exposed to temozolomide chemotherapy in the laboratory. The mutation blocks the ability of cancer cells to repair themselves after being damaged by chemotherapy, resulting in significantly less tumor growth and better patient outcomes. This mutation seems like a good thing to have because it makes cancer cells die more easily when exposed to chemotherapy.

However, we know that having an IDH1 mutation is like having a double-edged sword. After a while, the cancers begin to grow again and are resistant to chemotherapy. Why? Because the IDH1 mutation causes "downstream effects" or "aftershocks."

The cancer cell develops "epigenetic changes" that create dysfunctional Krebs cycle members (intermediates). The mitochondrial damage continues. If you are hungry for greater detail, read on.

When IDH becomes defective, the Krebs cycle cannot move properly to make AKG, and we will see AKG supplies fall. As AKG drops, we run out of the stress-reducing protector, NADPH, which changes cells into cancers. The defective (mutated) IDH1 also damages tumor-suppressor genes, so we lose our natural ability to suppress cancer. IDH1 mutations can also rearrange the DNA proteins (epigenetic change) and 'shut off' the maturation process. Cells with IDH1 mutations cannot make normal AKG and instead make a mutated version called *2-hydroxyglutarate*. Because AKG is low, the Krebs cycle can no longer function normally, so the cell turns towards glucose for alternative fuel. As the amounts of defective AKG accumulate, the cell activates the pro-cancer pathways (PI3K/Akt, and mTOR pathways). It opens new glucose docking stations (GLUT receptors) to create an energy-rich environment conducive to new cancer growth.

Because of these 'downstream effects,' according to several researchers, targeting IDH1 mutations (a type of chemotherapy called IDH inhibitor) can be a possible cancer treatment. (See: Tran, *et al.*, 2020; Dang, *et al.* 2016; Lu, *et al.*, 2012; Reitman & Yan, 2010.)

Glutamine uses transporters to enter the cell.

Glutamine cannot just flow freely into our cells. The entryway is tightly controlled. Special proteins called glutamine transporters are located on the cell membrane's surface. These proteins control the entry and exit of glutamine into and out of cells. Most transporters allow glutamine into cells, but only a few will allow glutamine to exit. Many transporters live in the liver, kidney, brain, and placenta cells.

Overactive glutamine transporters will allow glutamine to reach more cancers. By blocking some, we can starve glutamine-hungry cancers (Bhutia & Ganapathy, 2016). Let's look at some of these transporters.

Types of glutamine transporters

SLC1A5 (a.k.a. ASCT2) and SLC7A5 are two examples of glutamine transporters seen as active in many cancers, such as prostate, breast, colon, lung, brain, and retinoblastoma (Bhutia & Ganapathy, 2016). The retinoblastoma tumor suppressor gene encourages more glutaminase enzyme activity and activates the SLC1A5/ASCT2 transporters (Reynolds, *et al.*, 2014). The major glutamine transporter types in mammals appear to belong to the SLC38 family (Bhutia & Ganapathy, 2016).

This knowledge is important for the future development of drugs that target glutamine transporters or if you are searching for clinical trials (Bhutia & Ganapathy, 2016; Bhutia, *et al.*, 2015). Go to www.clinicaltrials.gov and type in the keywords to search for trials. For example, use glutamine transporters, SLC1A5, SLC7A5, and ASCT2.

Glutamine also makes lactic acid.

Glutamine enters the Krebs cycle through the AKG step. The cycle rotates and makes ATP energy. Some of that glutamine will detour into a different pathway to make lactate (lactic acid), another cancer fuel. The rest of the glutamine is excreted in the urine (Zielke, *et al.*, 1980).

Glutamine and oncogenes

C-Myc is a pro-cancer gene (oncogene) that helps cancers use glutamine by allowing more of it to enter cancer cells. How? C-Myc increases glutamine transporter proteins (SLC1A5/ASCT2) that sit on the cells. As cancers multiply and crowd each other out, oxygen levels fall, and C-Myc binds to glutamine receptors to let glutamine in (van Geldermalsen, *et al.*, 2016).

C-Myc also allows glutamine to enter the Krebs cycle to make energy by boosting the glutaminase (GLS) enzyme, which breaks down glutamine (Gln) to become glutamate (Glu). In turn, glutamate (Glu) becomes AKG (α-ketoglutarate), which then enters the Krebs cycle. C-Myc also boosts levels of *glutamine synthetase* (GS), the enzyme that makes glutamine (Gln) (Bott, *et al.*, 2015). Several cancers, such as pancreatic and esophagus, have high levels of C-Myc (Madden, *et al.*, 2021). We still do not have a clinically approved drug that will target C-Myc. Research is ongoing.

Glutamine ferments too.

Glucose and glutamine (Gln) can ferment to make lactic acid (lactate) to fuel cancers (Zielke, *et al.*, 1980; Martinez-Outschoorn, *et al.*, 2011). We can trace this pathway from glutamine (Gln) to glutamate (Glu)—AKG—succinate—malate—pyruvate until it eventually leads to lactate.

Aside from serving as cancer fuel, lactate can activate glutamine metabolism, C-Myc oncogenes, boost glutamine receptors, and participate in gluconeogenesis (GNG), to make more glucose (de la Cruz-López, *et al.*, 2019).

Breast cancers with higher lactate levels had more aggressive cancers, higher blood LDH levels, and worse prognoses (Cheung, *et al.*, 2020).

Glutaminase and new cancer blood vessels—*Angiogenesis:*

Glutamine, just like glucose, can help cancers sprout new

blood vessels. Its enzymes—GLS and GS—help build and maintain blood vessels for cancer growth. This GLS enzyme can delay the aging of the cells that line the blood vessels. The other enzyme, GS, is also linked to new blood vessel growth (Huang, *et al.*, 2017; Eelen, *et al.*, 2018).

Sirtuins proteins (SIRTs) and glutamine:

If you follow longevity news, you are likely familiar with SIRTs. As we age, our SIRT levels drop, and so do our *nicotinamide* (NAD+) levels. NAD+ was first discovered in 1906 as an enhancer to speed up alcohol fermentation. However, NAD+ is a very important signaling molecule because it controls the speed by which we age. Old age decreases NAD+ and SIRT. Proof of this was seen in animal studies where supplemental NAD+ appeared to prolong life.

There are seven versions of SIRT. Inside the mitochondria, we have SIRT 3, 4, and 5.

Sirtuin 4 (SIRT4):

SIRT4 is a glutamine 'switch' that can silence or foster glutamine metabolism. It blocks (switches off) the GLS enzyme, which changes glutamine (Gln) to glutamate (Glu), and activates (switches on) the pro-cancer AKT/GSK3β/cyclinD1 pathway (Cui, *et al.*, 2021).

SIRT4 levels are high in the brain, especially in embryos or newborns, but drop as babies develop and drop further as we age.

SIRT4 stops glutamine entry into the Krebs cycle.

Glutamate dehydrogenase (GDH) enzymes provide the 'grease' to change glutamate into AKG, the step before AKG enters the Krebs cycle. This step is also tightly monitored by SIRT4. SIRT4 keeps us healthy by blocking GDH and preventing glutamine from becoming ATP energy.

Remember, the pathway to make ATP begins with glutamine:

Glutamine (Gln) ➡ Glutamate (Glu) ➡AKG ➡ Krebs cycle ➡ ATP energy.

GDH greases the step between glutamate and AKG. SIRT4 puts a 'brake' on this step. To keep healthy, we need to keep our SIRT4 levels steady.

Under normal conditions, SIRT4 maintains and protects our metabolic processes against cancer, fatty liver, obesity, and type 2 diabetes.

Lab studies showed that when SIRT4 was low, colorectal cancers grew (Cui, *et al.*, 2021).

The supplement *nicotinamide riboside* (NR)(which later turns into NAD+) increased SIRT4 levels in mice. Although this sounds intriguing, we still need more research to investigate whether NR can help prevent human cancer by boosting SIRTs (Fernandez-Marcos & Serrano, 2013).

We also need to exercise caution because SIRT4 can

transform into a protector of cancer cells under extreme conditions such as radiation or chemotherapy, allowing them time to acquire defects and grow aggressively.

SIRT4 also blocks fatty acid oxidation (breakdown) and slows the glucose pathway by blocking the PDH gatekeeper enzyme. PDH takes the acetyl-CoA from glucose and feeds it into the Krebs cycle to make energy. By blocking this, SIRT4 can also fight cancer (Mathias, *et al.*, 2014).

We know SIRT4 is good because it keeps genes stable, maintains normal insulin signals, and regulates the Krebs cycle and fat metabolism. SIRT4 can also reduce stress, prolong life, and delay cancer. Another way to increase SIRT4 levels is by fasting (Wood, *et al.*, 2018).

The other versions of SIRTs—SIRT 1-3 and 5-7—have different functions which are not pertinent to our venture here.

Glutamine pathway crosses with mTORC pathways.

mTORC pathways are cancer growth signals that work with glutaminase (GLS) enzymes to make cancers grow. Advanced papillary thyroid cancers have elevated GLS activity. GLS inhibitors are potential cancer treatments that can help stop cancer growth and invasion by simultaneously deactivating the mTORC1 and blocking the glutamine pathway (Saladini, *et al.*, 2019). I will discuss glutaminase inhibitors in more detail in the next chapter.

Which cancers favor glutamine?

Many blood cancers and solid tumors have abnormal glutamine metabolism. Examples include *chronic lymphocytic leukemia* (CLL), chronic myelogenous leukemia (Poteti, *et al.*, 2021), acute myelogenous leukemia (Ashkan, 2015; Goto, *et al.*, 2014); pancreatic (Son, *et al.*, 2013), prostate (Albertelli, *et al.*, 2013), and papillary thyroid cancer 3 (Kim, *et al.*, 2016). There are probably more, as we currently do not have a way of testing people's cancers for glutamine metabolism abnormalities.

The great debate: Is glutamine your friend or enemy?

At the start of this chapter, I explained the many benefits of glutamine. Glutathione is also a product of glutamine. It is an antioxidant that can protect against cancer by neutralizing stress-inducing ROS.

We also know that glutamine can be our enemy, fueling cancer growth by using special pathways in the cell that may be linked to glucose and/or fat pathways.

Most people think that to fight glutamine-addicted cancer, we need to cut out all glutamine, but we cannot avoid glutamine; it is everywhere—in our muscles, in our organs, and almost all foods contain glutamine. We also need glutamine because, without it, we will easily get infections, lose energy, and die.

Are glutamine supplements safe to use in cancer patients?

Compared to patients not on glutamine, colorectal cancer patients who underwent radical surgery and took supplements had surgical wounds that leaked less and healed faster (Yang, *et al.*, 2021).

A study of sixty-five breast cancer patients received doxifluridine (no longer used) chemotherapy. Thirty-three received glutamine at 10 grams three times a day for eight consecutive days in between chemotherapy sessions, and the other group of thirty-two patients received maltodextrin. There was no difference in side effects, diarrhea, or tumor growth (Bozetti, *et al.*, 1997).

A study of nine newly diagnosed inflammatory breast cancer patients received glutamine at a dose of 0.5 grams for every kilogram of body weight per day in addition to methotrexate and doxorubicin (in common use) chemotherapy. None of the patients had severe chemotherapy toxic side effects. All patients except one responded to chemotherapy; median survival was thirty-five months (Rubio, *et al.*, 1998).

Another study of rectal cancer patients given oral glutamine supplements during radiation and chemotherapy showed no difference in preventing inflammation or diarrhea. More importantly, glutamine did not worsen tumor growth (Rotovnik, *et al.*, 2010; Vidal-Casariego, *et al.*, 2015).

In a study of *non-small cell lung cancer* (NSCLC), patients with radiation esophagitis (swelling of the esophagus after radiation) were given glutamine supplements to help heal them. Glutamine did not worsen the cancers (Topkan, *et al.*, 2012).

Glutamine shrinks tumors.

Radiation therapy can easily damage the delicate cells of the gut. Glutamine supplements given to a group of esophageal cancer patients undergoing chemotherapy plus radiation helped protect against gut barrier breakdown and preserved immunity by maintaining blood lymphocyte counts. Cachectic (rapid muscle wasting) rats injected with breast cancer cells were given glutamine injections. This slowed down the muscle wasting, helped their intestinal cells recover, and shrank their tumors (Martins, *et al.*, 2016)!

In rats carrying sarcoma tumors, glutamine supplementation plus methotrexate were injected into their body cavities/peritoneum. The results showed that methotrexate levels were higher inside the tumor and made the tumors shrink (Klimberg, *et al.*, 1992). GLS activity was also suppressed.

More recently, a mouse model of BRAFV600-positive melanoma, given glutamine supplements, showed improved tumor control and prolonged survival. Glutamine also helped the treatment (BRAF inhibitor) work better. But how?

The cancer had low levels of AKG. The glutamine supplement helped replenish the tumor's depleted AKG. When AKG was restored, an epigenetic change happened—the cancer cells removed excess methyl groups from the DNA. Removal of excess methyl groups (demethylation) allowed full gene expression, blocking cancer-signaling pathways (Ishak, *et al.*, 2020).

A study investigated whether glutamine could prevent breast cancer in rats. *Dimethylbenzaanthracene* (DMBA) is a lab supplement that blocks glutathione. When fed to young adult rats, they developed breast cancer because they lost their antioxidant protection. The investigators also gave glutamine to rats, some receiving four weeks, while others received eleven weeks of glutamine (Kaufmann, *et al.*, 2003). Those who received glutamine for a longer period had double the amount of the antioxidant glutathione. Glutamine prevented cancer from forming, and the longer the glutamine was given, the greater the protection.

Strangely, the reverse was seen when the cells of acute myelogenous leukemias (a type of blood cancer) were deprived of glutamine and glutathione. Researchers found that these glutamine-dependent blood cancers also had overactive GLS, the enzyme that makes glutamine. The activity of these glutamine-related enzymes appears to be an important clue that tells us whether or not a cancer is addicted to glutamine (Matre, *et al.*, 2016).

These case reports are both intriguing and encouraging. The timing of glutamine supplementation in humans with active cancer needs further investigation via well-designed randomized control trials.

Possible reasons for glutamine supplement benefit:

Our immune system has *T-lymphocytes* (T Cells), special white blood cells that provide immunity. T cells help clear abnormal cells from the body and lessen cancer risk. Glutamine is one of many amino acids that can help maintain our immune system (Calder &

Yaqoob, 1999).

When infections overwhelm the body, some may die of low blood pressure due to failure of blood vessels during shock. Glutamine helps keep the blood vessels active by boosting heat shock proteins (HSP) to lower inflammation (Jing, *et al.*, 2007).

How to effectively block glutamine:

With Glutamine blockers:

You will learn more about glutamine blockers in the next chapter.

With glutamine supplements:

Not for the faint of heart. We saw many cases of glutamine supplementation that did not fuel cancer growth. Could it be because the presence of glutamine itself might serve as negative feedback against GLS activity? Could the effect on T cell activation and improved cellular stress response overshadow cancer's glutamine hunger? Could the benefit of glutamine supplementation on gut health affect whether cancers develop or grow? Are we seeing tumor control because of a predominant anti-inflammatory gut-related benefit from the glutamine?

Another study of mice with colitis and colorectal cancers received a glutamine-rich diet. Their symptoms and tumor sizes were reduced. Glutamine dampened the inflammation by lowering NF-κB, *cyclooxygenase-2* (COX2), and inducible *nitric oxide synthase* (NOS) activity, resulting in cancer cell deaths (Tian, *et al.*, 2013).

Lastly, dietary glutamine supplements shrank a mouse melanoma by *hypomethylating* H3K4me3. Hypomethylation is a way of changing the gene expression (epigenetic) to suppress cancer activity. The researchers found that hypomethylation helped improve survival, delayed tumor growth, and improved the effectiveness of BRAF inhibitors in a BRAF-positive mouse. Glutamine supplementation replenished the depleted glutamine and AKG stores in the tumor without fueling the cancer (Ishak, *et al.*, 2020).

Chapter Summary/Key Takeaways:

Glucose-deprived cancers rewire themselves to use glutamine after exposure to low oxygen.

Once transformed into glutamine addicts, cancers can make energy by entering the Krebs cycle through the glutamine(Gln)-glutamate(Glu)-AKG pathway, going clockwise. When oxygen is very low, glutamine can also turn cancers into fat addicts using the reverse Krebs cycle, where glutamine enters through the same AKG step but goes counterclockwise toward the fat production pathway.

We cannot underestimate the damaging effects of lactate. Lactate allows new blood vessel formation, increased invasiveness, and pro-cancer epigenetic changes. Oncogenes and mutated tumor suppressors favor overexpression of glutamine transporters and enzymes. These mechanisms are complex and intertwined but open many possibilities for treatment. Both glucose and glutamine will also turn into lactate.

This chapter has also introduced you to the favorable side of glutamine. Alpha-ketoglutarate (AKG) is a form of beneficial glutamine that can potentially improve longevity. Glutamine itself can maintain cell integrity and immunity and protect against cancers.

The exact role of glutamine in cancer as an enemy or friend is still not firmly established. A unifying explanation is still awaited.

The next chapter will explore treatment strategies that may help fight cancer by targeting glutamine metabolism.

End Notes

Albertelli MA, O'Mahony OA, Brogley M, Tosoian J, Steinkamp M, Daignault S, Wojno K, Robins DM. Glutamine tract length of human androgen receptors affects hormone-dependent and -independent prostate cancer in mice. *Hum Mol Genet.* 2008 Jan 1;17(1): pp. 98-110. doi: 10.1093/hmg/ddm287. Epub 2007 Sep 29. PMID: 17906287.

Asadi Shahmirzadi A, Edgar D, Liao CY, Hsu YM, Lucanic M, Asadi Shahmirzadi A, Wiley CD, Gan G, Kim DE, Kasler HG, Kuehnemann C, Kaplowitz B, Bhaumik D, Riley RR, Kennedy BK, Lithgow GJ. Alpha-Ketoglutarate, an Endogenous Metabolite, Extends Lifespan and Compresses Morbidity in Aging Mice. *Cell Metab*. 2020 Sep 1;32(3): pp. 447-456.e6. doi: 10.1016/j.cmet.2020.08.004. PMID: 32877690; PMCID: PMC8508957.

Ashkan Emadi; Exploiting AML vulnerability: glutamine dependency. *Blood.* 2015; 126 (11): e1269–1270. doi: https://doi.org/10.1182/blood-2015-07-659508.

Bozzetti F, Biganzoli L, Gavazzi C, Cappuzzo F, Carnaghi C, Buzzoni R, Dibartolomeo M, Baietta E. Glutamine supplementation in cancer patients receiving chemotherapy: a double-blind randomized study. *Nutrition.* 1997 Jul-Aug;13(7-8): e748-51. doi: 10.1016/s0899-9007(97)83038-9. PMID: 9263281.

Bhutia YD, Ganapathy V. Glutamine transporters in mammalian cells and their functions in physiology and cancer. *Biochim Biophys Acta.* 2016 Oct;1863(10): e2531-9. doi: 10.1016/j.bbamcr.2015.12.017. Epub 2015 Dec 24. PMID: 26724577; PMCID: PMC4919214.

Bhutia, Y.D., Babu, E., Ramachandran, S., & Ganapathy, V. (2015). Amino Acid transporters in cancer and their relevance to "glutamine addiction": novel targets for the design of a new class of anticancer drugs. *Cancer Research,* 75 9, e1782-8.

Bott AJ, Peng IC, Fan Y, Faubert B, Zhao L, Li J, Neidler S, Sun Y, Jaber N, Krokowski D, Lu W, Pan JA, Powers S, Rabinowitz J, Hatzoglou M, Murphy DJ, Jones R, Wu S, Girnun G, Zong WX. Oncogenic Myc Induces Expression of Glutamine Synthetase through Promoter Demethylation. *Cell Metab.* 2015 Dec 1;22(6): e1068-77. doi: 10.1016/j.cmet.2015.09.025. Epub 2015 Oct 23. PMID: 26603296; PMCID: PMC4670565.

Calder PC, Yaqoob P. Glutamine and the immune system. *Amino Acids.* 1999;17(3): pp. 227-41. doi: 10.1007/BF01366922. PMID: 10582122.

Cheung SM, Husain E, Masannat Y, Miller ID, Wahle K, Heys SD, He J. Lactate concentration in breast cancer using advanced magnetic resonance spectroscopy. *Br J Cancer.* 2020 Jul;123(2): pp. 261-267. doi: 10.1038/s41416-020-0886-7. Epub 2020 May 19. PMID: 32424149; PMCID: PMC7374160.

Cui Y, Bai Y, Yang J, Yao Y, Zhang C, Liu C, Shi J, Li Q, Zhang J, Lu X, Zhang Y. SIRT4 is the molecular switch mediating cellular proliferation in colorectal cancer through GLS mediated activation of AKT/GSK3β/CyclinD1 pathway. *Carcinogenesis.* 2021 Apr 17;42(3): pp. 481-492. doi: 10.1093/carcin/bgaa134. PMID: 33315089.

Dang L, Yen K, Attar EC. IDH mutations in cancer and progress toward development of targeted therapeutics. *Ann Oncol.* 2016 Apr;27(4): pp. 599-608. doi: 10.1093/annonc/mdw013. PMID: 27005468.

Durán RV, Oppliger W, Robitaille AM, Heiserich L, Skendaj R, Gottlieb E, Hall MN. Glutaminolysis activates Rag-mTORC1 signaling. *Mol Cell.* 2012 Aug 10;47(3): pp. 349-58. doi: 10.1016/j.molcel.2012.05.043. Epub 2012 Jun 29. PMID: 22749528.

de la Cruz-López, K. G., Castro-Muñoz, L. J., Reyes-Hernández, D. O., García-Carrancá, A., & Manzo-Merino, J. (2019, October 15). Lactate in the regulation of tumor microenvironment and therapeutic approaches. *Frontiers.* https://www.frontiersin.org/journals/oncology/articles/10.3389/fonc.2019.01143/full

Eelen G, Dubois C, Cantelmo AR, Goveia J, Brüning U, DeRan M, Jarugumilli G, van Rijssel J, Saladino G, Comitani F, Zecchin A, Rocha S, Chen R, Huang H, Vandekeere S, Kalucka J, Lange C, Morales-Rodriguez F, Cruys B, Treps L, Ramer L, Vinckier S, Brepoels K, Wyns S, Souffreau J, Schoonjans L, Lamers WH, Wu Y, Haustraete J, Hofkens J, Liekens S, Cubbon R, Ghesquière B, Dewerchin M, Gervasio FL, Li X, van Buul JD, Wu X, Carmeliet P. Role of glutamine synthetase in angiogenesis beyond glutamine synthesis. *Nature.* 2018 Sep;561(7721): pp. 63-69. doi: 10.1038/s41586-018-0466-7. Epub 2018 Aug 29. PMID: 30158707.

Fernandez-Marcos PJ, Serrano M. Sirt4: the glutamine gatekeeper. *Cancer Cell.* 2013 Apr 15;23(4): pp. 427-8. doi: 10.1016/j.ccr.2013.04.003. PMID: 23597559; PMCID: PMC4851233.

Goto M, Miwa H, Shikami M, Tsunekawa-Imai N, Suganuma K, Mizuno S, Takahashi M, Mizutani M, Hanamura I, Nitta M. Importance of glutamine metabolism in leukemia cells by energy production through TCA cycle and by redox homeostasis. *Cancer Invest.* 2014 Jul;32(6): pp. 241-7. doi: 10.3109/07357907.2014.907419. Epub 2014 Apr 24. PMID: 24762082.

Harrison AP, Pierzynowski SG. Biological effects of 2-oxoglutarate with particular emphasis on the regulation of protein, mineral and lipid absorption/metabolism, muscle performance, kidney function, bone formation and cancerogenesis, all viewed from a healthy ageing perspective state of the art—review article. *J Physiol Pharmacol.* 2008 Aug;59 Suppl 1: pp. 91-106. PMID: 18802218.

Huang H, Vandekeere S, Kalucka J, Bierhansl L, Zecchin A, Brüning U, Visnagri A, Yuldasheva N, Goveia J, Cruys B, Brepoels K, Wyns S, Rayport S, Ghesquière B, Vinckier S, Schoonjans L, Cubbon R, Dewerchin M, Eelen G, Carmeliet P. Role of glutamine and interlinked asparagine metabolism in vessel formation. *EMBO J.* 2017 Aug 15;36(16): e2334-52. doi: 10.15252/embj.201695518. Epub 2017 Jun 28. PMID: 28659375; PMCID: PMC5556263.

Ishak Gabra MB, Yang Y, Li H, Senapati P, Hanse EA, Lowman XH, Tran TQ, Zhang L, Doan LT, Xu X, Schones DE, Fruman DA, Kong M. Dietary glutamine supplementation suppresses epigenetically-activated oncogenic pathways to inhibit melanoma tumour growth. *Nat Commun.* 2020 Jul 3;11(1): e3326. doi: 10.1038/s41467-020-17181-w. PMID: 32620791; PMCID: PMC7335172.

Ishak Gabra, M.B., Yang, Y., Li, H. *et al.* Dietary glutamine supplementation suppresses epigenetically-activated oncogenic pathways to inhibit melanoma tumour growth. *Nat Commun.* 11, e3326 (2020). https://doi.org/10.1038/s41467-020-17181-w

Kaufmann Y, Luo S, Johnson A, Babb K, Klimberg VS. Timing of oral glutamine on DMBA-induced tumorigenesis. *J Surg Res.* 2003 May 1;111(1): pp. 158-65. doi: 10.1016/s0022-4804(03)00090-8. PMID: 12842461.

Kim HM, Lee YK, Koo JS. Expression of glutamine metabolism-related proteins in thyroid cancer. *Oncotarget.* 2016 Aug 16;7(33): e53628-41. doi: 10.18632/oncotarget.10682. PMID: 27447554; PMCID: PMC5288210.

Klimberg VS, Pappas AA, Nwokedi E, Jensen JC, Broadwater JR, Lang NP, Westbrook KC. Effect of supplemental dietary glutamine on methotrexate concentrations in tumors. *Arch Surg.* 1992 Nov;127(11): e1317-20. doi: 10.1001/archsurg.1992.01420110063013. PMID: 1444793.

Jin L, Li D, Alesi GN, Fan J, Kang HB, Lu Z, Boggon TJ, Jin P, Yi H, Wright ER, Duong D, Seyfried NT, Egnatchik R, DeBerardinis RJ, Magliocca KR, He C, Arellano ML, Khoury HJ, Shin DM, Khuri FR, Kang S. Glutamate dehydrogenase 1 signals through antioxidant glutathione peroxidase 1 to regulate redox homeostasis and tumor growth. *Cancer Cell.* 2015 Feb 9;27(2): pp. 257-70. doi: 10.1016/j.ccell.2014.12.006. PMID: 25670081; PMCID: PMC4325424.

Jing L, Wu Q, Wang F. Glutamine induces heat-shock protein and protects against Escherichia coli lipopolysaccharide-induced vascular hyporeactivity in rats. *Crit Care.* 2007;11(2):R34. doi: 10.1186/cc5717. PMID: 17346354; PMCID: PMC2206450.

Kaufmann Y, Luo S, Johnson A, Babb K, Klimberg VS. Timing of oral glutamine on DMBA-induced tumorigenesis. *J Surg Res.* 2003 May 1;111(1): pp. 158-65. doi: 10.1016/s0022-4804(03)00090-8. PMID: 12842461.

Lu C, Ward PS, Kapoor GS, Rohle D, Turcan S, Abdel-Wahab O, Edwards CR, Khanin R, Figueroa ME, Melnick A, Wellen KE, O'Rourke DM, Berger SL, Chan TA, Levine RL, Mellinghoff IK, Thompson CB. IDH mutation impairs histone demethylation and results in a block to cell differentiation. *Nature.* 2012 Feb 15;483(7390): pp. 474-8. doi: 10.1038/nature10860. PMID: 22343901; PMCID: PMC3478770.

Madden SK, de Araujo AD, Gerhardt M, Fairlie DP, Mason JM. Taking the Myc out of cancer: toward therapeutic strategies to directly inhibit c-Myc. *Mol Cancer.* 2021 Jan 4;20(1): p. 3. doi: 10.1186/s12943-020-01291-6. PMID: 33397405; PMCID: PMC7780693.

Martinez-Outschoorn UE, Prisco M, Ertel A, Tsirigos A, Lin Z, Pavlides S, Wang C, Flomenberg N, Knudsen ES, Howell A, Pestell RG, Sotgia F, Lisanti MP. Ketones and lactate increase cancer cell "stemness," driving recurrence, metastasis and poor clinical outcome in breast cancer: achieving personalized medicine via Metabolo-Genomics. *Cell Cycle.* 2011 Apr 15;10(8): e1271-86. doi: 10.4161/cc.10.8.15330. PMID: 21512313; PMCID: PMC3117136.

Martins HA, Sehaber CC, Hermes-Uliana C, Mariani FA, Guarnier FA, Vicentini GE, Bossolani GD, Jussani LA, Lima MM, Bazotte RB, Zanoni JN. Supplementation with L-glutamine prevents tumor growth and cancer-induced cachexia as well as restores cell proliferation of intestinal mucosa of Walker-256 tumor-bearing rats. *Amino Acids.* 2016 Dec;48(12): e2773-84. doi: 10.1007/s00726-016-2313-1. Epub 2016 Aug 18. PMID: 27539646.

Mathias RA, Greco TM, Oberstein A, Budayeva HG, Chakrabarti R, Rowland EA, Kang Y, Shenk T, Cristea IM. Sirtuin 4 is a lipoamidase regulating pyruvate dehydrogenase complex activity. *Cell.* 2014 Dec 18;159(7): e1615-25. doi: 10.1016/j.cell.2014.11.046. PMID: 25525879; PMCID: PMC4344121.

Matre P, Velez J, Jacamo R, Qi Y, Su X, Cai T, Chan SM, Lodi A, Sweeney SR, Ma H, Davis RE, Baran N, Haferlach T, Su X, Flores ER, Gonzalez D, Konoplev S, Samudio I, DiNardo C, Majeti R, Schimmer AD, Li W, Wang T, Tiziani S, Konopleva M. Inhibiting glutaminase in acute myeloid leukemia: metabolic dependency of selected AML subtypes. *Oncotarget.* 2016 Nov 29;7(48): e79722-35. doi: 10.18632/oncotarget.12944. PMID: 27806325; PMCID: PMC5340236.

Nguyen TL, Durán RV. Glutamine metabolism in cancer therapy. *Cancer Drug Resist.* 2018;1: pp. 126-38. http://dx.doi.org/10.20517/cdr.2018.08.

Poteti M, Menegazzi G, Peppicelli S, Tusa I, Cheloni G, Silvano A, Mancini C, Biagioni A, Tubita A, Mazure NM, Lulli M, Rovida E, Dello Sbarba P. Glutamine Availability Controls BCR/Abl Protein Expression and Functional Phenotype of Chronic Myeloid Leukemia Cells Endowed with Stem/Progenitor Cell Potential. *Cancers (Basel)*. 2021 Aug 30;13(17): e4372. doi: 10.3390/cancers13174372. PMID: 34503182; PMCID: PMC8430815.

Rubio IT, Cao Y, Hutchins LF, Westbrook KC, Klimberg VS. Effect of glutamine on methotrexate efficacy and toxicity. *Ann Surg.* 1998 May;227(5): e772-8; discussion 778-80. doi: 10.1097/00000658-199805000-00018. PMID: 9605669; PMCID: PMC1191365.

Rotovnik Kozjek N, Kompan L, Soeters P, Oblak I, Mlakar Mastnak D, Možina B, Zadnik V, Anderluh F, Velenik V. Oral glutamine supplementation during preoperative radiochemotherapy in patients with rectal cancer: a randomised double blinded, placebo controlled pilot study. *Clin Nutr.* 2011 Oct;30(5): e567-70. doi: 10.1016/j.clnu.2011.06.003. Epub 2011 Jul 5. PMID: 21733605.

Reitman ZJ, Yan H. Isocitrate dehydrogenase 1 and 2 mutations in cancer: alterations at a crossroads of cellular metabolism. *J Natl Cancer Inst.* 2010 Jul 7;102(13): e932-41. doi: 10.1093/jnci/djq187. Epub 2010 May 31. PMID: 20513808; PMCID: PMC2897878.

Reynolds MR, Lane AN, Robertson B, Kemp S, Liu Y, Hill BG, Dean DC, Clem BF. Control of glutamine metabolism by the tumor suppressor Rb. *Oncogene.* 2014 Jan 30;33(5): e556-66. doi: 10.1038/onc.2012.635. Epub 2013 Jan 28. PMID: 23353822; PMCID: PMC3918885.

Saladini S, Aventaggiato M, Barreca F, Morgante E, Sansone L, Russo MA, Tafani M. Metformin Impairs Glutamine Metabolism and Autophagy in Tumour Cells. *Cells.* 2019 Jan 14;8(1): p. 49. doi: 10.3390/cells8010049. PMID: 30646605; PMCID: PMC6356289.

Son J, Lyssiotis CA, Ying H, Wang X, Hua S, Ligorio M, Perera RM, Ferrone CR, Mullarky E, Shyh-Chang N, Kang Y, Fleming JB, Bardeesy N, Asara JM, Haigis MC, DePinho RA, Cantley LC, Kimmelman AC. Glutamine supports pancreatic cancer growth through a KRAS-regulated metabolic pathway. *Nature.* 2013 Apr 4;496(7443): pp. 101-5. doi: 10.1038/nature12040. Epub 2013 Mar 27. Erratum in: *Nature.* 2013 Jul 25;499(7459): pp. 101-5. PMID: 23535601; PMCID: PMC3656466.

Tian Y, Wang K, Wang Z, Li N, Ji G. Chemopreventive effect of dietary glutamine on colitis-associated colon tumorigenesis in mice. *Carcinogenesis.* 2013 Jul;34(7): e1593-600. doi: 10.1093/carcin/bgt088. Epub 2013 Mar 7. Erratum in: Carcinogenesis. 2013 Dec;34(12):2929. PMID: 23471883.

Topkan E, Parlak C, Topuk S, Pehlivan B. Influence of oral glutamine supplementation on survival outcomes of patients treated with concurrent chemoradiotherapy for locally advanced non-small cell lung cancer. *BMC Cancer.* 2012 Oct 31;12: e502. doi: 10.1186/1471-2407-12-502. PMID: 23113946; PMCID: PMC3529187.

Tran TQ, Hanse EA, Habowski AN, Li H, Ishak Gabra MB, Yang Y, Lowman XH, Ooi AM, Liao SY, Edwards RA, Waterman ML, Kong M. α-Ketoglutarate attenuates Wnt signaling and drives differentiation in colorectal cancer. *Nat Cancer.* 2020 Mar;1(3): pp. 345-58. doi: 10.1038/s43018-020-0035-5. Epub 2020 Mar 20. PMID: 32832918; PMCID: PMC7442208.

van Geldermalsen M, Wang Q, Nagarajah R, Marshall AD, Thoeng A, Gao D, Ritchie W, Feng Y, Bailey CG, Deng N, Harvey K, Beith JM, Selinger CI, O'Toole SA, Rasko JE, Holst J. ASCT2/SLC1A5 controls glutamine uptake and tumour growth in triple-negative basal-like breast cancer. *Oncogene.* 2016 Jun 16;35(24): e3201-8. doi: 10.1038/onc.2015.381. Epub 2015 Oct 12. PMID: 26455325; PMCID: PMC4914826.

Yang T, Yan X, Cao Y, Bao T, Li G, Gu S, Xiong K, Xiao T. Meta-analysis of Glutamine on Immune Function and Post-Operative Complications of Patients With Colorectal Cancer. *Front Nutr.* 2021 Dec 6;8: e765809. doi: 10.3389/fnut.2021.765809. PMID: 34938760; PMCID: PMC8686683.

Vidal-Casariego A, Hernando-Martín M, Calleja-Fernández A, Cano-Rodríguez I, Cordido F, Ballesteros-Pomar MD. Tissue effects of glutamine in rectal cancer patients treated with preoperative chemoradiotherapy. *Nutr Hosp.* 2015 Apr 1;31(4): e1689-92. doi: 10.3305/nh.2015.31.4.8521. PMID: 25795959.

Wood JG, Schwer B, Wickremesinghe PC, Hartnett DA, Burhenn L, Garcia M, Li M, Verdin E, Helfand SL. Sirt4 is a mitochondrial regulator of metabolism and lifespan in Drosophila melanogaster. *Proc Natl Acad Sci USA*. 2018 Feb 13;115(7): e1564-9. doi: 10.1073/pnas.1720673115. Epub 2018 Jan 29. PMID: 29378963; PMCID: PMC5816209.

Yücel B, Ada S. Leukemia Cells Resistant to Glutamine Deprivation Express Glutamine Synthetase Protein. *Turk J Haematol.* 2022 Feb 23;39(1): pp. 22-28. doi: 10.4274/tjh.galenos.2021.2021.0054. Epub 2021 Apr 22. PMID: 33882633; PMCID: PMC8886269.

Zielke HR, Sumbilla CM, Sevdalian DA, Hawkins RL, Ozand PT. Lactate: a major product of glutamine metabolism by human diploid fibroblasts. *J Cell Physiol.* 1980 Sep;104(3): e433-41. doi: 10.1002/jcp.1041040316. PMID: 7419614.

Chapter Eleven

Targeting Glutamine

It seems all too simple. If glutamine feeds cancer, then we must stop eating glutamine. Right? This, unfortunately, won't be effective.

Glutamine is a non-essential amino acid and is made naturally in our body. We can't escape it. Even if we choose to be picky about our food, we still cannot avoid glutamine. It is present in almost everything we eat and within our major organs (heart, lungs, brain, etc.).

Glutamine, however, is also metabolized (broken down) in our body. Cancers appear to grow when the internal machinery of glutamine metabolism is moving rapidly or overactive.

Cancers often begin with addiction to glucose. The glucose breakdown (glycolysis) pathway normally feeds into the Krebs cycle, followed by the OXPHOS pathway, to make energy. In cancers, pyruvate (the last molecule of glycolysis) stops right before entering the Krebs cycle (pyruvate does not become acetyl-CoA). Pyruvate instead makes a 'detour' towards lactate. That is bad news for cancers that supposedly still have a semi-functioning Krebs cycle. The cancer tries to keep the Krebs cycle running by recruiting glutamine to compensate for the absence of acetyl-CoA (Erickson & Corinne, 2010), as displayed in Figure 8 (page 54).

Glutamine, like glucose, can enter the Krebs cycle and provide the necessary carbons and nitrogens for energy production to build cancer cell parts.

In short, glutamine metabolism becomes active in cancers when glucose breakdown is followed by lactate accumulation.

Glutamine itself can also transform into lactate, which makes the surrounding environment ideal for cancer metastasis (spread to other organs). Lactate maintains low oxygen conditions and promotes pro-tumor signaling (Yangzom, *et al.*, 2014).

How can we slow down these processes?

Glutamine-fighting strategies:

Use enzymes to deplete glutamine.

1. *Asparaginase* is an enzyme that is also a chemotherapy drug for leukemia. It is extracted from *Escherichia coli bacteria* and fights cancers by depleting glutamine. In scientific words, asparaginase has glutaminase (GLS) activity (see next point). This enzyme can break down glutamine (Gln) into glutamate (Glu) (glutamic acid). This step comes right before glutamate changes to AKG to enter the Krebs cycle. With time, as this reaction repeats itself,

glutamine levels will drop.

Asparaginase also blocks mTOR signals (Yangzom, *et al.*, 2014). It starves acute myelogenous leukemia cells of protein (Yangzom, *et al.*, 2014; Samudio & Konopleva, 2013).

Asparaginase can make cancer proteins dysfunctional, causing leukemia cells to die. However, only acute lymphoblastic leukemia (ALL) can be treated with asparaginase since it isn't FDA-approved for AML or other cancers (Chen, *et al.*, 2020).

2. *Glutaminase* (GLS) as an anticancer enzyme: In 1964, Greenberg used GLS in mice with *lymphosarcoma* and found it to have anticancer activity (Greenberg, *et al.*, 1964, e957-63; Ramadanm, *et al.*, 1964).

   GLS works because it turns glutamine (Gln) into glutamate (Glu) (glutamic acid). Repeat this process many times, and we will soon run out of glutamine (Gln). However, this causes severe intestinal side effects such as diarrhea, loss of the gut lining, ulcers, and cell necrosis, making this drug too toxic for clinical use (Souba, 1993).

Use glutamine lookalikes (analogues):

One way to fool a cancer is to impersonate one of its fuels. We can use glutamine impersonators to trick the metabolism and fight cancer (Souba, 1993).

1. *6-diazo-5-oxo-Lnorleucine* (L-DON) is isolated from Streptomyces bacteria and resembles glutamine. It has anti-cancer activity in leukemia, colon, and breast cancer mice models. There was no response in lung cancer, melanoma (a skin cancer), or ependymoblastoma (a type of brain cancer). Unfortunately, when fed to mice, L-DON caused fatal toxicity to the gut, nervous tissue, and bone marrow; therefore, researchers halted production, and L-DON was not available for patient use (Souba, 1993). I know DON is the talk of the town on social media because patients ask me where they can get this. It is currently not available for human consumption. At doses potent enough to kill cancer, it will also probably kill you. We still need more research to make this safe, and clinical trials are needed to get this FDA-approved.

2. *Azaserine* is another glutamine lookalike that competes with glutamine for metabolic cell-building pathways (Souba, 1993; National Center for Biotechnology Information, 2022). However, lab studies of rats also show azaserine to be carcinogenic and cause the growth of new pancreatic cancer (Appel, *et al.*, 1990).

3. *Acivicin* is a natural amino acid product extracted from Streptomyces bacteria that looks like glutamine and has activity against *hepatocellular* (liver cancer). <u>It does cause severe toxicities to the nervous system</u>; therefore, clinical studies are no longer available (Souba, 1993).

Nitrogen scavenging helps eliminate glutamine.

Nitrogen scavengers can help glutamine quickly exit in the urine:

1. *Phenylbutyrate* is FDA-approved to treat high ammonia levels in children with urea cycle (kidney-related) disorders. It is good for lowering ammonia and getting rid of glutamine. Phenylbutyrate converts to *phenylacetate* (an acid) and combines with glutamine to make *phenylacetylglutamine,* which then passes through urine (Iannitti & Palmieri, 2011). Its anti-cancer properties deserve further research.

2. *Sodium phenylbutyrate* (SPB) was added to prostate cancer cells in the lab. SPB-treated cells had more 'cell killing' due to blocking the *survivin* pathway. *Survivin* is a cancer protein that controls cell division and death. It protects cancers and is present in nearly all cancers (breast, colon, lung; ovarian, liver, uterus; blood cancers, glioblastoma; meningioma, astrocytoma, bladder; prostate, skin cancers, sarcoma, and melanoma). Survivin is usually detected in early stages and seen in cancer stem cells. Urine tests can detect bladder cancer relapse, while RT-PCR (reverse transcriptase polymerase chain reaction) blood tests can detect leukemia and breast cancer cells (Smith, *et al.*, 2001; Yie, *et al.*, 2006).

Target the glutaminase enzyme.

When the cell's mitochondria are damaged, cancers use glucose as the primary energy source because their regular energy maker, the Krebs cycle, is out of commission.

However, some greedy cancers want more energy. They rewire themselves to recruit glutamine and change it into AKG—a version of glutamine. This AKG enters the Krebs cycle through the AKG 'side door.' However, you also need two enzymes to change glutamine to AKG—glutaminase and glutaminase dehydrogenase.

CB-839 (telaglenastat) is a glutaminase (GLS) inhibitor. It blocks the transition from glutamine (Glu) to glutamate (Gln). This is a crucial step. Many cancers, such as B-cell lymphomas, prostate, pancreatic, and breast cancers, are examples of cancers with overactive GLS.

Interestingly, CB-839 had anti-tumor effects in triple-negative breast cancer cells but no effect in estrogen receptor-positive breast cancer lines (Gross, *et al.*, 2014; Erickson & Cerione, 2010).

Check clinicaltrials.gov to search for CB-839 trials or any trial that uses GLS inhibitors for your type of cancer.

Block glutamine transporters.

Normal cells do not possess as many transporters as cancers do; therefore, blocking transporters sounds like a clever idea to starve glutamine-hungry cancers without harming normal cells (Yangzom, *et al.*, 2014).

Blocking glutamine's uptake/entry into the cell also blocks the mTOR growth pathways.

1. *Solute carrier transporters* (SLC) and *alanine, serine, and cysteine-preferring transporter 2* (ASCT) are words and letters you will recognize in many publications on glutamine transporters. Cancers with too many glutamine transporters usually have a poor prognosis. Silencing the transporter genes can slow down triple-negative breast cancers and uterine, prostate, stomach, and melanoma skin cancers (van Geldermalsen, *et al.*, 2016; Wang, *et al.*, 2015; Marshall, *et al.*, 2017; Ye, *et al.*, 2018; Schulte, *et al.*, 2018).

2. *Benzylserine* (BenSer) is a SLC1A5/ASCT2 inhibitor that fights gastric (stomach) and breast cancers. BenSer, however, is only available for laboratory use and is not approved for humans (van Geldermalsen, *et al.*, 2018).

3. *V-9302* is another glutamine transporter blocker effective against triple-negative breast cancer (Edwards, *et al.*, 2021).

Target the hypoxia-inducible factor (HIF)—GDH pathway.

Remember that HIF-1α is a special pro-cancer protein that depends on oxygen. One job of HIF-1α is to make glutamine more accessible to the cell. You will learn more about HIF-1α in Chapter Twelve.

Many human lung cancers live in previously damaged lungs since oxygen cannot travel as freely to reach the bloodstream. Poor oxygen conditions will stabilize HIF-1α and use more glutamine by overexpressing the GDH enzymes. Human lung cancer cells resistant to *cisplatin chemotherapy* may depend on glutamine (Lee, *et al.*, 2016; Jiang, *et al.*, 2017).

Can we find a drug to target HIF-1α? Is there any treatment to fix the problem of having low oxygen? Hyperbaric oxygen (HBO) research is robust in animals and lab setups but poorly researched in humans. Research for drugs that target HIF-1-α isn't active now. This, indeed, is another area of research that needs a boost.

Get rid of defective p53 or try to reactivate it.

Roughly 50% of all tumors have a defective tumor suppressor protein 53 (TP53 or p53). It is the most common defect in cancers (Wang & Sun, 2010). TP53 keeps cell DNA stable; we need p53 to keep our bodies cancer-free. As we age or get exposed to the damaging effects of the environment, our p53 might also become defective. Once faulty, cancers may develop. We go to the doctor, and they, of course, offer us treatment. Usually, that might include chemotherapy. If you have a defective p53, you will have a higher chance of seeing no response to the chemotherapy. Or, if the cancers do respond to therapy, sooner or later, relapse is seen. The p53 is no longer doing its essential job, and cancers begin to grow.

Cancers require large amounts of glutamine to keep multiplying and to fight oxidative stress. In poor blood supply, the cancer's glutamine content dries out quickly. However, if the cancer also has defective p53, the cancer will survive even if glutamine supplies are down. In a 2010 study, human lymphoma cells died after glutamine withdrawal but only after the defective p53 protein was eliminated (Tran, *et al.*, 2010).

Unfortunately, no official treatment for fixing a defective p53 protein is available. However, researchers are aware of this void and are racing to try and find a solution. Off-label options include metformin, which does have anti-p53 activity (Wang & Sun, 2010).

Potential therapies to fight an abnormal p53:

1. *Pifithrin-alpha* (PFT-α) is an example of a p53 inhibitor studied in the lab but not used clinically. It can, however, be purchased for lab research (Bassi, *et al.*, 2002).

2. *Metformin* targets the bulky *mitochondrial complex I* protein at the ETC's first step. It is vital to the energy-making machinery of the cell. Without complex 1, the mitochondria cannot make energy from glucose. Therefore, metformin fights cancer by preventing glucose from being processed in the mitochondria.

You might be wondering, *Didn't Warburg say that cancer has non-working mitochondria?*

You are right. Warburg did say that. However, Weinhouse and others who came after him challenged Warburg's theory, stating that in addition to glycolysis, some cancers also have some functioning OXPHOS in their defective mitochondria (Warburg, 1956).

Assuming this might be true, we take a two-pronged attack on cancer, which includes starving the cells of glucose plus the simultaneous attack on the complex I protein to hit the remaining OXPHOS.

Metformin can also fight cancers for the following reasons: Cancers can grow freely by up-regulating the TP53. Secondly, it inhibits insulin, which cancers need to succeed. Lastly, metformin can inhibit the HIF proteins, which trigger cancer growth, by stopping the signals that activate HIF (Wheaton, *et al.*, 2014).

Assuming this might be true, a two-pronged attack, which includes starving the cells of glucose and a simultaneous attack on the complex I protein, to hit the remaining OXPHOS will kill the cancer.

Public health studies show that cancer patients who take metformin appear to survive longer than those who do not.

However, some glucose-loving cancers may rewire and use glutamine! In some lab and animal experiments of prostate cancer, when metformin blocks complex 1, the cancer, realizing it lost its energy from glucose, turns to glutamine as a second energy source. Therefore, a two-pronged attack of blocking glutamine, in addition to glucose, might be helpful. Anti-glutamine therapy plus metformin (anti-glucose) may double the potential anti-cancer effects (Fendt, *et al.*, 2013).

3. *Other Anti p53 therapies* still under investigation include small molecules, gene therapy, and peptides (Wang & Sun, 2010).

Blocking the production of glutamine itself

Up to this point, we have talked about blocking glutaminase (GLS), the enzyme that helps change glutamine (Gln) to glutamate (Glu) before it enters the Krebs cycle as AKG.

Another way is to start earlier in the pathway and stop the glutamine production. Nip it in the bud!

I am referring to the glutamine enzyme, GS (glutamine synthetase), which can recycle glutamate back into glutamine. Several scientists studied GS to see if it can fight cancer by stopping glutamine production.

Some cancers have high levels of GS. Gliomas, luminal breast cancers, liver (hepatocellular) cancer, ovarian, non-small cell lung, pancreas, and sarcoma (Kim, *et al.*, 2021).

Knowing this, what drug is available to block GS? Unfortunately, I found very little research in this niche.

1. *Methionine sulfoximine* (MS) is the most popular anti-GS drug. It is an antituberculosis drug discovered in 1949. It blocks GS to stop cancers from making glutamine. However, it was too toxic to the nerves and brain (caused convulsions) and, therefore, never made its way to the clinic (Ghoddoussi, *et al.*, 2010).

2. *Phosphinothricin* is a weed killer that also blocks GS. Its chemical structure is likened to bone strengtheners or bisphosphonates and was originally studied as a bone-seeking radioisotope used in bone scans and showed some promise against breast and lung cancer cells in the lab (Sakr, *et al.*, 2018; Berlicki, 2008).

3. *Vitamin C* therapy, when added to oxygen therapy, apparently has anti-GS activity and, therefore, can fight cancer by blocking glutamine production (Long, *et al.*, 2021).

GS inhibitors theoretically stop glutamine production and might have anticancer benefits.

Chapter Summary/Key Takeaways:

There are many ways to adjust glutamine metabolism to fight cancer.

We discussed strategies such as targeting glutamine transport and production. These therapies are not yet available to the public.

Many anti-glutamine therapies can have severe side effects at higher doses; therefore, few, if any, are available for clinical use. We need to encourage future clinical trials to investigate some of these new approaches.

In the next chapter, we will discuss the *Hypoxia Inducible Factor (HIF)* and how it plays a role in cancer metabolism.

End Notes

Appel MJ, nan Garderen-Hoetmer A, Woutersen RA. Azaserine-induced pancreatic carcinogenesis in rats: promotion by a diet rich in saturated fat and inhibition by a standard laboratory chow. *Cancer Lett.* 1990 Dec 17;55(3): pp. 239-48. doi: 10.1016/0304-3835(90)90125-h. PMID: 2257542.

Bassi L, Carloni M, Fonti E, Palma de la Peña N, Meschini R, Palitti F. Pifithrin-alpha, an inhibitor of p53, enhances the genetic instability induced by etoposide (VP16) in human lymphoblastoid cells treated in vitro. *Mutat Res.* 2002 Feb 20;499(2): pp. 163-76. doi: 10.1016/s0027-5107(01)00273-1. PMID: 11827710.

Berlicki Ł. Inhibitors of glutamine synthetase and their potential application in medicine. *Mini Rev Med Chem.* 2008 Aug;8(9): e869-78. doi: 10.2174/138955708785132800. PMID: 18691144.

Chen T, Zhang J, Zeng H, Zhang Y, Zhang Y, Zhou X, Zhou H. Antiproliferative effects of L-asparaginase in acute myeloid leukemia. *Exp Ther Med.* 2020 Sep;20(3): e2070-78. doi: 10.3892/etm.2020.8904. Epub 2020 Jun 18. PMID: 32782519; PMCID: PMC7401243.

Edwards DN, Ngwa VM, Raybuck AL, Wang S, Hwang Y, Kim LC, Cho SH, Paik Y, Wang Q, Zhang S, Manning HC, Rathmell JC, Cook RS, Boothby MR, Chen J. Selective glutamine metabolism inhibition in tumor cells improves antitumor T lymphocyte activity in triple-negative breast cancer. *J Clin Invest.* 2021 Feb 15;131(4):e140100. doi: 10.1172/JCI140100. PMID: 33320840; PMCID: PMC7880417.

Erickson JW, Cerione RA. Glutaminase: a hot spot for regulation of cancer cell metabolism? *Oncotarget.* 2010 Dec;1(8): e734-40. doi: 10.18632/oncotarget.208. PMID: 21234284; PMCID: PMC3018840.

Fendt SM, Bell EL, Keibler MA, Davidson SM, Wirth GJ, Fiske B, Mayers JR, Schwab M, Bellinger G, Csibi A, Patnaik A, Blouin MJ, Cantley LC, Guarente L, Blenis J, Pollak MN, Olumi AF, Vander Heiden MG, Stephanopoulos G. Metformin decreases glucose oxidation and increases the dependency of prostate cancer cells on reductive glutamine metabolism. *Cancer Res.* 2013 Jul 15;73(14): e4429-38. doi: 10.1158/0008-5472.CAN-13-0080. Epub 2013 May 17. PMID: 23687346; PMCID: PMC3930683.

Ghoddoussi F, Galloway MP, Jambekar A, Bame M, Needleman R, Brusilow WS. Methionine sulfoximine, an inhibitor of glutamine synthetase, lowers brain glutamine and glutamate in a mouse model of ALS. *J Neurol Sci.* 2010 Mar 15;290(1-2): pp. 41-7. doi: 10.1016/j.jns.2009.11.013. Epub 2010 Jan 8. PMID: 20060132.

Greenberg DM, Bluenthal G, Ramadan ME. Effect of Administration of the Enzyme Glutaminase on the Growth of Cancer Cells. *Cancer Res.* 1964 Jul;24: e957-63. PMID: 14195348.

Gross MI, Demo SD, Dennison JB, Chen L, Chernov-Rogan T, Goyal B, Janes JR, Laidig GJ, Lewis ER, Li J, Mackinnon AL, Parlati F, Rodriguez ML, Shwonek PJ, Sjogren EB, Stanton TF, Wang T, Yang J, Zhao F, Bennett MK. Antitumor activity of the glutaminase inhibitor CB-839 in triple-negative breast cancer. *Mol Cancer Ther.* 2014 Apr;13(4): e890-901. doi: 10.1158/1535-7163.MCT-13-0870. Epub 2014 Feb 12. PMID: 24523301.

Iannitti T, Palmieri B. Clinical and experimental applications of sodium phenylbutyrate. *Drugs R D.* 2011 Sep 1;11(3): pp. 227-49. doi: 10.2165/11591280-000000000-00000. PMID: 21902286; PMCID: PMC3586072.

Jiang ZF, Wang M, Xu JL, Ning YJ. Hypoxia promotes mitochondrial glutamine metabolism through HIF1α-GDH pathway in human lung cancer cells. *Biochem Biophys Res Commun.* 2017 Jan 29;483(1): pp. 32-38. doi: 10.1016/j.bbrc.2017.01.015. Epub 2017 Jan 5. PMID: 28065856.

Kim GW, Lee DH, Jeon YH, Yoo J, Kim SY, Lee SW, Cho HY, Kwon SH. Glutamine Synthetase as a Therapeutic Target for Cancer Treatment. *Int J Mol Sci.* 2021 Feb 8;22(4): e1701. doi: 10.3390/ijms22041701. PMID: 33567690; PMCID: PMC7915753.

Lee YM, Lee G, Oh TI, Kim BM, Shim DW, Lee KH, Kim YJ, Lim BO, Lim JH. Inhibition of glutamine utilization sensitizes lung cancer cells to apigenin-induced apoptosis resulting from metabolic and oxidative stress. *Int J Oncol.* 2016 Jan;48(1): pp. 399-408. doi: 10.3892/ijo.2015.3243. Epub 2015 Nov 11. PMID: 26573871.

Long Y, Qiu J, Zhang B, He P, Shi X, He Q, Chen Z, Shen W, Li Z, Zhang X. Pharmacological Vitamin C Treatment Impedes the Growth of Endogenous Glutamine-Dependent Cancers by Targeting Glutamine Synthetase. *Front Pharmacol.* 2021 May 11;12: e671902. doi: 10.3389/fphar.2021.671902. PMID: 34054545; PMCID: PMC8150514.

Marshall AD, van Geldermalsen M, Otte NJ, Lum T, Vellozzi M, Thoeng A, Pang A, Nagarajah R, Zhang B, Wang Q, Anderson L, Rasko JEJ, Holst J. ASCT2 regulates glutamine uptake and cell growth in endometrial carcinoma. *Oncogenesis.* 2017 Jul 31;6(7): e367. doi: 10.1038/oncsis.2017.70. PMID: 28759021; PMCID: PMC5541720.

National Center for Biotechnology Information (2022). *PubChem Compound Summary for CID* 460129, *Azaserine.* Retrieved August 26, 2022 from https://pubchem.ncbi.nlm.nih.gov/compound/Azaserine.

Ramadanm, E.-D., F. Elasmar, and D.M. Greenberg, Purification and Properties of Glutaminase and Asparaginase from a Pseudomonad. I. Purification and Physical Chemical Properties. *Archives of Biochemistry and Biophysics*, 1964. 108(1): pp. 143-9. https://doi.org/10.1016/0003-9861(64)90365-0.

Sakr TM, Khedr MA, Rashed HM, Mohamed ME. In Silico-Based Repositioning of Phosphinothricin as a Novel Technetium-99m Imaging Probe with Potential Anti-Cancer Activity. *Molecules.* 2018 Feb 23;23(2): p. 496. doi: 10.3390/molecules23020496. PMID: 29473879; PMCID: PMC6017358.

Samudio I, Konopleva M. Asparaginase unveils glutamine-addicted AML. *Blood.* 2013 Nov 14;122(20): e3398-400. doi: 10.1182/blood-2013-09-526392. PMID: 24235130.

Schulte ML, Fu A, Zhao P, Li J, Geng L, Smith ST, Kondo J, Coffey RJ, Johnson MO, Rathmell JC, Sharick JT, Skala MC, Smith JA, Berlin J, Washington MK, Nickels ML, Manning HC. Pharmacological blockade of ASCT2-dependent glutamine transport leads to antitumor efficacy in preclinical models. *Nat Med.* 2018 Feb;24(2): pp. 194-202. doi: 10.1038/nm.4464. Epub 2018 Jan 15. PMID: 29334372; PMCID: PMC5803339.

Souba WW. Glutamine and cancer. *Ann Surg.* 1993 Dec;218(6): e715-28. doi: 10.1097/00000658- 199312000-00004. PMID: 8257221; PMCID: PMC1243066.

Smith SD, Wheeler MA, Plescia J, Colberg JW, Weiss RM, Altieri DC. Urine detection of survivin and diagnosis of bladder cancer. *JAMA.* 2001 Jan 17;285(3): pp. 324-8. doi: 10.1001/jama.285.3.324. PMID: 11176843.

Tran TQ, Lowman XH, Reid MA, Mendez-Dorantes C, Pan M, Yang Y, Kong M. Tumor-associated mutant p53 promotes cancer cell survival upon glutamine deprivation through p21 induction. *Oncogene.* 2017 Apr 6;36(14): e1991-2001. doi: 10.1038/onc.2016.360. Epub 2016 Oct 10. PMID: 27721412; PMCID: PMC5383530.

Van Geldermalsen M, Wang Q, Nagarajah R, Marshall AD, Thoeng A, Gao D, Ritchie W, Feng Y, Bailey CG, Deng N, Harvey K, Beith JM, Selinger CI, O'Toole SA, Rasko JE, Holst J. ASCT2/SLC1A5 controls glutamine uptake and tumour growth in triple-negative basal-like breast cancer. *Oncogene.* 2016 Jun 16;35(24): e3201-8. doi: 10.1038/onc.2015.381. Epub 2015 Oct 12. PMID: 26455325; PMCID: PMC4914826.

Van Geldermalsen M, Quek LE, Turner N, Freidman N, Pang A, Guan YF, Krycer JR, Ryan R, Wang Q, Holst J. Benzylserine inhibits breast cancer cell growth by disrupting intracellular amino acid homeostasis and triggering amino acid response pathways. *BMC Cancer.* 2018 Jun 26;18(1): e689. doi: 10.1186/s12885-018-4599-8. PMID: 29940911; PMCID: PMC6019833.

Wang Q, Hardie RA, Hoy AJ, van Geldermalsen M, Gao D, Fazli L, Sadowski MC, Balaban S, Schreuder M, Nagarajah R, Wong JJ, Metierre C, Pinello N, Otte NJ, Lehman ML, Gleave M, Nelson CC, Bailey CG, Ritchie W, Rasko JE, Holst J. Targeting ASCT2-mediated glutamine uptake blocks prostate cancer growth and tumour development. *J Pathol.* 2015 Jul;236(3): pp. 278-89. doi: 10.1002/path.4518. Epub 2015 Apr 7. PMID: 25693838; PMCID: PMC4973854.

Wang Z, Sun Y. Targeting p53 for Novel Anticancer Therapy. *Transl Oncol.* 2010 Feb;3(1): pp. 1-12. doi: 10.1593/tlo.09250. PMID: 20165689; PMCID: PMC2822448.

Warburg O. On respiratory impairment in cancer cells. *Science.* 1956 Aug 10;124(3215): pp. 269-70. PMID: 13351639.

Wheaton WW, Weinberg SE, Hamanaka RB, Soberanes S, Sullivan LB, Anso E, Glasauer A, Dufour E, Mutlu GM, Budigner GS, Chandel NS. Metformin inhibits mitochondrial complex I of cancer cells to reduce tumorigenesis. *Elife.* 2014 May 13;3: e02242. doi: 10.7554/eLife.02242. PMID: 24843020; PMCID: PMC4017650.

Yangzom D. Bhutia, Ellappan Babu, Puttur D. Prasad, Vadivel Ganapathy, The amino acid transporter SLC6A14 in cancer and its potential use in chemotherapy. *Asian Journal of Pharmaceutical Sciences.* Volume 9, Issue 6, 2014, pp. 293-303, ISSN 1818 0876,https://doi.org/10.1016/j.ajps.2014.04.004.

Ye J, Huang Q, Xu J, Huang J, Wang J, Zhong W, Chen W, Lin X, Lin X. Targeting of glutamine transporter ASCT2 and glutamine synthetase suppresses gastric cancer cell growth. *J Cancer Res Clin Oncol.* 2018 May;144(5): e821-33. doi: 10.1007/s00432-018-2605-9. Epub 2018 Feb 12. PMID: 29435734; PMCID: PMC5916984.

Yie, S.-M., Luo, B., Ye, N.-Y., Xie, K., & Ye, S.-R. (2006, November 3). Detection of survivin-expressing circulating cancer cells in the peripheral blood of breast cancer patients by a RT-PCR ELISA - Clinical & experimental metastasis. *SpringerLink.* https://link.springer.com/article/10.1007/s10585-006-9037-7#author-information. https://doi.org/10.1007/s10585-006-9037-7

Chapter Twelve

Hypoxia-Inducible Factor

HIF-1: The metabolic switch

Our kidneys have an 'oxygen sensor' which helps us adapt to changing oxygen levels in our surroundings.

Normally, cells die at extremely low oxygen levels.

Our cells will begin to self-destruct when oxygen levels almost reach zero (0-0.1%). This is a state of *anoxia* (literally meaning "no oxygen").

Simple enough? Cut off almost <u>all</u> the oxygen, and cells die! It sounds like a good way to fight cancer. Unfortunately, that isn't a good option for the rest of our body.

If we allow more oxygen (≥1%), we arrive at the state of *hypoxia* (low oxygen). This is not good news for us because, at this level, cancers live! Cancers love this sweet spot, hypoxia—just the right tiny level of oxygen, enough to tickle the cancers into action, but not so low that it kills them.

When cells enter hypoxia, they make a lot of pro-cancer signals. The immune system, which fights cancers, is put on pause. Programs that benefit cancers activate. Blood vessel growth, invasion, and division are all activated once oxygen levels drop.

Here is where the 'alphabet soup' begins. Oncologists love to identify these signals by giving them complicated letter names. The letters stand for the smaller parts that make up these signals.

There are PI3K/AKT signals, NF-κB, and mTOR signals, to name just a few (Benizri, *et al.*, 2008).

Numbers of GLUTs glucose transporters (proteins that allow glucose to pass into cells) also grow, and all those will fuel cancer (Chung, *et al.*, 2009; Alfarouk, 2016; Cairns, *et al.*, 2011).

As the HIF-1 metabolic switch moves, cells learn to escape death and multiply without boundaries. Stem cells are favored (Mathieu, *et al.*, 2011). A cancer is born (Benizri, *et al.*, 2008), as portrayed in Figure 10 (page 181).

Let us look closer at the HIF-1 protein, also called HIF-1α. It has a sibling called HIF-1β.

Alpha is found outside the nucleus, and beta is inside. You will later see why knowing the locations of HIF-1α and β will help us understand how the metabolic switch operates.

Figure 10 (for reference only; identical to Figure 6):
HIF1-alpha

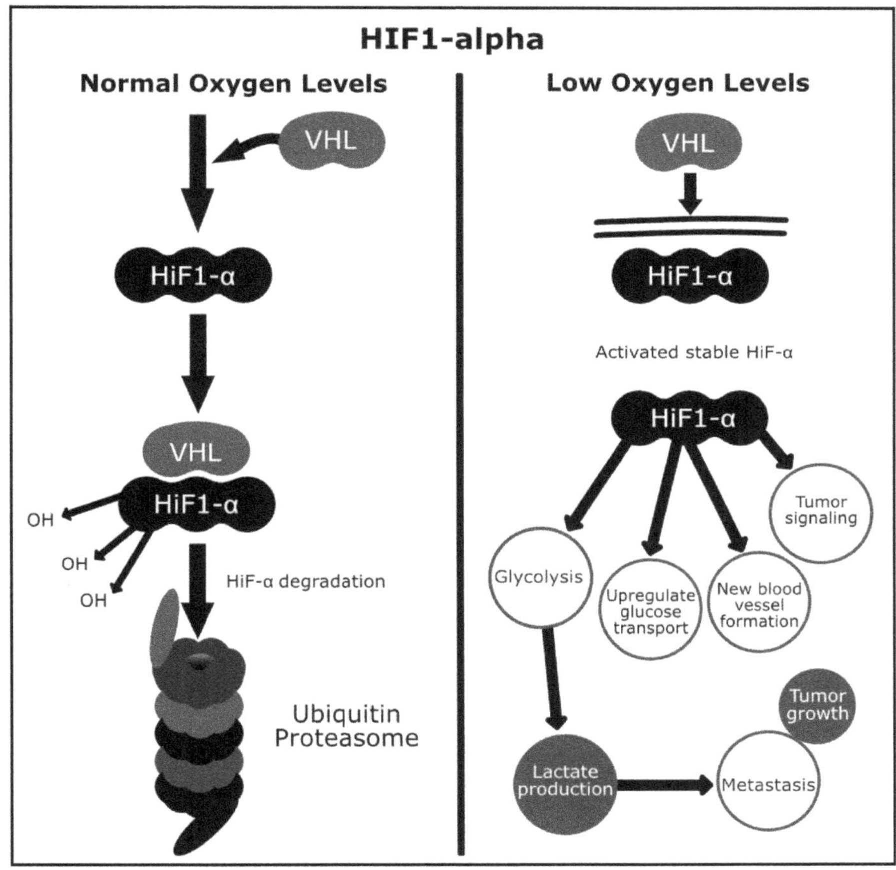

What controls HIF-1? – OXYGEN

HIF-1α can be troublesome because it can trigger harmful cancer signals.

Luckily, we can easily eliminate HIF-1α when oxygen levels are normal. HIF-1α first meets the very important *von Hipple Lindau*

(VHL) protein, after which the combo gets 'swept away and ground up' by the 'garbage disposal' called the *proteasome*, as shown in Figure 10 (page 181). Therefore, the VHL protein is a tumor suppressor because it keeps our body cancer-free.

Sometimes, things go wrong, and oxygen levels drop. For example, when people become anemic (low blood oxygen) or when cancers grow rapidly and crowd.

When oxygen drops, HIF-1α stops meeting VHL and instead meets HIF-1β. HIF-1α enters the nucleus to bind to HIF-1β. Together, they become a dangerous, stable, and active duo. The HIF-1(α/β) protein possesses many pro-cancer powers.

How does a stable HIF-1 turn on cancer?

The new stabilized combo version of HIF-1(α/β) can activate red blood cells and grow new blood vessels to supply nutrition for new cancers (Lerman, *et al.*, 2010).

In addition, HIF-1, in its stable form, will trigger more tumor-signaling pathways, growth factors, and glycolysis enzymes. There will also be more glucose transporters (GLUTS). Cancers of the ovary, colon, bladder, and brain love GLUTS. (See Yasuda, *et al.*, 2008; Wincewicz, *et al.*, 2007; Palit, *et al.*, 2005; Liu, *et al.*, 2009).

Now that cancers have come alive, HIF-1 can break the boundary—*epithelial-mesenchymal transition* or EMT—that keeps cancer cells in place and allows invasion of other body parts (Cane, *et al.*, 2010; Shang, *et al.*, 2017; Chen, *et al.*, 2016).

How does HIF-1 turn off the immune system?

We all have an immune system that protects us from cancers.

Our immune system normally has T cells, which 'arrest' cancer cells when they see them.

Before T cells can make an arrest, they need a very important 'witness.' The MHC (major histocompatibility gene complex) is that witness, which takes a piece of the cancer's protein (as evidence) to show to the T cells (the guards) so they can recognize the cancer.

Did I lose you there? Let me explain this again.

When oxygen is low (hypoxia), HIF-1 turns off the MHCs and, as a result, activates fewer T cells. With fewer T cells, cancers can escape and travel. The immune system is disarmed.

On the other hand, if we crank up the oxygen (60% or more), we see an anti-cancer effect! High oxygen levels encourage more MHC-1 expression—more eyewitnesses—therefore, we fight cancer better by improving the immune defense with more T cells activated (Sethumadhavan, *et al.*, 2017).

Iron, HIF-1, and cancer:

Iron can harm us because we accumulate HIF-1 by preventing the HIF—VHL—proteasome—destruction process.

Recall that to get rid of HIF-1, we need the HIF-1α to bind to VHL before it gets chewed up by the proteasome. Iron can interfere with the 'garbage disposal' (proteasome) and prevent it from doing its job, so we end up with too much HIF-1.

Potential treatment? Get rid of the iron. Iron chelators (absorbers of iron) like desferrioxamine or iron-displacing elements, like cobalt, can prevent free radical (unstable molecule) formation but can also allow the proteasome to eliminate the VHL—HIF-1α (Yu, *et al.*, 2006; Richardson, 2002; Greene, 2018).

IDH1 mutations, HIF-1 and cancer:

IDH1 mutations interfere with removing HIF-1 so that more HIF-1 can do more damage. The exact mechanism of how this happens isn't very clear (Han, *et al.*, 2020).

You may have heard of IDH1 mutations in aggressive gliomas (brain cancer). Many gliomas have IDH1 mutations (isocitrate dehydrogenase), which cause resistance to temozolomide chemotherapy (Han, *et al.*, 2020).

IDH1 is a normal Krebs cycle enzyme. When mutated (defective), IDH1 makes D2HG instead of the regular Krebs cycle step, AKG. The Krebs cycle cannot use D2HG to make energy; therefore, glutamine will rescue the Krebs cycle and keep it moving by providing the missing AKG (Metallo, *et al.*, 2012). Many brain cancers that have the IDH1 mutation also become dependent on glutamine (Metallo, *et al.*, 2012). After glutamine, the glioma makes its own fats and uses them (*de novo* lipogenesis). What a mess!

Turning off the switch: Potential anti-HIF-1 therapies

Targeting HIF-1a by targeting c-Myc.

C-Myc is a pro-cancer gene (oncogene) that can communicate with HIF-1α to promote cell growth. Strangely, c-Myc can also promote cell suicide by causing breaks in our DNA structure. What drives c-Myc to choose the pro-cancer versus the anticancer role? We don't know.

Normal or slow-dividing cancer cells have little to no c-Myc. However, in fast-growing cancers, c-Myc takes a sinister role. It begins special talks with the HIF-1α and the p53 to reprogram the cells into cancers (Zornig & Evan, 1996; Kumari, *et al.*, 2017; Yoo, *et al.*, 2009).

Unfortunately, we still do not have anti-HIF-1 therapies in the oncology clinic. Research is ongoing but slow.

One example of a c-Myc inhibitor effective in pediatric acute lymphoblastic leukemia (ALL) is inhibitor *10058F4*. However, drug development is still in the early stages (Sayyadi, *et al.*, 2020).

Dioscin is a natural product from traditional Chinese medicines with anti-c-Myc properties. Dioscin therapy slowed down cancers in a lab mouse with colorectal cancer by removing c-Myc (Wu, *et al.*, 2020).

A similar benefit was seen in hepatocellular (liver) cancer (Chen, *et al.*, 2019).

Anti-inflammatory agents:

Non-steroidal anti-inflammatory agents or NSAIDs like ibuprofen may have anti-cancer effects. Special activated white blood cells called *macrophages* can cause cancer by causing inflammation and oxidative stress, stabilizing and activating HIF-1α (Oda, *et al.*, 2006; Li, *et al.*, 2018; Palayoor, *et al.*, 2003).

NSAIDs can protect against prostate cancer by stopping macrophages to reduce HIF-1α and HIF-2α (Palayoor, *et al.*, 2003).

Gut microflora:

There is growing interest in gut microflora and its possible connection to cancer development (Adamczyk & Westendorf, 2018).

Intestinal bacteria cause chronic inflammation and injury to intestinal blood vessels and can activate the HIF1 protein. Subsequent signaling pathway activation leads to cancer and metastases (Koury, *et al.*, 2004).

Probiotics are live, friendly bacteria that can help decrease the population of harmful bacteria, improve intestinal tissue health, and regulate the immune system (Adamczyk & Westendorf, 2018; Williams, 2010).

Chromomycin A3 (ChA3) is an antibiotic that can kill cells with defective VHL tumor suppressors. This can effectively suppress the growth of cholangiocarcinoma (bile duct cancer) and clear cell renal (kidney) cancer (Sutphin, *et al.*, 2007; Saranaruk, *et al.*, 2020).

Unfortunately, when researchers tested this drug on cancer patients, the toxicity was severe and even led to two deaths. Chromomycin is still in production but is only used to stain DNA for lab experiments (Saranaruk, *et al.*, 2020).

Erythropoietin (EPO):

Anemia is a state of low oxygen that promotes cancers. Anemia develops when red blood cells contain very little *hemoglobin* (HgB), a protein that carries oxygen and gives red color to blood. Some tumors respond poorly to radiation because of their low oxygen content. How can we improve anemia? *Erythropoietin* (EPO) is a hormone that stimulates the bone marrow to make more red blood cells and, therefore, can improve oxygenation in the cell.

Can EPO fight cancer by improving the oxygen levels of tumors? To test this hypothesis, researchers made some mice anemic by exposing their entire bodies to radiation. Another group of mice received EPO hormone before the whole-body radiation. After total body radiation, they injected glioma tumors into their hind legs and then treated the legs with more radiation.

They found that the mice that received EPO fared better. They had better-oxygenated blood, and their tumors shrank more than the anemic mice without EPO; therefore, correcting anemia before radiation therapy may help the treatments work better (Kelleher, *et al.*, 1995; Stuben, *et al.*, 2001, 2003).

Hyperbaric oxygen:

Hyperbaric oxygen therapy (HBOT) involves breathing in 100% oxygen under pressurized conditions in an atmosphere greater than 1.4 (Lam, *et al.*, 2017).

Can we improve oxygen levels with HBOT?

Yes. Cancer cells treated with a combination of HBO and chemotherapy saw benefit. Cancer cells treated with HBO + radiation + chemotherapy similarly benefitted. There is fear that HBO might encourage cancer growth because of its effect on making new blood vessels; however, there is no evidence to support this (Feldmeier, *et al.*, 1994).

Digitalis as a HIF1 inhibitor:

We learned that HIF-1α promotes tumor growth proteins—VEGF and PDGF—that help grow red blood vessels and lymphatic vessels. Mouse models with breast cancer showed that the cardiac drug digitalis can prevent lymph vessel growth as well as lymphatic metastasis. How? Digitalis can activate the proteasome (the cell's garbage disposal), which may help us clean up HIF-1α (Busonero, 2020).

Another drug, *imatinib* (a tyrosine kinase inhibitor or cancer signal blocker), can also inhibit HIF-1α (Litz & Krystal, 2006).

Chapter Summary/Key Takeaways:

We learned that low oxygen levels could promote cancer while correct amounts of oxygen can be used to fight it. Oxygen-related proteins called hypoxia-inducible factors can cause cancer to grow, proliferate, metastasize, and avoid immune surveillance.

We saw how glycolysis, glutamine, and lactate production combined with hypoxia can promote cancer.

Using a metabolically targeted approach, we considered a few possible mechanisms of anticancer drug development. I explored potential ways to fight cancer, whether they follow the Warburg or the non-Warburg theory.

In the next chapter, we will learn more about mitochondrial experiments and how the results support the concepts behind the Warburg effect.

End Notes

Adamczyk, A., & Westendorf, A. M. (2018). Editorial: Cancer, drugs, and bugs—Bacteriotherapy on the rise? *Journal of Leukocyte Biology*, *103*(5), e795-797. https://doi.org/10.1002/JLB.5CE0118-018R.

Alfarouk KO. Tumor metabolism, cancer cell transporters, and microenvironmental resistance. *J Enzyme Inhib Med Chem.* 2016 Dec;31(6): e859-66. doi: 10.3109/14756366.2016.1140753. Epub 2016 Feb 10. PMID: 26864256.

Benizri E, Ginouvès A, Berra E. The magic of the hypoxia-signaling cascade. *Cell Mol Life Sci.* 2008 Apr;65(7-8): e1133-49. doi: 10.1007/s00018-008-7472-0. PMID: 18202826.

Busonero C, Leone S, Bianchi F, Maspero E, Fiocchetti M, Palumbo O, Cipolletti M, Bartoloni S, Acconcia F. Ouabain and Digoxin Activate the Proteasome and the Degradation of the ERα in Cells Modeling Primary and Metastatic Breast Cancer. *Cancers (Basel).* 2020 Dec 19;12(12): e3840. doi: 10.3390/cancers12123840. PMID: 33352737; PMCID: PMC7766733.

Cairns RA, Harris IS, Mak TW. Regulation of cancer cell metabolism. *Nat Rev Cancer.* 2011 Feb;11(2): pp. 85-95. doi: 10.1038/nrc2981. PMID: 21258394.

Cane G, Ginouvès A, Marchetti S, Buscà R, Pouysségur J, Berra E, Hofman P, Vouret-Craviari V. HIF-1alpha mediates the induction of IL-8 and VEGF expression on infection with Afa/Dr diffusely adhering E. coli and promotes EMT-like behaviour. *Cell Microbiol.* 2010 May 1;12(5): e640-53. doi: 10.1111/j.1462-5822.2009.01422.x. Epub 2009 Dec 21. PMID: 20039880.z

Chen B, Zhou S, Zhan Y, Ke J, Wang K, Liang Q, Hou Y, Zhu P, Ao W, Wei X, Xiao J. Dioscin Inhibits the Invasion and Migration of Hepatocellular Carcinoma HepG2 Cells by Reversing TGF-β1-Induced Epithelial-Mesenchymal Transition. *Molecules.* 2019 Jun 14;24(12): e2222. doi: 10.3390/molecules24122222. PMID: 31197076; PMCID: PMC6630778.

Chen Y, Shi Y, Dai G. [Role of HIF-induced EMT in invasion and metastasis of tumor]. Zhong Nan Da Xue Xue Bao Yi Xue Ban. 2016 Aug;41(8): e872-8. Chinese. doi: 10.11817/j.issn.1672-7347.2016.08.017. PMID: 27600018.

Chung FY, Huang MY, Yeh CS, Chang HJ, Cheng TL, Yen LC, Wang JY, Lin SR. GLUT1 gene is a potential hypoxic marker in colorectal cancer patients. *BMC Cancer.* 2009 Jul 20;9: p. 241. doi: 10.1186/1471-2407-9-241. PMID: 19619276; PMCID: PMC3087329.

Feldmeier JJ, Heimbach RD, Davolt DA, Brakora MJ, Sheffield PJ, Porter AT. Does hyperbaric oxygen have a cancer-causing or -promoting effect? A review of the pertinent literature. *Undersea Hyperb Med.* 1994 Dec;21(4): pp. 467-75. PMID: 8000286.

Greene CJ, Sharma NJ, Fiorica PN, Forrester E, Smith GJ, Gross KW, Kauffman EC. Suppressive effects of iron chelation in clear cell renal cell carcinoma and their dependency on VHL inactivation. *Free Radic Biol Med.* 2019 Mar;133: pp. 295-309. doi: 10.1016/j.freeradbiomed.2018.12.013. Epub 2018 Dec 13. PMID: 30553971.

Han, S., Liu, Y., Cai, S.J. et al. IDH mutation in glioma: molecular mechanisms and potential therapeutic targets. *Br J Cancer.* 122, e1580–89 (2020). https://doi.org/10.1038/s41416-020-0814-x.

Kelleher DK, Matthiensen U, Thews O, Vaupel P. Tumor oxygenation in anemic rats: effects of erythropoietin treatment versus red blood cell transfusion. *Acta Oncol.* 1995;34(3): pp. 379-84. doi: 10.3109/02841869509093993. PMID: 7779426.

Koury J, Deitch EA, Homma H, Abungu B, Gangurde P, Condon MR, Lu Q, Xu DZ, Feinman R. Persistent HIF-1alpha activation in gut ischemia/reperfusion injury: potential role of bacteria and lipopolysaccharide. *Shock.* 2004 Sep;22(3): pp. 270-7. doi: 10.1097/01.shk.0000135256.67441.3f. PMID: 15316398.

Kumari A, Folk WP, Sakamuro D. The Dual Roles of MYC in Genomic Instability and Cancer Chemoresistance. *Genes (Basel).* 2017 Jun 7;8(6): p. 158. doi: 10.3390/genes8060158. PMID: 28590415; PMCID: PMC5485522.

Lam G, Fontaine R, Ross FL, Chiu ES. Hyperbaric Oxygen Therapy: Exploring the Clinical Evidence. *Adv Skin Wound Care.* 2017 Apr;30(4): pp. 181-190. doi: 10.1097/01.ASW.0000513089.75457.22. PMID: 28301358.

Lerman OZ, Greives MR, Singh SP, Thanik VD, Chang CC, Seiser N, Brown DJ, Knobel D, Schneider RJ, Formenti SC, Saadeh PB, Levine JP. Low-dose radiation augments vasculogenesis signaling through HIF-1-dependent and -independent SDF-1 induction. *Blood.* 2010 Nov 4;116(18): e3669-76. doi: 10.1182/blood-2009-03-213629. Epub 2010 Jul 14. PMID: 20631377.

Li J, Zhang J, Xie F, Peng J, Wu X. Macrophage migration inhibitory factor promotes Warburg effect via activation of the NFκB/ HIF1α pathway in lung cancer. *Int J Mol Med.* 2018 Feb;41(2): e1062-1068. doi: 10.3892/ijmm.2017.3277. Epub 2017 Nov 22. PMID: 29207023.

Litz J, Krystal GW. Imatinib inhibits c-Kit-induced hypoxia-inducible factor-1alpha activity and vascular endothelial growth factor expression in small cell lung cancer cells. *Mol Cancer Ther.* 2006 Jun;5(6): e1415-22. doi: 10.1158/1535-7163.MCT-05-0503. PMID: 16818499.

Liu Y, Li YM, Tian RF, Liu WP, Fei Z, Long QF, Wang XA, Zhang X. The expression and significance of HIF-1alpha and GLUT-3 in glioma. *Brain Res.* 2009 Dec 22;1304: pp. 49-54. doi: 10.1016/j.brainres.2009.09.083. Epub 2009 Sep 25. PMID: 19782666.

Oda T, Hirota K, Nishi K, Takabuchi S, Oda S, Yamada H, Arai T, Fukuda K, Kita T, Adachi T, Semenza GL, Nohara R. Activation of hypoxia-inducible factor 1 during macrophage differentiation. *Am J Physiol Cell Physiol.* 2006 Jul;291(1): C104-13. doi: 10.1152/ajpcell.00614.2005. Epub 2006 Feb 15. Erratum in: *Am J Physiol Cell Physiol.* 2021 Apr 1;320(4): C666-C667. PMID: 16481368.

Mathieu J, Zhang Z, Zhou W, Wang AJ, Heddleston JM, Pinna CM, Hubaud A, Stadler B, Choi M, Bar M, Tewari M, Liu A, Vessella R, Rostomily R, Born D, Horwitz M, Ware C, Blau CA, Cleary MA, Rich JN, Ruohola-Baker H. HIF induces human embryonic stem cell markers in cancer cells. *Cancer Res.* 2011 Jul 1;71(13): e4640-52. doi: 10.1158/0008-5472.CAN-10-3320. Epub 2011 Jun 28. PMID: 21712410; PMCID: PMC3129496.

Metallo, C., Gameiro, P., Bell, E. et al. Reductive glutamine metabolism by IDH1 mediates lipogenesis under hypoxia. *Nature.* 481, pp. 380–384 (2012). https://doi.org/10.1038/nature10602.

Palayoor ST, Tofilon PJ, Coleman CN. Ibuprofen-mediated reduction of hypoxia-inducible factors HIF-1alpha and HIF-2alpha in prostate cancer cells. *Clin Cancer Res.* 2003 Aug 1;9(8): e3150-7. PMID: 12912967.

Palit V, Phillips RM, Puri R, Shah T, Bibby MC. Expression of HIF-1alpha and Glut-1 in human bladder cancer. *Oncol Rep.* 2005 Oct;14(4): e909-13. doi: 10.3892/or.14.4.909. PMID: 16142350.

Richardson, D.R. (2002). Therapeutic Potential of Iron Chelators in Cancer Therapy. In: Hershko, C. (eds) *Iron Chelation Therapy. Advances in Experimental Medicine and Biology*, vol 509. Springer, Boston, MA. https://link.springer.com/chapter/10.1007/978-1-4615-0593-8_12 .

Saranaruk P, Kariya R, Sittithumcharee G, Boueroy P, Boonmars T, Sawanyawisuth K, Wongkham C, Wongkham S, Okada S, Vaeteewoottacharn K. Chromomycin A3 suppresses cholangiocarcinoma growth by induction of S phase cell cycle arrest and suppression of Sp1related antiapoptotic proteins. *Int J Mol Med.* 2020 Apr;45(4): e1005-16. doi: 10.3892/ijmm.2020.4482. Epub 2020 Jan 29. PMID: 32124934; PMCID: PMC7053871.

Sayyadi M, Safaroghli-Azar A, Safa M, Abolghasemi H, Momeny M, Bashash D. NF-κB-dependent Mechanism of Action of c-Myc Inhibitor 10058-F4: Highlighting a Promising Effect of c-Myc Inhibition in Leukemia Cells, Irrespective of p53 Status. *Iran J Pharm Res.* 2020 Winter;19(1): pp. 153-165. doi: 10.22037/ijpr.2020.112926.14018. PMID: 32922477; PMCID: PMC7462502.

Sethumadhavan S, Silva M, Philbrook P, Nguyen T, Hatfield SM, Ohta A, Sitkovsky MV. Hypoxia and hypoxia-inducible factor (HIF) downregulate antigen-presenting MHC class I molecules limiting tumor cell recognition by T cells. *PLoS One.* 2017 Nov 20;12(11): e0187314. doi: 10.1371/journal.pone.0187314. PMID: 29155844; PMCID: PMC5695785.

Sutphin PD, Chan DA, Li JM, Turcotte S, Krieg AJ, Giaccia AJ. Targeting the loss of the von Hippel-Lindau tumor suppressor gene in renal cell carcinoma cells. *Cancer Res.* 2007 Jun 15;67(12): e5896-905. doi: 10.1158/0008-5472.CAN-07-0604. PMID: 17575159.

Shang Y, Chen H, Ye J, Wei X, Liu S, Wang R. HIF-1α/Ascl2/miR-200b regulatory feedback circuit modulated the epithelial-mesenchymal transition (EMT) in colorectal cancer cells. *Exp Cell Res.* 2017 Nov 15;360(2): pp. 243-56. doi: 10.1016/j.yexcr.2017.09.014. Epub 2017 Sep 9. PMID: 28899657.

Stüben G, Pöttgen C, Knühmann K, Schmidt K, Stuschke M, Thews O, Vaupel P. Erythropoietin restores the anemia-induced reduction in radiosensitivity of experimental human tumors in nude mice. Int J Radiat Oncol Biol Phys. 2003 Apr Wu Z, Han X, Tan G, Zhu Q, Chen H, Xia Y, Gong J, Wang Z, Wang Y, Yan J. Dioscin Inhibited Glycolysis and Induced Cell Apoptosis in Colorectal Cancer via Promoting c-myc Ubiquitination and Subsequent Hexokinase-2 Suppression. *Onco Targets Ther.* 2020 Jan 6;13: pp. 31-44. doi: 10.2147/OTT.S224062. PMID: 32021252; PMCID: PMC6954095.

Stüben G, Thews O, Pöttgen C, Knühmann K, Vaupel P, Stuschke M. Recombinant human erythropoietin increases the radiosensitivity of xenografted human tumours in anaemic nude mice. *J Cancer Res Clin Oncol.* 2001;127(6): pp. 346-50. doi: 10.1007/s004320000215. PMID: 11414194.

Williams NT. Probiotics. *Am J Health Syst Pharm.* 2010 Mar 15;67(6): pp. 449-58. doi: 10.2146/ajhp090168. PMID: 20208051. 1;55(5): e1358-62. doi: 10.1016/s0360-3016(03)00012-9. PMID: 12654448.

Wincewicz A, Sulkowska M, Koda M, Sulkowski S. Clinicopathological significance and linkage of the distribution of HIF-1alpha and GLUT-1 in human primary colorectal cancer. *Pathol Oncol Res.* 2007;13(1): pp. 15-20. doi: 10.1007/BF02893436. Epub 2007 Mar 27. PMID: 17387384.

Wu Z, Han X, Tan G, Zhu Q, Chen H, Xia Y, Gong J, Wang Z, Wang Y, Yan J. Dioscin Inhibited Glycolysis and Induced Cell Apoptosis in Colorectal Cancer via Promoting c-myc Ubiquitination and Subsequent Hexokinase-2 Suppression. *Onco Targets Ther.* 2020 Jan 6;13: pp. 31-44. doi: 10.2147/OTT.S224062. PMID: 32021252; PMCID: PMC6954095.

Yasuda M, Miyazawa M, Fujita M, Kajiwara H, Iida T, Hirasawa T, Muramatsu T, Murakami M, Mikami M, Saitoh K, Shimizu M, Takekoshi S, Osamura RY. Expression of hypoxia inducible factor-1alpha (HIF-1alpha) and glucose transporter-1 (GLUT-1) in ovarian adenocarcinomas: difference in hypoxic status depending on histological character. *Oncol Rep.* 2008 Jan;19(1): pp. 111-16. PMID: 18097583.

Yoo YG, Hayashi M, Christensen J, Huang LE. An essential role of the HIF-1alpha-c-Myc axis in malignant progression. *Ann N Y Acad Sci.* 2009 Oct;1177: pp. 198-204. doi: 10.1111/j.1749-6632.2009.05043.x. PMID: 19845622.

Yu Y, Wong J, Lovejoy DB, Kalinowski DS, Richardson DR. Chelators at the cancer coalface: desferrioxamine to Triapine and beyond. *Clin Cancer Res.* 2006 Dec 1;12(23): e6876-83. doi: 10.1158/1078-0432.CCR-06-1954. PMID: 17145804.

Zörnig M, Evan GI. Cell cycle: on target with Myc. *Curr Biol.* 1996 Dec 1;6(12): e1553-56. doi: 10.1016/s0960-9822(02)70769-0. PMID: 8994810.

Chapter Thirteen

Mitochondrial Transfer Experiments

We traditionally believe that our nucleus acts as the control center of our cells. The Warburg hypothesis states that the mitochondria, not the nucleus, dictate how cancers behave.

Israel and Schaeffer (1987) fused cells containing cancerous nuclei with cells with a normal cytoplasm. The cells created were completely normal (pp. 627-32). Figure 11 displays this cytoplasmic fusion (page 200).

Mice with melanoma spreading to their lungs received injections of normal mitochondria from normal mice, and their tumors shrank (Fu, *et al.*, 2019).

Fibroblasts are special cells that connect our tissues. They are rich in mitochondria—ideal donors for mitochondrial experiments. Fibroblasts share similar behavioral features with our *mesenchymal stromal cells* (MSCs).

Figure 11

Cytoplasmic Fusion

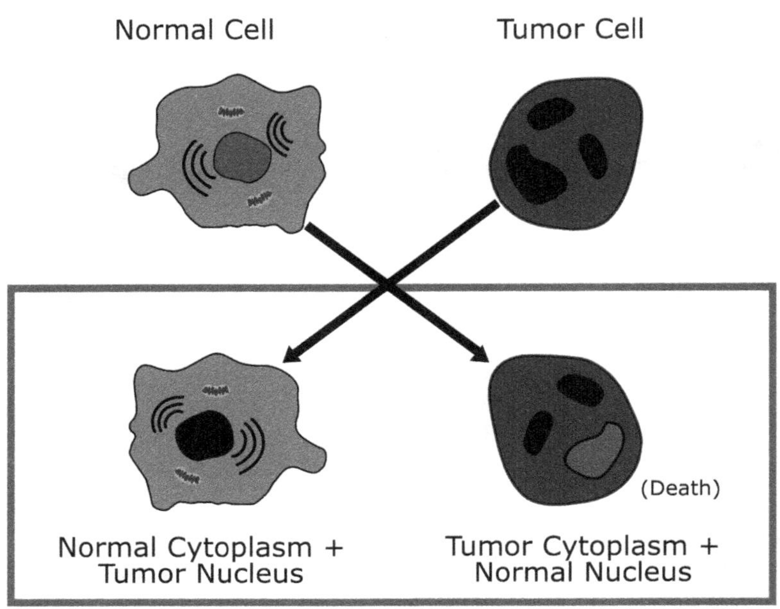

Normal cytoplasm combined with malignant whole cells will create a cell containing both normal and cancerous cytoplasm.

MSCs are cells in our bone marrow and fat tissues that can travel and become replacements for damaged tissues.

Imagine what can happen if we reprogram these cancerous MSCs and 'normalize' them with normal mitochondrial injections.

When melanoma mice were injected with normal mitochondria under the skin, their fibroblasts' glycolytic enzyme (HK2 and LDH) levels and glucose transporters decreased (Fu, *et al.*,

2019; Shay, 1983). In other words, the melanoma cells lost some of their cancer properties and were turning normal again.

Mitochondrial injections could potentially rescue and restore aerobic respiration of damaged mitochondria by converting them into normal ones.

The reasoning behind the anti-cancer effects of cell fusion:

Israel and Shaeffer (1987) suggested that "epigenetic changes in nuclear DNA" were responsible for the anticancer effects of normal cytoplasmic transfer (pp. 627-32).

The mitochondrial transplant or cytoplasmic transfer made the DNA behave differently by making epigenetic (subtle structural) changes to the DNA without changing the main internal gene pattern. Epigenetic change is like watching the Titanic, the 1998 movie, and then the new version 25 years later. The film uses the same story, but some actors are different, and the movie is unique. DNA can undergo epigenetic changes, and although it's the same DNA, the epigenetically changed version is different. With DNA, you change the DNA parts but keep the DNA sequence intact.

Conversely, cancerous cytoplasm (containing defective mitochondria), when inserted into a normal cell with a normal nucleus, can change DNA methylation patterns and steer the nuclear gene expression toward cancer (Shay, 1983), as portrayed in Figure 11 (page 200).

Another explanation could be that the immune system springs into action when cancer cells fuse with non-cancerous cytoplasm. The histocompatibility antigens (MHC1 [major histocompatibility complex class 1], antigen proteins found on cancer cell surfaces) will take the cancer and expose its location to the immune system. Once the immune system recognizes the cancer cells, they are destroyed. When we suppress the histocompatibility antigens, we allow cancer cells to escape detection.

How can we use this knowledge in the clinic? One way would be to immunize (vaccinate) using tumor cells that contain normal levels of Class 1 antigens. This approach may convince the immune system to reject tumors (Vogel, *et al.*, 1987).

Interestingly, other researchers have felt that the cell fusion process, not the mitochondrial transfer, was responsible for tumor suppression (Israel & Schaeffer, 1987; Shay, 1983; Vogel, *et al.*, 1987).

Chapter Summary/Key Takeaways:

We were taught in medical school that the nucleus is the cell's control center. Since the nucleus is key to normal cell control, any defect inside may cause cancer.

Newer research challenges this well-known theory. Perhaps the control center isn't at the nucleus after all. Is it in the mitochondria?

We need more research on how to target the mitochondria as a means of fighting cancer. After all, we might be looking at the wrong tree!

The next chapter discusses an emerging topic: Do fats really feed cancer?

End Notes

Fu A, Hou Y, Yu Z, Zhao Z, Liu Z. Healthy mitochondria inhibit the metastatic melanoma in lungs. *Int J Biol Sci.* 2019 Oct 15;15(12): e2707-718. doi: 10.7150/ijbs.38104. PMID: 31754341; PMCID: PMC6854369.

Israel BA, Schaeffer WI. Cytoplasmic suppression of malignancy. *In Vitro Cell Dev Biol.* 1987 Sep;23(9): e627-32. doi: 10.1007/BF02621071. PMID: 3654482.

Shay JW. Cytoplasmic modification of nuclear gene expression. *Mol Cell Biochem.* 1983;57(1): pp. 17-26. doi: 10.1007/BF00223521. PMID: 6358857.

Vogel J, Tanaka K, Hoekzema GS, Jay G. Experimental strategies for modification of histocompatibility antigens in tumor cells. *Cancer Metastasis Rev.* 1987;6(4): e677-83. doi: 10.1007/BF00047474. PMID: 3327636.

Chapter Fourteen

Cancers and Fat Synthesis

In previous chapters, we saw that glutamine can enter the Krebs cycle to make energy, but what about fats? Indeed, this adds to some concern. If cancers feed on glucose, glutamine, and fats, is nothing safe to eat left?

I am not aware of any way by which fats can ferment to turn into energy or enter the Krebs cycle to make energy. When the Krebs cycle is dysfunctional, excess glucose and glutamine components can head to the fat-making pathway to make fat for cancer-building material.

Unfortunately, many people are confused when they try to understand scientific articles. They misinterpret and conclude that fats are cancer food, and they begin to eat more carbohydrates and avoid dietary fat. They should be avoiding excess glucose and/or protein.

The more excess carbohydrates you eat, the more fat your

body makes. Yes, your body can 'make' fat using materials from glucose and glutamine. You don't necessarily have to fear eating fat if it is done in the proper context. For example, overeating fat and plenty of carbohydrates is expected in the standard American diet. Many doctors recognize this diet (high fat, high carbohydrate) as unhealthy and pro-inflammatory. The ketogenic diet (KD) is not the same as a standard American diet. In a KD, you must limit carbohydrates so that your body will use that fat for energy, and then, out of that fat, you will make ketones too. Ketones will serve as another energy source and can be anti-inflammatory.

Most modern-day Americans love to eat lots of carbohydrates <u>and</u> add fat to that combination. This is when you might get into trouble. The energy is harvested immediately from the heavy carbohydrate load, and the excess carbohydrates will turn into excess body fat.

We already saw how cancers changed normal glucose metabolism and tweaked it to their growth advantage. We also read about glutamine in previously glucose-hungry cancers. Most people with cancer do not have to avoid dietary fat. However, there are several recent publications about faulty fat metabolism in cancers.

Fat metabolism can satisfy cancer's greedy needs for cell building. Read on to learn more about the internal abnormalities of fat metabolism in cancers.

Types of fat:

Aside from the word <u>fat</u>, we also hear other fancy words such as *fatty acids, glycerol,* and *triglycerides*. These are all members of the fat family but with different names and chemical structures.

Fatty acids are building blocks that make up fat. Eating excess carbohydrates or protein leads to excess fatty acids. Fatty acids are used to build cells—yes, even cancer cells!

Cancers also use fatty acids as 'secondary signal messengers' to 'talk' to one another. When it is time to store an energy source, the fatty acids assemble into three groups to join glycerol (a sweet fat) to make triglycerides. Glycerol is a small, 3-carbon molecule, a slightly sticky, sweet-tasting compound that contains three O-H (Oxygen and Hydrogen) groups. Triglycerides are three fatty acids and one glycerol backbone. *Palmitate* is a crucial fatty acid needed to make new cell membranes of ordinary and cancer cells. Palmitate can also be externally sourced from the fruit of oil palms and other foods in our diet. Glucose and glutamine can also become palmitate through *de novo* fatty acid synthesis.

Aggressive cancers can rely on overactive fat-making.

Cancers in the lab 'appear to consume fat.' In a 1953 study of Ehrlich ascites tumor cells, scientists observed that fat levels in the ascites fluid dropped when fat was given to the cancer (Mather & Spectors, 1978).

Does this mean that cancers consume fat? Remember, what goes on in the lab dish cannot precisely duplicate what truly goes on in the human body. Many errors can occur, starting with the lab's temperature, the glucose content of the jelly that goes into the lab dish cultures, the acidity of the media, and so forth.

Fat, like carbohydrates, is a form of energy for normal and cancerous cells. However, the source of the fat differs between normal cells and cancer cells.

Normal cells prefer 'dietary fat.' Under normal conditions, our regular cells are satisfied with dietary fat and do not need to make more. During times of carbohydrate excess—when we overeat—our body changes surplus carbohydrates into stored fat.

Cancer cells are different. They need plenty of energy and, at first, will prefer glucose. Later, as cancers grow, some will 'rewire' and look for more nutrition. Glutamine and fats are possible sources.

Cancer cells don't like to use dietary fat. Fats can't be fermented to make adequate energy to fuel cancers. As cancers multiply and crowd each other, their blood supply and oxygen levels soon lag and cannot sustain them. The poor blood vessel network also means dietary fat cannot be absorbed well. Cancers make their fats because dietary fat is insufficient to meet their needs. This special fat-making process, unique to most cancers, is called *de novo* (new) *fatty acid synthesis* (Menendez & Colomer, 2005).

The raw ingredients for *de novo* fatty acid synthesis (FAS) are usually glucose and glutamine. We normally activate FAS when our body senses that we are low in fat stores. Cancers do not care, and they make fat regardless of how much fat is already around. Cancers use carbon atoms from glucose and glutamine to build palmitate, a fatty acid (Kuhadja, 2000). The overactive enzyme protein FASN (fatty acid synthase) helps grease this biochemical reaction. There are other enzymes involved. I won't get into those details, but if you want to know more, you can read until this chapter's end. Scientists are studying how to slow down or block these hyperactive fat-related biochemical pathways to fight cancer. Unfortunately, this is still considered early research.

Once the fat is made, cancer cells need to break it down before they can harvest the energy. The long-chain fatty acids become smaller fat chains through fatty acid oxidation. As fat breaks down, we release ATP energy (Mathur & Spector, 1978). Aggressive cancers also use fat to build cell membranes, stockpile energy, and send pro-cancer messages to nearby cells.

When oxygen falls, acidity rises, and the cancer senses danger. To survive, cancers might 'epigenetically' affect their genes to perform in a way that favors fat production. Increased fatty acid synthesis (FAO) is needed to sustain high turnover and growth (Menendez & Decker, 2005).

De novo fat synthesis also provides cancers with raw materials such as cholesterol, fatty acids, and triglycerides to form membranes to protect themselves against *oxidative damage* (damage from hyperactive oxygen molecules) (Röhrig & Schulze, 2016).

Cancer cells eventually transform into three-dimensional structures and form fatty acids before oncogene activation (Corces & Corces, 2016; Liberti & Locasale, 2016). *De novo* fat synthesis becomes important for many poor prognosis cancers such as leukemia, breast, glioma; pancreatic, colorectal, lung; ovarian, endometrial, thyroid; stomach, Wilms, and prostate. All these cancers have high levels of fat-making enzymes, such as FASN, compared to their normal tissue. (See: Menendez, *et al.*, 2005; Zhao, *et al.*, 2006; Nishi, *et al.*, 2016; Del Cornò, *et al.*, 2019; Swinnen, *et al.*, 2000; Guo, *et al.*, 2019; Liberti & Locasale, 2016). *Acute myelogenous leukemia* (AML) cells appear to depend heavily on *de novo* fat synthesis (Zeng & Lu, *et al.*, 2022.) AML is challenging to treat, and relapses are common.

Sugar and fat work together to support cancers. The Warburg effect (sugar) maintains fat synthesis by providing raw material (metabolites) to feed into the other pathways (fat-making pathway, glutamine pathway) (Liberti & Locasale, 2016).

Finally, we also have cancer stem cells, which rely on fat. They are not actively dividing, at least not yet. Slow-dividing cells sometimes respond poorly to chemotherapy. Because stem cells don't reproduce rapidly, they don't respond as well to chemotherapy as active cancer cells. Because some stem cells rely on fat, targeting FAS could help stop cancer stem cell growth (Liberti & Locasale, 2016; Skubitz, *et al.*, 2019).

Should we avoid eating fat?

This topic confuses most laypeople. Due to the anti-fat publicity from the 1980s and 1990s, we learned to avoid eating fat. But we also avoid sugar because we hear it feeds cancer, and we begin to avoid eating protein and meat because we see a social media reel or video that tells us to avoid all animal products. As a result, we avoid many nutrients—carbs, protein, and fats—and end up with a "malnutrition diet." Beginners often need clarification on what a ketogenic diet (KD) really means. Ketogenic dieters may eat a lot of fat but must remember to reduce carbs. They need to know that to follow a KD correctly, a high-fat diet must be combined with a low-carbohydrate content. A common beginner's mistake: Eating high-fat diets without cutting out carbohydrates will not make one enter ketosis.

In contrast, a standard American diet is also high-fat but combined with moderate to high amounts of carbohydrates. This combination of high fat and high carbohydrates can be highly inflammatory. We must be careful when reading scientific articles that blame dietary fat alone on cancer. Most of these publications do not use KDs as their study diets, but rather those in composition to the standard American diets that are mistakenly labeled as ketogenic.

We covered a lot of material. Unless you are a scientist looking for material to begin a new experiment, all you need to remember from this chapter is to avoid excess calories and combining too much fat with excess carbohydrates. The combination (fat + carbs) can lead to trouble. Consuming fat by itself is not to be feared in most cancer cases. See this book's Appendices for the acceptable and unacceptable foods while on Keto, and a sample diet.

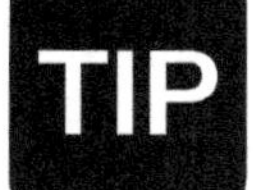

The amount of dietary fat alone is usually not a cause of worry. Most cancers make their own fat because of an overactive *de novo* fatty acid synthesis. The faulty fat metabolism lies in the pathways. We need more clinical trials to target these pathways.

De novo **fatty acid synthesis:**

Warning: Highly technical material ahead.

Here, we dive deeper into the details and learn how to target cancer fat metabolism. If you are satisfied knowing that cancer prefers to make its fat, you may skip this next portion and proceed to the next chapter.

What steps come before the start of *de novo* fat synthesis? The following is a 'simplified' explanation of the biochemical pathways involved in cancer fat metabolism. Knowing the paths may help you locate suitable trials to enroll in if you are searching for clinical trials.

1. The first step is during *de novo* fatty acid synthesis. The growth factors turn on multiple cell signals. Some growth factors are made of steroids, some from protein. Example of growth factors: *Epidermal growth factor* (EGF) works with androgens (male hormones in the prostate) to send signals—*HER2/neu* (HRAS) (Kharmate, *et al.*, 2016).

2. In the second step, the growth factors turn on cancer signals. These signal pathways go by fancy, sometimes difficult-to-remember names. A famous one is the MAPK (mitogen-activated protein kinase) PI3K/Akt pathways (Kharmate, *et al.*, 2016; Guo, *et al.*, 2019).

3. Within the third step, the growth factors and signals activate a protein called SREBP-1c (sterol regulatory element-binding protein-1c) (Guo, *et al.*, 2019).

This is a major event!

Sterol regulatory element-binding protein (SREBP):

SREBP's job is to build the codes of the enzymes that make cholesterol, fat, triglycerides, and phospholipids. One critical enzyme that is overactive in many cancers is FASN.

Aside from its involvement with cancer, SREBP also creates cellular stress that increases the risk of developing obesity, high cholesterol, kidney disease, fatty liver, or cancer (Shimano & Sato, 2017).

How do glucose and insulin play a role in fat-making?

SREBP obeys glucose through insulin. When blood glucose levels are high, the enzyme *pancrease* releases insulin to activate SREBP, which tells the cell to use glucose—to activate glycolysis. At the same time, it switches on the signals to start making FAS. SREBP, therefore, starts <u>both</u> glycolysis and *de novo* fat synthesis. It is no wonder, therefore, why aggressive cancers of the liver, breast, and glioma have very active SREBP-1 proteins.

How does an overactive fat pathway promote cancer?

Now that the SREBP engine is running, we need some 'grease,' the enzymes to speed up the process. I will briefly explain to you how glucose connects to fat metabolism. Remember acetyl-CoA? It came from glucose. Acetyl-CoA must somehow get to the fat pathway by turning itself into palmitate. The following will explain how this happens.

There are at least three important enzymes involved, in the following order:

- Citrate lyase (ACYL)
- Acetyl-CoA carboxylase (ACC)
- Fatty acid synthase (FASN)

Dietary glucose enters the Krebs cycle as acetyl-CoA, producing citric acid or citrate.

Citrate lyase (ACYL) enzymes change the citrate into acetyl-CoA. Excessive amounts (overexpression) of ATP citrate lyase (ACLY) enzymes in aggressive cancers exist. The acetyl-CoA carboxylase (ACC) enzyme takes acetyl-CoA from the ACLY reaction and changes it to malonyl-CoA.

Finally, the third enzyme, FASN, takes acetyl-CoA plus malonyl-CoA and converts them to palmitate, which is sixteen carbon chains long and is very cancer-promoting. It is the final step in the fatty acid synthesis pathway but the first step towards many other forms of fatty acids (Song, *et al.*, 2018).

The process of making palmitate is also highly cancer-promoting, as you will see next (Qu & Shen, 2015; Marteinn, *et al.*, 2020).

Palmitate, the end of the fat pathway, and how it leads to inflammation:

We now know that the FAS pathway ends with a final

product, palmitate. What is next?

Fats are great sources of energy. To use fat, one must break it down through *oxidation*—adding oxygen to the fat.

Unfortunately, the palmitate oxidation process itself causes damaging effects that lead to cancer. Oxidation activates inflammation pathways such as NLRP3 (NOD-like receptor family, pyrin domain-containing-3) and proteins such as interleukin-6 (IL-6) and tumor necrosis factor-alpha (TNF-α) (Song, *et al.*, 2018). Palmitate can be made into new proteins that activate more pro-cancer signals. Palmitate can drive up MMP enzymes, which break down cell membrane barriers to promote metastases (Tzeng, *et al.*, 2019). Palmitate worsens inflammation by boosting ROS and *cytokine* production.

All these effects can fuel cancer, and that is just the beginning!

When do normal cells make fats for themselves?

Normal cells have very few FASN enzymes because they do not need to make fats. Exceptions include liver cells, lactating breast, brain, and fatty tissue.

FASN acts as a housekeeper in the liver because when there are excess carbohydrates, FASN turns them into fatty acids and then reassembles them into groups of three triglycerides, which are stored as fat droplets. The brain needs new cells and maintains the existing ones for memory and intellectual functioning. FASN helps maintain brain stem cells to ensure proper lifetime performance. The breast tissue of lactating mothers needs FASN to make good-quality milk for their offspring.

Why do cancers need to make their own fat?

Fatty acid synthesis promotes 3D cancer structures.

The main job of the FASN enzyme is to consume Acetyl-CoA and change tumors from a 2-D structure into a 3-D structure (Bueno, *et al.* 2019).

Fats help cancers grow new blood vessels.

This is made possible through active, pro-blood vessel signals. Free fatty acids bind to *peroxisome proliferator-activated receptors* (PPAR), creating new blood vessels that help cancers grow (Del Cornò, *et al.*, 2019). Fatty acids also activate the *AMP-activated protein kinase* (AMPK) pathway as well as the *mammalian target of rapamycin* (mTOR)/*protein kinase-B signaling* (PKB) pathways (Madak-Erdogan, *et al.*, 2019; Watt, *et al.*, 2006). These signaling pathways control the formation and growth of new blood vessels that supply cancers (angiogenesis) (Li, *et al.*, 2019).

Fatty acid synthase (FASN):

FASN helps cancers spread or metastasize. FASN encourages the use of metalloproteinase (MMP-2 and MMP-9) more. MMP 'melts' the barriers separating cancer from normal cells. This showed increased metastases of liver and breast cancers. Omega 3 polyunsaturated fatty acids (PUFAs) can neutralize this effect by blocking MMP (Taguchi, *et al.*, 2014).

Fatty acids can turn on or turn off cancer-promoting genes with the help of STAT3 proteins (signal transducer and activator of transcription-3) (Niu, *et al.*, 2019).

Which cancers have high FASN activity?

Mantle cell lymphoma:

Cancers with excess cyclin D1 (cell cycle protein), such as mantle cell lymphoma, can make their fats by inhibiting PPAR-α, a fatty acid-oxidizing nuclear receptor. Blocking FASN can be an effective tool against mantle cell lymphoma (Dengler, *et al.*, 2011).

BRCA1 positive cancers:

BRCA1 is a tumor suppressor gene responsible for DNA repair. BRCA1 mutated cancers often follow aggressive courses. BRCA1-positive patients have a high risk of breast and ovarian cancers. BRCA1 interacts with one of the FASN enzymes, ACC. This interaction between ACC and BRCA1 possibly explains why these breast and ovarian cancers are genetically predisposed to overactive fat metabolism (Ortega, *et al.*, 2012).

***Hormone receptor-positive cancers (estrogen receptor* [ER] and *progesterone receptor* [PR]):**

Fatty acid synthesis (FAS) can regulate estrogen receptor signaling in breast, endometrial, and other cancers. FASN also affects the androgen (male hormone) receptor (AR) axis. FASN and AR are abundant in the prostate (Sena & Denmeade, 2021) and breast cancer cell lines (Menendez & Lulu, 2017).

Her2-neu positive breast cancer:

Her2-positive breast cancers tend to be aggressive and grow rapidly and are often seen with overactive fatty acid synthesis. 15-30% of breast and ovarian cancers and 10-30% of stomach and esophageal cancers have many copies of the HER2 oncogene (Iqbal & Iqbal, 2014). Eating foods high in PUFAs blocks FASN to help breast cancer cells respond better to Herceptin therapy (Tarantino, *et al.*, 2021; Yee, *et al.*, 2013).

Does my cancer love glucose, glutamine, fat, or ketones?

Wait. Hit the pause button!

I began this book by discussing cancers that love glucose. We then pivoted to the role of glutamine and discussed how cancers can start making their fat. Cancers do not rely on just one fuel. Most cancers are combinations of different cells; each cell may prefer a different food type. Glucose-loving cancer cells may coexist with glutamine or fat-loving cells within the same living space.

Let us review these key concepts again but in more detail.

Let us begin with glucose. Warburg states that most cancers have a fundamental defect in respiration or OXPHOS. Respiration and OXPHOS, as you recall, are found in the mitochondria. Therefore, most cancers are sugar-loving and make energy by breaking down glucose (glycolysis). They do not need to go through OXPHOS anymore since it is defective. This is Warburg's hypothesis.

Now, let us talk about glutamine. Later, cancers get used to sugar and 'rewire' themselves to 'like' other fuels, such as glutamine. Some authors claim that cancers can also consume fats. These authors also declare that cancers have some functional OXPHOS after all.

Was Warburg wrong? Do cancers really 'switch' from one type of metabolism to another? Do some cancers have intact mitochondria?

It is likely that instead of 'switching,' cancers may first develop an appetite for sugar. Followed later by glutamine. Whether the last two—lactate and ketones—are considered fuel for cancers is still highly debatable. Multiple papers support this idea, but there are also multiple papers that have contradictory evidence. We do know that they—lactate and ketones—are sometimes seen in abundant amounts around cancers. But their mere presence does not necessarily prove the existence of intact respiration.

The ketogenic paradox that I described earlier also cannot explain why patients continue to benefit from ketones and fasting despite laboratory experiments that suggest ketones are otherwise (Abolhassani, *et al.*, 2022).

Dr. Tom Seyfried (Boston College) (2014) is convinced that cancers do not feed on fats, nor do they feed on ketones, as several published papers claiming that cancers prefer ketones or fats failed to cite publications that show faulty respiration in cancers (pp. 515-27). It is also possible that commercially used culture media may also contain glucose, which could inadvertently skew the experimental results. Most significant cancers will have some defect in their seemingly functional mitochondria. Therefore, even those cancers that appear to consume fats or ketones will, in reality, not be able to produce enough energy to support hungry cancer (Seyfried, 2014).

Against Warburg's theory: Do fats and ketones really feed cancers?

There are now some researchers who claim that the idea of sugar-loving cancers is incorrect. They claim their mitochondria are normal and describe some cancers that don't ferment. Instead, these cancers prefer oxygen and mostly depend on fats to produce ATP energy.

This is against Warburg's original theory.

Weinhouse (1956) reports, "Because these cancers are using oxygen similar to non-cancer cells, these investigators concluded that cancers don't ferment glucose and must have intact and fully functional mitochondria" (p. 269). He, therefore, concluded that Warburg's theory about impaired respiration in cancers was wrong. He believed there were cancers with fully functional mitochondria with enough normal OXPHOS activity and respiration to provide energy themselves (Weinhouse, 1956).

Later papers suggesting that cancers can survive using fatty acids and intact OXPHOS support Weinhouse's idea. Subsequent publications, however, contradict this idea by failing to show that cancers can use fatty acids to make adequate ATP energy to support themselves (Seyfried, 2014; Bloch-Frankenthal, *et al.*, 1965; Kuok, *et al.*, 2019).

Supporting Warburg's theory: Cancers love glucose and cannot rely on fats or ketones.

In an elegant compilation of cancers and mitochondrial defects, Seyfried's 2014 paper showed that <u>all major cancers</u> have documented abnormalities in mitochondrial structure, function, and number (pp. 515-27). Proof of oxygen consumption is not a substitute for proof of intact mitochondria. Many cancers treated with cyanide lose the ability to use oxygen yet remain alive. Per Seyfried (2014), these cancers must be getting their ATP energy from a source other than the oxygen requiring OXPHOS (pp. 515-27).

Warburg first described glucose-fermenting cancers as having a major breakdown in OXPHOS. So where will the damaged cancer get enough ATP energy to support itself?

In a previous chapter, we discussed how cancers can sense low oxygen conditions. As a response, the cancer begins making fats through the *de novo* fatty acid synthesis pathways, followed by fat accumulation. As levels of fatty acids rise, the fats will cause the mitochondria to swell, and inside, the ETC will desynchronize, causing it to 'uncouple.' Another way to describe this is to say that the mitochondrion "sprung a leak." With the main ATP machinery down, the cancer cell compensates by triggering more fermentation, increasing glycolysis, and using more glucose to make ATP. Glutamine is also recruited to ferment glucose eventually. This is the accelerated process of SLP. It is also known as the "missing link" to Warburg's original theory (Chinopoulos & Seyfried, 2018).

Originally, Warburg only mentioned that cancers have defective respiration, but he could not explain where they eventually got their energy. SLP now makes this explainable.

Because the accumulation of fatty acids triggered this chain reaction, it may appear that the cancer cells are using the fats for energy. Most of the ATP energy comes from the subsequent glycolysis and fermentation boost. Fats and ketones cannot feed cancer because they cannot enter this pathway to be directly fermented like glucose and glutamine can (Seyfried, 2014; Samudio, *et al.*, 2009; Valle, *et al.*, 2010; Vozza, *et al.*, 2014; Hess & Lehninger, 1964).

Chapter Summary/Key Takeaways:

We learned about the different fat forms and how fat benefits the normal cell. We also learned that most aggressive cancers prefer to make fats from glucose and glutamine. A minority of investigators believe that cancers can get their energy directly from dietary fats, but their evidence is weak. Most major cancers, even the ones that make a lot of fat, are still believed to have that one fundamental defect: a defect in respiration and overactive glucose metabolism. Cancers prefer to make their fats but continue relying on glucose.

The next chapter will explore ways to attack cancer by targeting specific parts of cancer fat metabolism.

End Notes

Abolhassani, Mohammad & E, Berg & G, Tenenbaum & Israël, Maurice. (2022). Inhibition of SCOT and Ketolysis Decreases Tumor Growth and Inflammation in the Lewis Cancer Model. *JOCR*. 3. e104. 10.17303/jocr.2022.3.104.

Bueno, M.J., Jimenez-Renard, V., Samino, S. *et al.* Essentiality of fatty acid synthase in the 2D to anchorage-independent growth transition in transforming cells. *Nat Commun,* 10, e5011 (2019). https://doi.org/10.1038/s41467-019-13028-1.

Bloch-Frankenthal, L., Langan, J., Morris, H.P., & Weinhouse, S. (1965). Fatty Acid Oxidation and Ketogenesis in Transplantable Liver Tumors. *Cancer Research*, 25, e732-6.

Corces MR, Corces VG. The three-dimensional cancer genome. *Curr Opin Genet Dev.* 2016 Feb;36: e1-7. doi: 10.1016/j.gde.2016.01.002. Epub 2016 Feb 6. PMID: 26855137; PMCID: PMC4880523.

Chinopoulos C, Seyfried TN. Mitochondrial Substrate-Level Phosphorylation as Energy Source for Glioblastoma: Review and Hypothesis. *ASN Neuro*. 2018 Jan-Dec;10: 1759091418818261. doi:10.1177/1759091418818261. PMID: 30909720; PMCID: PMC6311572.

Del Cornò M, Baldassarre A, Calura E, Conti L, Martini P, Romualdi C, Varì R, Scazzocchio B, D'Archivio M, Masotti A, Gessani S. Transcriptome Profiles of Human Visceral Adipocytes in Obesity and Colorectal Cancer Unravel the Effects of Body Mass Index and Polyunsaturated Fatty Acids on Genes and Biological Processes Related to Tumorigenesis. *Front Immunol.* 2019 Feb 19;10: p. 265. doi: 10.3389/fimmu.2019.00265. PMID: 30838002; PMCID: PMC6389660.

Guo D, Prins RM, Dang J, Kuga D, Iwanami A, Soto H, Lin KY, Huang TT, Akhavan D, Hock MB, Zhu S, Kofman AA, Bensinger SJ, Yong WH, Vinters HV, Horvath S, Watson AD, Kuhn JG, Robins HI, Mehta MP, Wen PY, DeAngelis LM, Prados MD, Mellinghoff IK, Cloughesy TF, Mischel PS. EGFR signaling through an Akt-SREBP-1-dependent, rapamycin-resistant pathway sensitizes glioblastomas to antilipogenic therapy. *Sci Signal.* 2009 Dec 15;2(101): ra82. doi: 10.1126/scisignal.2000446. PMID: 20009104; PMCID: PMC2978002.

Guo W, Abudumijiti H, Xu L, Hasim A. CD147 promotes cervical cancer migration and invasion by up-regulating fatty acid synthase expression. *Int J Clin Exp Pathol.* 2019 Dec 1;12(12): e4280-88. PMID: 31933828; PMCID: PMC6949868.

Iqbal N, Iqbal N. Human Epidermal Growth Factor Receptor 2 (HER2) in Cancers: Overexpression and Therapeutic Implications. *Mol Biol Int.* 2014;2014:e852748. doi: 10.1155/2014/852748. Epub 2014 Sep 7. PMID: 25276427; PMCID: PMC4170925.

Kuhajda FP. Fatty-acid synthase and human cancer: new perspectives on its role in tumor biology. *Nutrition.* 2000 Mar;16(3): pp. 202-8. doi: 10.1016/s0899-9007(99)00266-x. PMID: 10705076.

Kuok IT, Rountree AM, Jung SR, Sweet IR. Palmitate is not an effective fuel for pancreatic islets and amplifies insulin secretion independent of calcium release from endoplasmic reticulum. *Islets.* 2019;11(3): pp. 51-64. doi: 10.1080/19382014.2019.1601490. Epub 2019 May 14. PMID: 31084524; PMCID: PMC6548485.

Kharmate G, Hosseini-Beheshti E, Caradec J, Chin MY, Tomlinson Guns ES. Epidermal Growth Factor Receptor in Prostate Cancer Derived Exosomes. *PLoS One.* 2016 May 6;11(5): e0154967. doi: 10.1371/journal.pone.0154967. *Erratum in: PLoS One.* 2016;11(6): e0157392. PMID: 27152724; PMCID: PMC4859494.

Lehninger, V. A. L. (1965). The Mitochondrion: Molecular basis of structure and function. (B. Hess, Ed.). *Angewandte Chemie, 77*(8), p. 390. https://doi.org/10.1002/ange.19650770829

Li Y, Sun R, Zou J, Ying Y, Luo Z. Dual Roles of the AMP-Activated Protein Kinase Pathway in Angiogenesis. *Cells.* 2019 Jul 19;8(7): e752. doi: 10.3390/cells8070752. PMID: 31331111; PMCID: PMC6678403.

Liberti MV, Locasale JW. The Warburg Effect: How Does it Benefit Cancer Cells? Trends Biochem Sci. 2016 Mar;41(3):211-218. doi: 10.1016/j.tibs.2015.12.001. Epub 2016 Jan 5. Erratum in: Trends Biochem Sci. 2016 Mar;41(3):287. Erratum in: *Trends Biochem Sci.* 2016 Mar;41(3): p. 287. PMID: 26778478; PMCID: PMC4783224.

Ortega FJ, Moreno-Navarrete JM, Mayas D, García-Santos E, Gómez-Serrano M, Rodriguez-Hermosa JI, Ruiz B, Ricart W, Tinahones FJ, Frühbeck G, Peral B, Fernández-Real JM. Breast cancer 1 (BrCa1) may be behind decreased lipogenesis in adipose tissue from obese subjects. *PLoS One.* 2012;7(5): e33233. doi: 10.1371/journal.pone.0033233. Epub 2012 May 30. PMID: 22666314; PMCID: PMC3364252.

Madak-Erdogan Z, Band S, Zhao YC, Smith BP, Kulkoyluoglu-Cotul E, Zuo Q, Santaliz Casiano A, Wrobel K, Rossi G, Smith RL, Kim SH, Katzenellenbogen JA, Johnson ML, Patel M, Marino N, Storniolo AMV, Flaws JA. Free Fatty Acids Rewire Cancer Metabolism in Obesity-Associated Breast Cancer via Estrogen Receptor and mTOR Signaling. *Cancer Res.* 2019 May 15;79(10): e2494-510. doi: 10.1158/0008-5472.CAN-18-2849. Epub 2019 Mar 12. PMID: 30862719.

Marteinn Thor Snaebjornsson, Sudha Janaki-Raman, Almut Schulze,Greasing the Wheels of the Cancer Machine: The Role of Lipid Metabolism in Cancer, *Cell Metabolism*, 2020; 31(1): pp. 62-76.

Mathur SN, Spector AA. Effects of dietary fat composition on the Ehrlich ascites tumor fluid lipoproteins. *J Lipid Res.* 1978 May;19(4): pp. 457-66. PMID: 207800.

Menendez JA, Decker JP, Lupu R. In support of fatty acid synthase (FAS) as a metabolic oncogene: extracellular acidosis acts in an epigenetic fashion activating FAS gene expression in cancer cells. *J Cell Biochem.* 2005 Jan 1;94(1): pp. 1-4. doi: 10.1002/jcb.20310. PMID: 15523670.

Menendez JA, Colomer R, Lupu R. Why does tumor-associated fatty acid synthase (oncogenic antigen-519) ignore dietary fatty acids? *Med Hypotheses.* 2005;64(2): pp. 342-9. doi: 10.1016/j.mehy.2004.07.022. PMID: 15607569.

Menendez JA, Oza BP, Colomer R, Lupu R. The estrogenic activity of synthetic progestins used in oral contraceptives enhances fatty acid synthase-dependent breast cancer cell proliferation and survival. *Int J Oncol.* 2005 Jun;26(6): e1507-15. PMID: 15870863.

Menendez JA, Lupu R. Fatty acid synthase (FASN) as a therapeutic target in breast cancer. *Expert Opin Ther Targets.* 2017 Nov;21(11):e1001-16. doi: 10.1080/14728222.2017.1381087. Epub 2017 Sep 21. PMID: 28922023.

Michael A. Dengler, Matthias Gutekunst, Stephanie Kopacz, Heike Horn, Ute Hofmann, Matthias Schwab, German Ott, Heiko van der Kuip, Walter E. Aulitzky; Cyclin D1 Over-Expressing Mantle Cell Lymphoma Cells Are Hypersensitive to Inhibition of Fatty Acid Synthase (FASN). *Blood.* 2011; 118 (21): e1656. doi: 10.1182/blood.V118.21.1656.1656

Momcilovic M, Jones A, Bailey ST, Waldmann CM, Li R, Lee JT, Abdelhady G, Gomez A, Holloway T, Schmid E, Stout D, Fishbein MC, Stiles L, Dabir DV, Dubinett SM, Christofk H, Shirihai O, Koehler CM, Sadeghi S, Shackelford DB. In vivo imaging of mitochondrial membrane potential in non-small-cell lung cancer. *Nature.* 2019 Nov;575(7782): pp. 380-84. doi: 10.1038/s41586-019-1715-0. Epub 2019 Oct 30. *Erratum in: Nature.* 2020 Jan;577(7791):e7. PMID: 31666695; PMCID: PMC7328016.

Niu J, Sun Y, Chen B, Zheng B, Jarugumilli GK, Walker SR, Hata AN, Mino-Kenudson M, Frank DA, Wu X. Fatty acids and cancer-amplified ZDHHC19 promote STAT3 activation through S-palmitoylation. *Nature.* 2019 Sep;573(7772): pp. 139-43. doi: 10.1038/s41586-019-1511-x. Epub 2019 Aug 28. *Retraction in: Nature.* 2020 Jul;583(7814): p. 154. PMID: 31462771; PMCID: PMC6728214.

Nishi K, Suzuki K, Sawamoto J, Tokizawa Y, Iwase Y, Yumita N, Ikeda T. Inhibition of Fatty Acid Synthesis Induces Apoptosis of Human Pancreatic Cancer Cells. *Anticancer Res.* 2016 Sep;36(9): e4655-60. doi: 10.21873/anticanres.11016. PMID: 27630308.

Qu M, Shen W. [Role of PI3K/Akt pathway in endoplasmic reticulum stress and apoptosis induced by saturated fatty acid in human steatotic hepatocytes]. Zhonghua Gan Zang Bing Za Zhi. 2015 Mar;23(3): pp. 194-9. Chinese. doi: 10.3760/cma.j.issn.1007-3418.2015.03.008. PMID: 25938832.

Röhrig F, Schulze A. The multifaceted roles of fatty acid synthesis in cancer. *Nat Rev Cancer.* 2016 Nov;16(11): e732-49. doi: 10.1038/nrc.2016.89. Epub 2016 Sep 23. PMID: 27658529.

Samudio I, Fiegl M, Andreeff M. Mitochondrial uncoupling and the Warburg effect: molecular basis for the reprogramming of cancer cell metabolism. *Cancer Res.* 2009 Mar 15;69(6): e2163-6. doi: 10.1158/0008-5472.CAN-08-3722. Epub 2009 Mar 3. PMID: 19258498; PMCID: PMC3822436.

Sena LA, Denmeade SR. Fatty Acid Synthesis in Prostate Cancer: Vulnerability or Epiphenomenon? *Cancer Res.* 2021 Sep 1;81(17): e4385-93. doi: 10.1158/0008-5472.CAN-21-1392. Epub 2021 Jun 18. PMID: 34145040; PMCID: PMC8416800

Seyfried TN, Flores RE, Poff AM, D'Agostino DP. Cancer as a metabolic disease: implications for novel therapeutics. *Carcinogenesis.* 2014 Mar;35(3): e515-27. doi: 10.1093/carcin/bgt480. Epub 2013 Dec 16. PMID: 24343361; PMCID: PMC3941741.

Shimano H, Sato R. SREBP-regulated lipid metabolism: convergent physiology - divergent pathophysiology. *Nat Rev Endocrinol.* 2017 Dec;13(12): e710-30. doi: 10.1038/nrendo.2017.91. Epub 2017 Aug 29. PMID: 28849786.

Siyue Du, Nicole Wagner, Kay-Dietrich Wagner, "The Emerging Role of PPAR Beta/Delta in Tumor Angiogenesis," *PPAR Research*, vol. 2020, Article ID 3608315, pp. 1-16, 2020. https://doi.org/10.1155/2020/3608315.

Skubitz, K.M., Wilson, J.D., Cheng, E.Y. *et al.* Effect of chemotherapy on cancer stem cells and tumor-associated macrophages in a prospective study of preoperative chemotherapy in soft tissue sarcoma. *J Transl Med.* 17, p. 130 (2019). https://doi.org/10.1186/s12967-019-1883-6.

Song Z, Xiaoli AM, Yang F. Regulation and Metabolic Significance of *De Novo* Lipogenesis in Adipose Tissues. *Nutrients*. 2018; 10(10): e1383. https://doi.org/10.3390/nu10101383.

Swinnen JV, Vanderhoydonc F, Elgamal AA, Eelen M, Vercaeren I, Joniau S, Van Poppel H, Baert L, Goossens K, Heyns W, Verhoeven G. Selective activation of the fatty acid synthesis pathway in human prostate cancer. *Int J Cancer.* 2000 Oct 15;88(2): pp. 176-9. doi: 10.1002/1097-0215(20001015)88:2 <176::aid-ijc5>3.0.co;2-3. PMID: 11004665.

Taguchi A, Kawana K, Tomio K, Yamashita A, Isobe Y, Nagasaka K, Koga K, Inoue T, Nishida H, Kojima S, Adachi K, Matsumoto Y, Arimoto T, Wada-Hiraike O, Oda K, Kang JX, Arai H, Arita M, Osuga Y, Fujii T. Matrix metalloproteinase (MMP)-9 in cancer-associated fibroblasts (CAFs) is suppressed by omega-3 polyunsaturated fatty acids in vitro and in vivo. *PLoS One.* 2014 Feb 27;9(2): e89605. doi: 10.1371/journal.pone.0089605. PMID: 24586907; PMCID: PMC3937340.

Tarantino P, Morganti S, Curigliano G. Targeting HER2 in breast cancer: new drugs and paradigms on the horizon. *Explor Target Antitumor Ther.* 2021;2(2): pp. 139-55. doi: 10.37349/etat.2021.00037. Epub 2021 Apr 30. PMID: 36046143; PMCID: PMC9400740.

Tzeng HT, Chyuan IT, Chen WY. Shaping of Innate Immune Response by Fatty Acid Metabolite Palmitate. *Cells.* 2019 Dec 13;8(12): e1633. doi: 10.3390/cells8121633. PMID: 31847240; PMCID: PMC6952933.

Valle A, Oliver J, Roca P. Role of uncoupling proteins in cancer. *Cancers (Basel).* 2010 Apr 16;2(2): e567-91. doi: 10.3390/cancers2020567. PMID: 24281083; PMCID: PMC3835092.

Vozza A, Parisi G, De Leonardis F, Lasorsa FM, Castegna A, Amorese D, Marmo R, Calcagnile VM, Palmieri L, Ricquier D, Paradies E, Scarcia P, Palmieri F, Bouillaud F, Fiermonte G. UCP2 transports C4 metabolites out of mitochondria, regulating glucose and glutamine oxidation. *Proc Natl Acad Sci U S A.* 2014 Jan 21;111(3): e960-5. doi: 10.1073/pnas.1317400111. Epub 2014 Jan 6. PMID: 24395786; PMCID: PMC3903233.

Watt MJ, Steinberg GR, Chen ZP, Kemp BE, Febbraio MA. Fatty acids stimulate AMP-activated protein kinase and enhance fatty acid oxidation in L6 myotubes. *J Physiol.* 2006 Jul 1;574(Pt 1): pp. 139-47. doi: 10.1113/jphysiol.2006.107318. Epub 2006 Apr 27. PMID: 16644805; PMCID: PMC1817791.

Weinhouse S., On respiratory impairment in cancer cells. *Science.* 1956 Aug 10;124(3215): pp. 267-9. doi: 10.1126.science.124.3215.267. PMID: 13351638.

Yee LD, Agarwal D, Rosol TJ, Lehman A, Tian M, Hatton J, Heestand J, Belury MA, Clinton SK. The inhibition of early stages of HER-2/neu-mediated mammary carcinogenesis by dietary n-3 PUFAs. *Mol Nutr Food Res.* 2013 Feb;57(2): pp. 320-7. doi: 10.1002/mnfr.201200445. Epub 2012 Dec 5. PMID: 23213007; PMCID: PMC3855004.

Zeng, P., Lu, W., Tian, J. *et al.* Reductive TCA cycle catalyzed by wild-type IDH2 promotes acute myeloid leukemia and is a metabolic vulnerability for potential targeted therapy. *J Hematol Oncol.* 15, p. 30 (2022). https://doi.org/10.1186/s13045-022-01245-z.

Zhao W, Kridel S, Thorburn A, Kooshki M, Little J, Hebbar S, Robbins M. Fatty acid synthase: a novel target for antiglioma therapy. *Br J Cancer*. 2006 Oct 9;95(7): e869-78. doi: 10.1038/sj.bjc.6603350. Epub 2006 Sep 12. PMID: 16969344; PMCID: PMC2360524.

Chapter Fifteen

Targeting Fatty Acid Synthesis

Cancers need plenty of fat to create building materials for themselves. To make fat through *de novo* fatty synthesis, we need enzymes. Studies show that blocking fatty acid synthesis's main enzymes (ACC and FASN) can slow down cancer.

How do we stop fatty acid synthesis (FAS)?

Fasting or exercise can activate the AMPK pathway to limit FAS, increase fatty acid breakdown (oxidation), improve insulin sensitivity, and maybe blunt cancer growth. Researchers are trying to make a drug to activate AMPK and stop FAS (Smith & Steinberg, 2017).

Potential risks:

There are some risks involved with blocking these pathways. Fat pathways are important for fetal development and muscle building. We need the fat-making pathway to make healthy platelets, which help us stop bleeding when we receive a cut (Batchuluun, *et al.*, 2022).

Potential treatments:

This list is meant to be incomplete, yet I include as much potentially useful information as possible. Some items here are commercially available, some by prescription, while others are experimental. You can check out clinicaltrials.gov and search for clinical trials using the information here to guide your keyword search, and some of the data here will help you find available resources. Many clinical trials of ACC inhibitors can be found on the website clinicaltrials.gov.

A. Betulin, fatostatin, and xanthohumol

Betulin is an extract isolated from birch, Platanus, and eucalyptus tree bark sap. It has anti-tumor activity against many cancers, including melanoma, leukemia, myeloma, breast, lung, liver, colon, prostate, cervical, ovarian, head and neck (Lou, *et al.*, 2021). Xanthohumol is another natural extract derived from hops, while fatostatin is lab-created (Girisa, *et al.*, 2021).

All are powerful blockers of the SREBP central protein, a key player in *de novo* fatty acid synthesis in many cancers (Tang, *et al.*, 2011; Li, *et al.*, 2014; Costa, *et al.*, 2017).

B. Cerulenin

It is a natural anti-fungal antibiotic that effectively stops FAS. It does so by blocking the malonyl-CoA step and preventing HMG-CoA synthase of the cholesterol pathway. It also inhibits FASN by competing with its activity.

Cerulenin was effective against laboratory breast, colon, and ovarian cancer cell lines (Thupari, *et al.*, 2001; Pizer, *et al.*, 1996; Huang *et al.*, 2000). It enhanced the potency of *oxaliplatin chemotherapy* for human colon cancer cells. In colon cancer mice models, cerulenin prevented liver metastases while shrinking existing liver metastases (Huang, *et al.*, 2000; Murata, *et al.*, 2010).

Cerulenin is very effective in slowing cancer growth and promoting cancer death. However, this drug is very unstable in animals and humans because it loses potency when exposed to high temperatures or humidity. Therefore, it is not currently available for use outside the laboratory (Omura, 1976; Sukjoi, *et al.*, 2021). While cerulenin is not typically found in food, some plants, like cerulenin, produce natural compounds that can inhibit FAS. Some excellent examples are Chinese herbs, such as parasitic Loranthus, polygonum multiflorum, ginkgo leaf; maple leaf, night kodo, galanga; spices, and other plant-based foods (Tian, *et al.*, 2011).

C. 5-tetradecyloxy-2-furoic acid (TOFA)

TOFA can also inhibit FASN and slow down large-cell lung cancer and colon cancer cell lines by targeting ACC (Wang, *et al.*, 2009). In a lab experiment of pancreatic cancer cells, treatment with TOFA blocked FASN and starved them of fatty acids, resulting in a significant number of dying cancer cells (Nishi, *et al.* 2016). Food normally does not contain TOFA. It is mainly used in industrial applications, such as pesticide and specialty chemical production, food processing, and preservation. Adding TOFA to food is highly unlikely and could be toxic to normal cells.

D. Soraphen A

The antifungal Soraphen A was able to limit the activity of the fat enzyme, ACC, to chemically inhibit cancer stem cells (Wang, *et al.*, 2009). ACC usually changes acetyl-CoA to malonyl-CoA to control FAS and oxidation. It is very effective as a fungicide. Research towards human use is currently under clinical trials for treating metabolic diseases such as diabetes, obesity, and cancer (Naini, *et al.*, 2019; Corominas-Faja, *et al.*, 2014). Trials use a synthetic soraphen version.

Check out your medicine cabinet.

Note: Some are prescriptions, so check with your doctor first.

The anti-diabetic drug Metformin and the anti-cholesterol

drugs or statins both have anti-FASN activity (Xiong, *et al.*, 2021).

A. Statins

There are reports that cholesterol-reducing agents may decrease colon, prostate, and breast cancer incidence. In a study of 1953 colorectal cancer patients, statins given for five years were matched to a control group of 2015 patients (non-use of statins). After adjusting for aspirin and non-steroidal inflammatory drug NSAID use, there was a significant decrease in the relative risk of colorectal cancer (odds ratio: 0.50; 95 percent confidence interval, 0.40 to 0.63). This translated to a 47 percent relative decrease in colorectal cancer (Poynter, *et al.*, 2005; Demierre, *et al.*, 2005).

Statins lower cholesterol production by blocking the HMG-CoA enzyme (β-Hydroxy β-methylglutaryl-CoA reductase). While it wasn't clear why blocking the cholesterol pathway would also block the fatty acid pathway, Trub (2022) explained that blocking the cholesterol pathway with statins will modify the proteins of the FASN enzyme itself to change its activity (e2542).

Another explanation is that blocking cholesterol production limits farnesyl-PPi and geranyl-PPi, activating metabolites of pro-cancer genes (oncogenes) such as HRAS and KRAS.

Carroll (2018) described a link between FAS and cholesterol synthesis to lowering inflammation, *toll-like receptor*

(TLR) signaling, and macrophage activation (e5509-21). Macrophages are inflammatory white blood cells. The FASN *inhibitor C75* might help stop TLR signals (Carroll, *et al.*, 2018).

Statins can also change the behavior of our T-cells (immune system white blood cells) from a pro-inflammatory to an anti-inflammatory profile (Demierre, *et al.*, 2005).

B. Niacin

Niacin is similar to statins and can treat high cholesterol and triglycerides. It is a form of vitamin B3, structurally similar to NAD+. Side effects such as diarrhea, rash, and skin flushing can be limiting. It blocks FAS by activating AMPK pathways and the ACC enzyme, reducing mTOR signals and the SREBP. We know that SREBP later controls the other enzymes of fat metabolism. Therefore niacin could potentially 'turn off' most fat pathways fueling cancer (Wang, *et al.*, 2020).

C. Aspirin

Aspirin is a common over-the-counter medication and has antiplatelet functions. Platelets have some role in controlling inflammation, blood vessel growth, and cancer metastases. In a lab study, Aspirin slowed down fat metabolism in liver cancer cells by reducing the activity of another fat-related enzyme, *acyl-CoA synthetase* (ACSL1), an early enzyme involved in the fatty acid breakdown pathway.

When this pathway was hit, it also slowed down NF-κB pathway (Yang, *et al.*, 2017).

One must be aware that Aspirin can increase bleeding; hence, it should be used with caution if one has a history of active bleeding (i.e., ulcers and bleeding disorders) or is already on blood thinners.

D. Orlistat (Xenical)

Orlistat is currently sold as a weight loss drug. It can block FASN and has anti-cancer benefits in prostate cancer. Up to 50% of breast cancers have elevated FASN, also seen with high HER2/neu oncogene levels. Orlistat can potentially suppress HER2/neu oncogene expression. Currently, orlistat pills are FDA-approved for weight loss but not for cancer therapy. We still don't know the best dose that will be effective against cancer. More research is needed to clarify this drug's potential benefits (Menendez, *et al.*, 2005c).

E. NMN supplements and nicotinamide riboside (NR)

Both NMN supplements and NR can suppress fat synthesis by boosting levels of SIRT1 proteins. High levels of SIRT1 can have similar benefits to fasting. It may help regulate fat synthesis, decrease oxidative stress, improve insulin sensitivity, and protect beta cells of the pancreas to help prevent diabetes. It helps keep DNA stable and lowers the risk of dementia, heart disease, cancer, and other diseases (Hwang & Song, 2017).

Sometimes, it's what you don't eat that counts.

1. *Fasting and caloric restriction* increase a special anti-aging protein, SIRT. Boosted SIRT1 (sirtuin 1) protein levels will lead to loss of SREBP-1. Since SREBP is a major regulator of fat metabolism, losing the SREBP-1 protein will suppress fat and cholesterol production. SIRT proteins come in seven types (SIRT1-7). SIRT1, in particular, helps prolong life by keeping fat metabolism under control, protecting cells from stressful events, and keeping DNA stable, all of which can help prevent cancer (Elibol & Kilic, 2018).

2. *Caloric restriction (CR)* is similar to the effects of fasting and will both change the gut bacterial population. CR causes a boost in the gut's Lactobacillus probiotic population, which controls fat metabolism in an anti-inflammatory environment (Tanca, *et al.*, 2018).

3. *Low carbohydrate diets.* Insulin promotes the FAS pathway through the PI3K/Akt pathway. High carbohydrate diets trigger the body to make fats (Hudgins, 1996).

Search your grocery store or your garden!

A. Hydroxycitrate, or hydroxycitric acid

Hydroxycitrate or hydroxycitric acid is the active ingredient in the rind of the Garcinia cambogia fruit. It inhibits FAS by pushing the Krebs cycle to use up acetyl-CoA so that less acetyl-CoA will be available for FAS.

Hydroxycitrate also directly competes with ATP citrate lyase (ACLY) (the enzyme that changes citrate to oxaloacetate, then to acetyl-CoA), the goal being to limit the amount of acetyl-CoA entering the fat synthesis pathway (Li, *et al.*, 2017).

B. Fish oil

Fish oil contains omega-3 fatty acids that reverse the FAS process by boosting the malonyl-CoA decarboxylase enzyme. Omega-3 oil reduces the amounts of inflammatory proteins such as TNF-α and IL-1β. It blunts the ability of white blood cells to secrete *arachidonic acid* (proinflammatory omega-6 member). It helps reduce the clotting agent, thromboxane A2, protecting us against strokes and heart attacks. An omega-3-derived metabolite effectively killed leukemia stem cells grown in mice (Surette, 2008; Hegde, *et al.*, 2011).

C. Soy protein

Soy protein increases cholesterol metabolism, eliminates cholesterol through the feces, and reduces cholesterol absorption. (See Surette, 2008; Pang, *et al.*, 2016; Flavin, *et al.*, 2010; Takahashi, *et al.*, 2019; Nelson Hayes, *et al.*, 2018.)

D. Quercetin

Quercetin is another natural flavonoid with anti-fat pathway activity. It is abundant in vegetables and fruits and can potentially suppress cancer stem cells and prevent metastases in prostate cancers. In a study, Quercetin significantly suppressed the expression of the ACC enzyme and SBERPs and suppressed the AMPK pathway (the main signaling pathway of lipid/fat synthesis) (Wang, *et al.*, 2021).

Cancers that love to metastasize have overactive MMP enzymes. Both luteolin and quercetin can stop MMP as well as blunt the Akt/mTOR signaling pathways (Wang, *et al.*, 2021; Tsai, *et al.*, 2016).

E. Luteolin (3', 4', 5, 7-Tetrahydroxyflavone)

Luteolin is another natural flavonoid in many herbs, vegetables, and fruits. It fights cancer by arresting the cancer's cell growth cycle and triggering the cell death (apoptosis) pathways. Luteolin can also reverse the EMT and keep cancers within their boundaries, preventing metastases. In glioma (brain cancer), luteolin can increase ROS stress to reach levels lethal to the cancer (Imran, *et al.*, 2019).

F. Pycnogenol

Pycnogenol is an extract of the French maritime pine tree. It is a blend of bioflavonoids, and like Orlistat, it is also an anti-obesity drug; however, it has fewer side effects. It can break down tissue fat stores and prevent fat accumulation by blocking FAS. Pycnogenol can lower total cholesterol and boost HDL (good) cholesterol. It has anticancer benefits because it can block inflammation (Ho, *et al.*, 2014).

G. Apigenin

Apigenin is also found in many plants and herbs and is plentiful in chamomile tea, red wine, grapefruit; parsley, onions, wheat sprouts; tea, and oranges. It can decrease anxiety, but in higher doses, it makes people drowsy. Parsley juice can increase levels of the antioxidant glutathione and superoxide dismutase, which can help protect us against damaging oxidants and prevent cancer. Apigenin can inhibit FASN and decrease *low-density lipoproteins* (LDL) (Shukla & Gupta, 2010). Cervical, colon, blood; prostate, lung, skin; ovarian, thyroid, endometrial; gastric, liver, adrenal, neuroblastoma, and breast cancers all had some benefits from apigenin (Shukla & Gupta, 2010).

H. Epigallocatechin gallate (EGCG)

EGCG, or *green tea extracts*, have polyphenols that can inhibit FASN enzymes, reduce cell signaling, and produce cell death (apoptosis) in breast cancers (Shukla & Gupta, 2010).

I. Kaempferol

Kaempferol is another natural anticancer flavonoid. It is found in kale, beans, spinach, broccoli, coffee and tea. It has multiple other benefits and acts upon multiple pathways. It is an antioxidant that protects our normal cells from free radical damage. Radicals cause cancer! Kaempferol stops VEGF to prevent cancers from growing new blood vessels. It is also anti-inflammatory and anti-cancer and can stop the HIF1, NF-κB, AKT, and insulin pathways, preventing fatty liver. Kaempferol can cause cancer cell death or apoptosis, which is believed to be due to its ability to stop the fat synthesis pathway (Brusselmans, *et al.*, 2005; Chen & Chen, 2012; Liu, *et al.*, 2021).

The following dietary fatty acids may suppress some solid cancers that have overactive fatty acid synthase activity.

A. Omega-3 fatty acid

Omega-3 fatty acids, or *docosahexaenoic acid* (DHA), are found in breast colostrum and seafood. DHA can degrade male hormone receptors (androgen receptors) to delay prostate cancer growth (Hu, *et al.*, 2015). DHA can control gene transcription and promote cell death of human colon cancers grown in the lab (Narayanan, *et al.*, 2001). DHA can also significantly increase BRCA1 proteins in rat mammary tissue, decreasing the risk of tumor formation by 30% ($p=0.007$) (Gao, *et al.*, 2013).

B. Alpha-linolenic acid

Alpha-linolenic acid is a plant-based omega-3 essential fatty acid found in chia, flax, walnut seeds, and hemp.

C. Gamma linolenic acid

Gamma linolenic acid is an omega-6 fatty acid found in trace amounts in nuts, green leafy vegetables, and breast milk. These omega fats can inhibit cancers at higher than naturally occurring body levels by slowing down FASN activity (Menendez, *et al.*, 2005a).

D. SPARC proteins

Secreted acidic proteins rich in cysteine (SPARC) make cancers mobile and prone to spread elsewhere. Eating foods rich in gamma-linolenic acid can also reduce the secretion of SPARC proteins and protect against the spread of cancer (Watkins, *et al.*, 2005).

E. Oleic acid

There is also a benefit in decreasing Her2neu activity in breast cancers (Menendez, *et al.*, 2005b). Oleic acid, found in olive oil, can also decrease Her2neu activity and help make Herceptin therapy more effective (Menendez, *et al.*, 2005d).

F. Resveratrol

Resveratrol is a polyphenol supplement that imitates the benefits of fasting. Both resveratrol and fasting can increase SIRTs (SIRT1, SIRT3, and SIRT5) protein levels, decrease SREBP, and restrict fat synthesis. You can buy resveratrol over-the-counter (Walker, *et al.*, 2010).

G. Curcumin

Curcumin, a yellow-colored polyphenol, is commonly added to food as a seasoning. It is extracted from the rhizome root turmeric and has anti-growth effects on human breast cancer cells. Her2-positive breast cancers are known to have higher levels of FASN activity, which curcumin can block (Younesian, *et al.*, 2017).

Chapter Summary/Key Takeaways:

We learned about fat metabolism and how cancers use fats to their advantage. Since cancers don't directly feed on fats, we should not fear dietary fat. Instead, we should look for ways to attack cancer's faulty fat metabolism from within. How do we do this? By targeting enzymes and pathways related to fat metabolism and aging. Indeed, fatty acid synthesis plays many roles in transforming normal cells into cancers. Fat can be your enemy but also your friend. At the same time, these cancers also continue to feed on glucose. Recognizing this scenario may lead us to develop metabolic-based strategies to improve cancer treatment outcomes.

End Notes

Batchuluun, B., Pinkosky, S.L. & Steinberg, G.R. Lipogenesis inhibitors: therapeutic opportunities and challenges. *Nat Rev Drug Discov.* 21, pp. 283–305 (2022). https://doi.org/10.1038/s41573-021-00367-2.

Brusselmans K, Vrolix R, Verhoeven G, Swinnen JV. Induction of cancer cell apoptosis by flavonoids is associated with their ability to inhibit fatty acid synthase activity. *J Biol Chem.* 2005 Feb 18;280(7): e5636-45. doi: 10.1074/jbc.M408177200. Epub 2004 Nov 8. PMID: 15533929.

Calle, R.A., Amin, N.B., Carvajal-Gonzalez, S. *et al.* ACC inhibitor alone or co-administered with a DGAT2 inhibitor in patients with non-alcoholic fatty liver disease: two parallel, placebo-controlled, randomized phase 2a trials. *Nat Med.* 27, e1836–48 (2021). https://doi.org/10.1038/s41591-021-01489-1.

Chen AY, Chen YC. A review of the dietary flavonoid, kaempferol on human health and cancer chemoprevention. *Food Chem.* 2013 Jun 15;138(4): e2099-107. doi: 10.1016/j.foodchem.2012.11.139. Epub 2012 Dec 28. PMID: 23497863; PMCID: PMC3601579.

Carroll RG, Zasłona Z, Galván-Peña S, Koppe EL, Sévin DC, Angiari S, Triantafilou M, Triantafilou K, Modis LK, O'Neill LA. An unexpected link between fatty acid synthase and cholesterol synthesis in proinflammatory macrophage activation. *J Biol Chem*. 2018 Apr 13;293(15): e5509-21. doi: 10.1074/jbc.RA118.001921. Epub 2018 Feb 20. PMID: 29463677; PMCID: PMC5900750.

Corominas-Faja B, Cuyàs E, Gumuzio J, Bosch-Barrera J, Leis O, Martin ÁG, Menendez JA. Chemical inhibition of acetyl-CoA carboxylase suppresses self-renewal growth of cancer stem cells. *Oncotarget.* 2014. Sep 30;5(18): e8306-16. doi: 10.18632/oncotarget.2059. PMID: 25246709; PMCID: PMC4226684.

Demierre MF, Higgins PD, Gruber SB, Hawk E, Lippman SM. Statins and cancer prevention. *Nat Rev Cancer.* 2005 Dec;5(12): e930-42. doi: 10.1038/nrc1751. PMID: 16341084.

Elibol B, Kilic U, High Levels of SIRT1 Expression as a Protective Mechanism Against Disease-Related Condition Front. *Endocrinol.*, 15 October 2018. Sec. Cellular Endocrinology. https://doi.org/10.3389/fendo.2018.00614.

Flavin R, Peluso S, Nguyen PL, Loda M. Fatty acid synthase as a potential therapeutic target in cancer. *Future Oncol.* 2010 Apr;6(4): e551-62. doi: 10.2217/fon.10.11. PMID: 20373869; PMCID: PMC3197858.

Gao YX, Zhang J, Wang C, Li L, Man Q, Song P, Meng L, Lie O, Frøyland L. The fatty acid composition of colostrum in three geographic regions of China. *Asia Pac J Clin Nutr.* 2013;22(2): pp. 276-82. doi: 10.6133/apjcn.2013.22.2.02. PMID: 23635374.

Girisa S, Saikia Q, Bordoloi D, Banik K, Monisha J, Daimary UD, Verma E, Ahn KS, Kunnumakkara AB. Xanthohumol from Hop: Hope for cancer prevention and treatment. *IUBMB Life*. 2021 Aug;73(8): e1016-44. doi: 10.1002/iub.2522. Epub 2021 Jul 6. PMID: 34170599.

Hegde S, Kaushal N, Ravindra KC, Chiaro C, Hafer KT, Gandhi UH, Thompson JT, van den Heuvel JP, Kennett MJ, Hankey P, Paulson RF, Prabhu KS. Δ12-prostaglandin J3, an omega-3 fatty acid-derived metabolite, selectively ablates leukemia stem cells in mice. *Blood.* 2011 Dec 22;118(26): e6909-19. doi: 10.1182/blood-2010-11-317750. Epub 2011 Oct 3. PMID: 21967980; PMCID: PMC3245211.

Ho JN, Kim OK, Nam DE, Jun W, Lee J. Pycnogenol supplementation promotes lipolysis via activation of cAMP-dependent PKA in ob/ob mice and primary-cultured adipocytes. *J Nutr Sci Vitaminol (Tokyo)*. 2014;60(6): pp. 429-35. doi: 10.3177/jnsv.60.429. PMID: 25866307.

Hu Z, Qi H, Zhang R, Zhang K, Shi Z, Chang Y, Chen L, Esmaeili M, Baniahmad A, Hong W. Docosahexaenoic acid inhibits the growth of hormone-dependent prostate cancer cells by promoting the degradation of the androgen receptor. *Mol Med Rep.* 2015 Sep;12(3): e3769-74. doi: 10.3892/mmr.2015.3813. Epub 2015 May 21. PMID: 25997493.

Huang P, Zhu S, Lu S, Li L, Dai Z, Jin Y. [Cerulenin inhibits growth of human colonic carcinoma in nude mice]. Zhonghua Bing Li Xue Za Zhi. 2000 Dec;29(6): pp. 435-8. Chinese. PMID: 11866947.

Hudgins LC, Hellerstein M, Seidman C, Neese R, Diakun J, Hirsch J. Human fatty acid synthesis is stimulated by a eucaloric low fat, high carbohydrate diet. *J Clin Invest.* 1996 May 1;97(9): e2081-91. doi: 10.1172/JCI118645. PMID: 8621798; PMCID: PMC507283.

Hwang ES, Song SB. Nicotinamide is an inhibitor of SIRT1 in vitro, but can be a stimulator in cells. *Cell Mol Life Sci.* 2017 Sep;74(18): e3347-62. doi: 10.1007/s00018-017-2527-8. Epub 2017 Apr 17. PMID: 28417163.

Nelson Hayes, C., Zhang, P., & Chayama, K. (2018). The role of lipids in hepatocellular carcinoma. *Hepatocellular Carcinoma*, *9*, pp. 95–110. https://doi.org/10.15586/hepatocellular carcinoma.2019.ch5.

Li L, Peng M, Ge C, Yu L, Ma H: (-)-Hydroxycitric Acid Reduced Lipid Droplets Accumulation Via Decreasing Acetyl-Coa Supply and Accelerating Energy Metabolism in Cultured Primary Chicken Hepatocytes. *Cell Physiol Biochem.* 2017;43: e812-31. doi: 10.1159/000481564.

Liu, P., Wu, P., Yang, B., Wang, T., Li, J., Song, X., & Sun, W. (2021). Kaempferol prevents the progression from simple steatosis to non-alcoholic steatohepatitis by inhibiting the NF-κB pathway in oleic acid-induced HepG2 cells and high-fat diet-induced rats. *Journal of Functional Foods*, 85, e104655. https://doaj.org/article/083b809a500946d189cd04c5c4cb1f0c.

Li X, Chen YT, Hu P, Huang WC. Fatostatin displays high antitumor activity in prostate cancer by blocking SREBP-regulated metabolic pathways and androgen receptor signaling. *Mol Cancer Ther.* 2014 Apr;13(4): e855-66. doi: 10.1158/1535-7163.MCT-13-0797. Epub 2014 Feb 3. PMID: 24493696; PMCID: PMC4084917.

Lou H, Li H, Zhang S, Lu H, Chen Q. A Review on Preparation of Betulinic Acid and Its Biological Activities. *Molecules.* 2021 Sep 14;26(18): e5583. doi: 10.3390/molecules26185583. PMID: 34577056; PMCID: PMC8468263.

Omura S. The antibiotic cerulenin, a novel tool for biochemistry as an inhibitor of fatty acid synthesis. *Bacteriol Rev.* 1976 Sep;40(3): e681-97. doi: 10.1128/br.40.3.681-697.1976. PMID: 791237; PMCID: PMC413976.

Menendez JA, Colomer R, Lupu R. Inhibition of fatty acid synthase-dependent neoplastic lipogenesis as the mechanism of gamma-linolenic acid-induced toxicity to tumor cells: an extension to Nwankwo's hypothesis. *Med Hypotheses.* 2005;64(2): pp. 337-41. doi: 10.1016/j.mehy.2004.06.032. PMID: 15607568.

Menendez JA, Lupu R, Colomer R. Exogenous supplementation with omega-3 polyunsaturated fatty acid docosahexaenoic acid (DHA; 22:6n-3) synergistically enhances taxane cytotoxicity and downregulates Her-2/neu (c-erbB-2) oncogene expression in human breast cancer cells. *Eur J Cancer Prev.* 2005 Jun;14(3): pp. 263-70. doi: 10.1097/00008469-200506000-00011. PMID: 15901996.

Menendez JA, Vellon L, Colomer R, Lupu R. Oleic acid, the main monounsaturated fatty acid of olive oil, suppresses Her-2/neu (erbB-2) expression and synergistically enhances the growth inhibitory effects of trastuzumab (Herceptin) in breast cancer cells with Her-2/neu oncogene amplification. *Ann Oncol.* 2005 Mar;16(3): pp. 359-71. doi: 10.1093/annonc/mdi090. Epub 2005 Jan 10. PMID: 15642702.

Menendez JA, Vellon L, Lupu R. Antitumoral actions of the anti-obesity drug orlistat (XenicalTM) in breast cancer cells: blockade of cell cycle progression, promotion of apoptotic cell death and PEA3-mediated transcriptional repression of Her2/neu (erbB-2) oncogene. *Ann Oncol.* 2005 Aug;16(8): e1253-67. doi: 10.1093/annonc/mdi239. Epub 2005 May 3. PMID: 15870086.

Muhammad Imran, Abdur Rauf, Tareq Abu-Izneid, Muhammad Nadeem, Mohammad Ali Shariati, Imtiaz Ali Khan, Ali Imran, Ilkay Erdogan Orhan, Muhammad Rizwan, Muhammad Atif, Tanweer Aslam Gondal, Mohammad S. Mubarak, Luteolin, a flavonoid, as an anticancer agent: A review, *Biomedicine & Pharmacotherapy*, Volume 112, 2019, e108612, ISSN 0753-3322,https://doi.org/10.1016/j.biopha.2019.108612.

Murata S, Yanagisawa K, Fukunaga K, Oda T, Kobayashi A, Sasaki R, Ohkohchi N. Fatty acid synthase inhibitor cerulenin suppresses liver metastasis of colon cancer in mice. 2010 Aug;101(8): e1861-5. doi: 10.1111/j.1349-7006.2010.01596.x. Epub 2010 Apr 21. PMID: 20491775.

Narayanan BA, Narayanan NK, Reddy BS. Docosahexaenoic acid regulated genes and transcription factors inducing apoptosis in human colon cancer cells. *Int J Oncol.* 2001 Dec;19(6): e1255-62. doi: 10.3892/ijo.19.6.1255. PMID: 11713597.

Naini, ArunA, Sasse, F., & Brönstrup, M. (2019). The Intriguing Chemistry and biology of soraphens. *Natural Product Reports*, 36(10), e1394–1411. https://doi.org/10.1039/c9np00008a.

Nishi K, Suzuki K, Sawamoto J, Tokizawa Y, Iwase Y, Yumita N, Ikeda T. Inhibition of Fatty Acid Synthesis Induces Apoptosis of Human Pancreatic Cancer Cells. *Anticancer Res.* 2016 Sep;36(9): e4655-60. doi: 10.21873/anticanres.11016. PMID: 27630308.

Pang LY, Hurst EA, Argyle DJ. Cyclooxygenase-2: A Role in Cancer Stem Cell Survival and Repopulation of Cancer Cells during Therapy. *Stem Cells Int.* 2016;2016: e2048731. doi: 10.1155/2016/2048731. Epub 2016 Nov 1. PMID: 27882058; PMCID: PMC5108861.

Pizer ES, Wood FD, Heine HS, Romantsev FE, Pasternack GR, Kuhajda FP. Inhibition of fatty acid synthesis delays disease progression in a xenograft model of ovarian cancer. *Cancer Res.* 1996 Mar 15;56(6): e1189-93. PMID: 8640795.

Poynter JN, Gruber SB, Higgins PD, Almog R, Bonner JD, Rennert HS, Low M, Greenson JK, Rennert G. Statins and the risk of colorectal cancer. *N Engl J Med.* 2005 May 26;352(21): e2184-92. doi: 10.1056/NEJMoa043792. PMID: 15917383.

Raquel Costa, Ilda Rodrigues, Luísa Guardão, Sílvia Rocha-Rodrigues, Carolina Silva, José Magalhães, Manuel Ferreira-de-Almeida, Rita Negrão, Raquel Soares,Xanthohumol and 8-prenylnaringenin ameliorate diabetic-related metabolic dysfunctions in mice, *The Journal of Nutritional Biochemistry*, Volume 45, 2017, pp. 39-47, ISSN 0955-2863,https://doi.org/10.1016/j.jnutbio.2017.03.006.

Sukjoi W, Ngamkham J, Attwood PV, Jitrapakdee S. Targeting Cancer Metabolism and Current Anti-Cancer Drugs. *Adv Exp Med Biol.* 2021; e1286: pp. 15-48. doi: 10.1007/978-3-030-55035-6_2. PMID: 33725343.

Shukla S, Gupta S. Apigenin: a promising molecule for cancer prevention. *Pharm Res.* 2010 Jun;27(6): e962-78. doi: 10.1007/s11095-010-0089-7. Epub 2010 Mar 20. PMID: 20306120; PMCID: PMC2874462.

Smith BK, Steinberg GR. AMP-activated protein kinase, fatty acid metabolism, and insulin sensitivity. *Curr Opin Clin Nutr Metab Care.* 2017 Jul;20(4): pp. 248-53. doi: 10.1097/MCO.0000000000000380. PMID: 28375880.

Surette ME. The science behind dietary omega-3 fatty acids. *CMAJ*. 2008 Jan 15;178(2): e177-80. doi: 10.1503/cmaj.071356. PMID: 18195292; PMCID: PMC2174995.

Tang JJ, Li JG, Qi W, Qiu WW, Li PS, Li BL, Song BL. Inhibition of SREBP by a small molecule, betulin, improves hyperlipidemia and insulin resistance and reduces atherosclerotic plaques. *Cell Metab.* 2011 Jan 5;13(1): pp. 44-56. doi: 10.1016/j.cmet.2010.12.004. Erratum in: Cell Metab. 2021 Jan 5;33(1):222. PMID: 21195348.

Tanca, A., Abbondio, M., Palomba, A. *et al.* Caloric restriction promotes functional changes involving short-chain fatty acid biosynthesis in the rat gut microbiota. *Sci Rep.* 8, e14778 (2018). https://doi.org/10.1038/s41598-018-33100-y.

Takahashi Y, Konishi T, Yamaki K. Tofu and fish oil independently modulate serum lipid profiles in rats: Analyses of 10 class lipoprotein profiles and the global hepatic transcriptome. *PLoS One.* 2019 Jan 17;14(1): e0210950. doi: 10.1371/journal.pone.0210950. PMID: 30653569; PMCID: PMC6336308.

Thupari JN, Pinn ML, Kuhajda FP. Fatty acid synthase inhibition in human breast cancer cells leads to malonyl-CoA-induced inhibition of fatty acid oxidation and cytotoxicity. *Biochem Biophys Res Commun.* 2001 Jul 13;285(2): pp. 217-23. doi: 10.1006/bbrc.2001.5146. Erratum in: Biochem Biophys Res Commun 2002 Jul 12;295(2): e570. PMID: 11444828.

Tian, Wx., Ma, Xf., Zhang, Sy. *et al.* Fatty acid synthase inhibitors from plants and their potential application in the prevention of metabolic syndrome. *Clin Oncol Cancer Res.* 8, pp. 1–9 (2011). https://doi.org/10.1007/s11805-011-0550-3.

Trub AG, Wagner GR, Anderson KA, Crown SB, Zhang GF, Thompson JW, Ilkayeva OR, Stevens RD, Grimsrud PA, Kulkarni RA, Backos DS, Meier JL, Hirschey MD. Statin therapy inhibits fatty acid synthase via dynamic protein modifications. *Nat Commun.* 2022 May 10;13(1): e2542. doi: 10.1038/s41467-022-30060-w. PMID: 35538051; PMCID: PMC9090928.

Tsai, P. H., Cheng, C. H., Lin, C. Y., Huang, Y. T., Lee, L. T., Kandaswami, C. C., … Lee, M. T. (2016). Dietary flavonoids luteolin and quercetin suppressed cancer stem cell properties and metastatic potential of isolated prostate cancer cells. *Anticancer Research*, 36(12), e6367–80. https://doi.org/10.21873/anticanres.11234.

Wang C, Xu C, Sun M, Luo D, Liao DF, Cao D. Acetyl-CoA carboxylase-alpha inhibitor TOFA induces human cancer cell apoptosis. *Biochem Biophys Res Commun.* 2009 Jul 31; 385(3): pp. 302-6. doi: 10.1016/j.bbrc.2009.05.045. Epub 2009 May 18. PMID: 19450551; PMCID: PMC2724073.

Wang M, Wang B, Wang S, Lu H, Wu H, Ding M, Ying L, Mao Y, Li Y. Effect of Quercetin on Lipids Metabolism Through Modulating the Gut Microbial and AMPK/PPAR Signaling Pathway in Broilers. *Front Cell Dev Biol.* 2021 Feb 9;9: e616219. doi: 10.3389/fcell.2021.616219. PMID: 33634119; PMCID: PMC7900412.

Wang J, Cao Y, Fu S, Li W, Ge Y, Cheng J, Liu J. Niacin inhibits the synthesis of milk fat in BMECs through the GPR109A-mediated downstream signalling pathway. *Life Sci.* 2020 Nov 1;260: e118415. doi: 10.1016/j.lfs.2020.118415. Epub 2020 Sep 9. PMID: 32918974.

Walker AK, Yang F, Jiang K, Ji JY, Watts JL, Purushotham A, Boss O, Hirsch ML, Ribich S, Smith JJ, Israelian K, Westphal CH, Rodgers JT, Shioda T, Elson SL, Mulligan P, Najafi-Shoushtari H, Black JC, Thakur JK, Kadyk LC, Whetstine JR, Mostoslavsky R, Puigserver P, Li X, Dyson NJ, Hart AC, Näär AM. Conserved role of SIRT1 orthologs in fasting-dependent inhibition of the lipid/cholesterol regulator SREBP. *Genes Dev.* 2010 Jul 1;24(13): e1403-17. doi: 10.1101/gad.1901210. PMID: 20595232; PMCID: PMC2895199.

Watkins G, Martin TA, Bryce R, Mansel RE, Jiang WG. Gamma-Linolenic acid regulates the expression and secretion of SPARC in human cancer cells. *Prostaglandins Leukot Essent Fatty Acids*. 2005 Apr;72(4): pp. 273-8. doi: 10.1016/j.plefa.2004.12.004. PMID: 15763439.

Xiong W, Sun KY, Zhu Y, Zhang X, Zhou YH, Zou X. Metformin alleviates inflammation through suppressing FASN-dependent palmitoylation of Akt. *Cell Death Dis.* 2021 Oct 12;12(10): e934. doi: 10.1038/s41419-021-04235-0. PMID: 34642298; PMCID: PMC8511025.

Yang G, Wang Y, Feng J, Liu Y, Wang T, Zhao M, Ye L, Zhang X. Aspirin suppresses the abnormal lipid metabolism in liver cancer cells via disrupting an NFκB-ACSL1 signaling. *Biochem Biophys Res Commun.* 2017 May 6;486(3): e827-32. doi: 10.1016/j.bbrc.2017.03.139. Epub 2017 Mar 27. PMID: 28359761.

Younesian O, Kazerouni F, Dehghan-Nayeri N, Omrani D, Rahimipour A, et al. Effect of Curcumin on Fatty Acid Synthase Expression and Enzyme Activity in Breast Cancer Cell Line SKBR3. *Int J Cancer Manag.* 2017;10(3): e8173. doi: 10.5812/ijcm.8173.

Chapter Sixteen

What About Weight Loss?

Many people feel that weight loss during a cancer diagnosis is bad. I hear many of my patients say, "I can't afford to lose weight."

We should worry about weight loss, especially at the end of life. Weight loss is often seen with terminal cancer. During the last weeks of life, the cancer takes over and takes energy not only from sugar but also from muscles and fat. The terminally ill cancer patient loses muscles from their skull temples, and limbs become thin and spindly as they waste away.

If cancer patients are already overweight, I would <u>not</u> be worried about weight loss. In fact, I encourage it.

The knee-jerk reaction to any weight loss is to load up on carbohydrates. It is as if *any* weight gain will bring back good health.

Weight gain is a sign of health, but that does not mean it is the correct treatment. Unfortunately, if your cancer depends on fat, any weight gain from carbs is likely going to end up as extra fat in the waistline and, worse, fat in the tissues. This is the type of weight gain that we must avoid.

Fixing severe weight loss or *cachexia:*

Sometimes, our goal is <u>not</u> to stop FAS but to preserve it. When patients become very thin due to advanced cancer, their fat and their muscles shrink when death is imminent. During scenarios like this, we need to try to improve muscle mass.

Unfortunately, we don't have any effective drug to treat cancer cachexia. Most of the time, doctors and nutritionists prescribe high-calorie and high-carbohydrate foods to correct weight loss. I have never seen anyone improve their cachexia using this approach!

Terminal cancer patients often have a profound loss of fat and muscle because of elevated inflammation markers such as IL-6 and TNF-α. The ideal way to treat cachexia is to target the underlying cause. In this case, it is inflammation.

NAD+ levels also decline in cancer, and since NAD+ is needed in SIRT proteins, the lifespan shortens with low NAD+. Experiments in lab mice with colon cancer implants showed that *nicotinamide riboside* (NR), or vitamin B3, can slow down fat and muscle loss and reverse cancer-related cachexia (Park, *et al.*, 2021). Since nicotinamide also boosts SIRT1 proteins, there might be potential for prolongation of lifespans. We need more research on whether nicotinamide can help improve cancer-related weight loss (Monfrecola, *et al.*, 2013; Hwang & Song, 2017).

Chapter Summary/Key Takeaways:

Fats are essential to cancers. We learned what they are and how the normal body uses fats. We peeked into how cancers can use *de novo* fat synthesis to their advantage.

We also learned some ways to fight cancer by targeting areas of fat metabolism. Current information on how cancers feed on fat is extensive yet spotty and often misunderstood.

Many areas still need more explanation. How can we truly 'switch off' the 'cancer switch'? It seems there is more than one switch and more than one pathway.

Why can we still not bring fatty acid inhibition strategies to the bedside? Research is badly needed to solidify our knowledge before this can become one of our current standards of care.

The next chapter will discuss *uncoupling proteins* and their importance in explaining the cancer switch.

End Notes

Hwang ES, Song SB. Nicotinamide is an inhibitor of SIRT1 in vitro, but can be a stimulator in cells. *Cell Mol Life Sci.* 2017 Sep;74(18): e3347-62. doi: 10.1007/s00018-017-2527-8. Epub 2017 Apr 17. PMID: 28417163.

Monfrecola G, Gaudiello F, Cirillo T, Fabbrocini G, Balato A, Lembo S. Nicotinamide downregulates gene expression of interleukin-6, interleukin-10, monocyte chemoattractant protein-1, and tumour necrosis factor-α gene expression in HaCaT keratinocytes after ultraviolet B irradiation. *Clin Exp Dermatol.* 2013 Mar;38(2): pp. 185-8. doi: 10.1111/ced.12018. PMID: 23397947.

Park JM, Han YM, Lee HJ, Park YJ, Hahm KB. Nicotinamide Riboside Vitamin B3 Mitigated C26 Adenocarcinoma-Induced Cancer Cachexia. *Front Pharmacol.* 2021 Jun 28;12: e665493. doi: 10.3389/fphar.2021.665493. PMID: 34262449; PMCID: PMC8273280.

Chapter Seventeen

Uncoupling Proteins and Cancer

Uncoupling proteins (UCPs) are attracting attention in medical news as a possible anti-cancer target. There is a potential to fight cancer using food and medications that target UCPs. Research is ongoing, and I do not see a drug commercially available soon. Still, because UCPs maintain a balance of energy within the cell, it has earned a place in this book as a chapter.

UCPs are unique proteins on inner mitochondrial membranes that act like maintenance men. Many different types of UCPs exist, but not all UCPs are cancer-related.

What do uncoupling proteins do?

Let us back up and review what usually happens in the mitochondria: Inside the mitochondria, the energy-making process involves several steps. Electrons made in the Krebs cycle go on to the ETC. The ETC is a string of proteins that sits on the inner mitochondrial membrane. A lot of energy is sitting right here on this chain. To transform into useful energy, a few steps must occur. Hydrogen particles H+ move away from the chain and pass through the inner membrane to enter the middle chamber (sandwiched between the inner and outer membrane). As hydrogen accumulates, the pressure inside the middle chamber rises. Excess hydrogen will return to the inner chamber by squeezing through the mushroom-shaped tunnel called ATP synthase. During that process, ATP energy is made.

Like ATP synthase, UCPs also sit on the mitochondrial membrane. Unlike ATP synthase, UCPs <u>do not</u> produce energy. As hydrogen exits the UCP, we lower the *mitochondrial membrane potential* (difference in electrical charges between inside and outside). When this electrical potential is low, the circuitry also drops. This pause interrupts or 'uncouples' the link between electron transport and ATP synthesis, and, as a result, the cell loses the drive needed to propel energy to OXPHOS. ATP energy production stops (Jacobson, *et al.*, 1985). Figure 12 shows this process (page 267).

How many types of UCPs are there?

There are at least five different types of UCPs. UCP1-5, depending on where they are located. The function may overlap across different UCPs. I'm listing them below to help familiarize you with them.

A. Uncoupling protein 1

UCP1 was the first UCP to be discovered. It is found in the brown fat tissue of both human babies and polar bears. We know that the mitochondria typically make energy through the OXPHOS process. The UCP will disconnect the link to OXPHOS and release heat instead of producing energy. Hibernating animals and polar bears have lots of brown fat and are rich in UCP1. They do not need to shiver to keep warm because the UCPs help cells create heat efficiently. UCP1s are also abundant in human infants. They preserve body heat without shivering, but unfortunately, we lose UCP1s as we age. Our UCP1-rich brown fat uses as much oxygen as the brain yet rarely develops cancer despite being metabolically active (Schrauwen & Hesselink, 2022).

Figure 12

Oxidative Phosphorylation

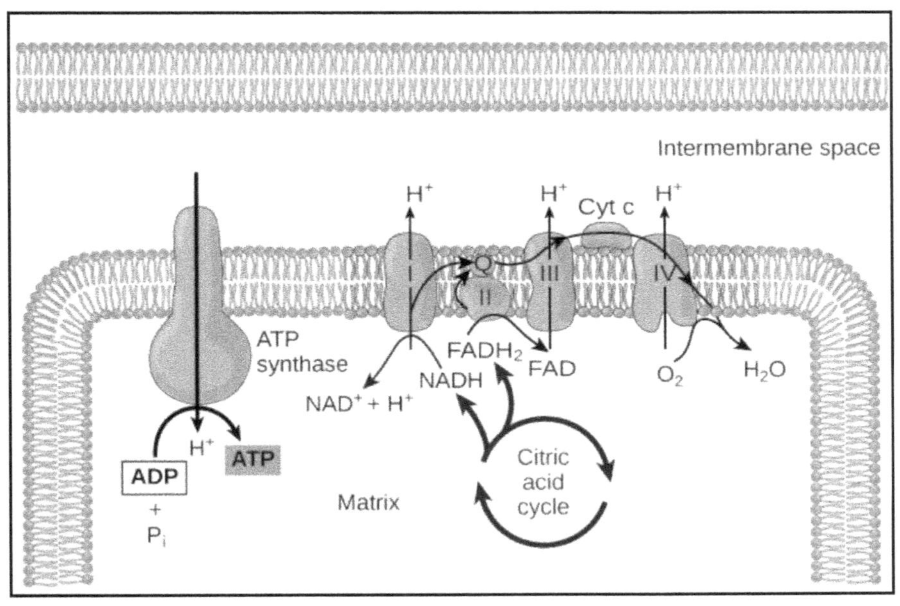

Image modified from "Oxidative phosphorylation: Figure 1" by OpenStax College, Biology (CC BY 3.0). Access for free at https://openstax.org/books/biology/pages/1-introduction

In oxidative phosphorylation, the pH gradient formed by the electron transport chain is used by ATP synthase to form ATP.

B. Uncoupling protein 2

UCP2s are structurally similar to UCP1 and can prevent cancer development by releasing any accumulated oxidative stress pressure, shielding cells from damaging oxygen molecules known as ROS. UCP2 monitors the situation inside the mitochondria and diffuses the build-up of ROS.

Where do ROS come from? Imagine a fireworks display where a few stray sparks land outside the designated area, potentially causing damage. This analogy highlights the localized nature of ROS production and its potential for harm if not controlled. Similarly, you may recall that ATP production typically starts from the Krebs cycle (the Ferris wheel) and then on to the ETC found in the mitochondria. During ATP energy production—ETC, for example—we make oxygen molecules hyperactive and produce ROS. Please review Chapter Two if this is not clear.

When ROS levels rise excessively, mitochondrial UCP2 becomes a portal that allows hydrogen protons to 'leak out' excess metabolic energy and prevent damage. This 'proton leak' will stop the production of ATP energy in the mitochondria and, therefore, stop making ROS.

Like ATP synthase, UCP2 acts like a pressure release valve to allow hydrogen passage, but unlike ATP synthase, UCPs don't make ATP energy.

To simplify this, pretend we make energy with a fancy

energy drink machine. The process is simple. To make a quality energy drink, we need the machine (mitochondria) and the ingredients (Krebs cycle and the ETC). The machine chops the ingredients in one chamber, passes them to a second chamber, and then out to a spout. After a few minutes, we have a nice, nutrient-packed energy drink.

One day, the machine springs a leak, and some liquid from chamber two disappears. The machine keeps running, but because of the leak, the engine does not have enough material; only a little is coming out from the spout (ATP synthase), producing only half the energy drinks as before. The machine starts to heat up because it is running half-empty.

Like the mitochondrion (the machine), we feed it stuff—hydrogen protons constantly move in. When protons start to leak out (uncouple), but the electron transport and ATP synthase machinery keep going, the empty machinery (mitochondria) will soon produce heat instead of energy.

Because it takes "two (machine + ingredients) to tango," the machine gives up because it has lost its partner (the ingredients). Hopefully, the cancer with uncoupled mitochondria will die because it isn't making enough energy.

Remember, to make energy, there must be a big difference in pressures between the inside and outside chambers of the mitochondria. If there is an uncoupling (a leak), the pressure is lost, and we don't make energy.

With insufficient uncoupling, pressure builds up, and oxidative stress accumulates. Extra stress from too many hyperactive oxygen molecules (HBOT), or ROS may lead to damaged mitochondria and, eventually, cancer.

We need more UCPs to lessen some damage by quenching ROS to increase lifespans (Schrauwen & Hesselink, 2022; Deng, *et al.*, 2012). Both UCP1 and 2 have a protective, anti-cancer effect in the early stages of cancer. They protect cells from ROS damage. UCPs activate the process of autophagy (cells' ability to remove damaged parts) by slowing stem cell activity in breast cancers (Yu, *et al.*, 2022).

Many published articles refer to the UCP2 because it is everywhere: muscle, kidney, GI tract, liver, pancreas, spleen, thymus, and brain. Of all the UCPs, UCP2 controls insulin and transforms normal cells into abnormal, glucose-loving cells (Warburg effect). UCP2 can cause a 'proton leak' in the mitochondria. Because fewer protons propel through the ATP synthase protein, OXPHOS becomes inefficient as the cell runs out of ATP energy. The cancerous cell survives by switching to glycolysis. Cancers make plenty of ROS, damaging DNA and promoting tumor growth. UCP2 can protect normal cells by keeping the levels of inflammation low—cell damage increases when we accumulate too much ROS. UCPs come to the rescue to cancel ROS damage. It acts as an antioxidant and protects the cell from ROS damage by lowering the mitochondrial potential (like battery power) and decreasing the proton pressure difference between the inner and outer chambers of the mitochondria. Think of the UCP as an escape valve that releases pressure by causing a leak in the membrane of the mitochondria. The release of stress will tone down the inflammation from the ROS and rescue the cell from further damage.

The benefits of UCP2's are not limited to preventing cancer. They can also prevent heart disease and atherosclerosis (Pierelli, *et al.*, 2017) and delay aging. Low levels of UCP2 predispose aging blood vessels to a higher risk of stroke and heart attacks. UCP2 can communicate with the insulin/IGF aging pathway and affect our risk of developing diabetes (Hirose, *et al.*, 2016).

Drugs such as berberine, fenofibrate, and sitagliptin can boost UCP2 levels, and so do extracts from foods in the cabbage family, mustards, and cruciferous vegetables (e.g., cauliflower, Brussels sprouts, kale, cress, and bok choy) (Robbins & Zhao, 2011).

C. UCP 3, 4 and 5

UCP3 is another protein similar to UCP1 and 2, found in human skeletal muscle and brown fat tissues. UCP3 has a role in transporting fatty acids into the mitochondria and protecting cells against inflammation and stress (Erlanson-Albertsson, 2002; Schrauwen & Hesselink, 2022). UCP3 has anti-cancer activity, too. It acts as a negative feedback sensor. If something is wrong (e.g., UCP3 senses that cancers are developing), UCP3 activates AMPK pathways to block the HIF-1α protein (Schrauwen &

Hesselink, 2022. (Remember, the HIF-1α protein switches on when oxygen is low and wakes cancer signals).

UCP3s can also limit glycolysis, control cell division, and promote fatty acid oxidation (FAO) (breakdown). Ultimately, glycolysis slows, and OXPHOS returns to normal functioning (Samudio, *et al.*, 2009).

UCP4 and 5 are found mainly in the brain. Some UCP5 are in the testes and pituitary. Scientists think they may help protect from inflammation and stress, but their roles could be better defined (Erlanson-Albertsson, 2002; Schrauwen & Hesselink, 2022).

UCPs and cancer: more unanswered questions

Up to this point, UCPs seem to be protective against cancers. We learned that UCPs protect normal cells by stamping out harmful oxidative stress.

Some authors, however, reported conflicting results in the lab. They observed that many aggressive cancers have overexpression of UCP2.

Do the levels of UCP2 matter?

Will too many UCPs cause, rather than prevent, cancer?

Esteves (2015) states, "UCP2 modifies metabolic substrate orientation through modulation of metabolite compartmentalization involved in mitochondrial anaplerotic metabolism" (e975024).

In plain language, when the UCP2 causes a proton leak, it allows some of the key members of the Krebs cycle (e.g. oxaloacetate) to leave the mitochondria. As a result, OXPHOS and ATP production inside the mitochondria slows down, and glycolysis takes over. This is a proposed explanation of how cancers use UCPs to switch to glycolysis (Vozza, *et al.*, 2014).

Uncoupling may boost the enzymes of glycolysis while preventing glucose oxidation. Energy production moves towards glycolysis and away from OXPHOS. Glucose addiction develops, as well as more glutamine and FAS (Pecqueur, *et al.*, 2017).

UCP2s can also block the p53 cell death (apoptosis) pathway, allowing cancers to grow and proliferate (Robbins & Zhao, 2011).

UCP2 influences gene expression of oncogenes and tumor suppressor genes at extremely high levels. In lay terms, UCP2 may awaken our pro-cancer genes and put our tumor suppressor genes to sleep (Robbins & Zhao, 2011).

Is there a way to identify cancers with UCPs?

Esteves (2015) found two forms of UCP2s: Slow, low glycolytic cancers had high UCP2, while aggressive, highly glycolytic cancers had low UCP2 (e975024).

Cancers with <u>high</u> UCP2 mRNA levels:

- lymphomas
- lung
- breast
- colorectal

Cancers with low UCP2 mRNA levels:

- glioblastoma
- melanoma
- prostate
- liver

This observation may underlie some metabolic differences between these two groups. UCP2 involvement in tumorigenesis is cell type-dependent and may depend on the metabolism exhibited by normal cells before their transformation, as reflected by the endogenous protein level of UCP2 (Esteves, *et al.*, 2015).

Kuai (2010) described a relationship between UCP2 levels and tumor aggressiveness. Slow colon cancers had low UCP2, while aggressive, advanced-stage cancers had high UCP2 levels (e5773-8).

The type of cancer also seems to determine whether a tumor has high or low UCP. Colon cancer, breast, lung, neck, skin, pancreas, and prostate have high UCPs (Li, *et al.*, 2013). Other cancers have low levels of UCP2 (i.e., melanoma, glioblastoma, prostate, and liver) (Kuai, *et al.*, 2010).

Robbins (2011), however, noted that a study of colon cancer with high UCP levels also had high levels of oxidant levels; therefore, it was "hard to explain whether it is a cause or effect relationship between uncoupling and oxidative stress" (e5285-93).

UCP3 is implicated in cancer cachexia or muscle wasting due to its effect on fat metabolism (Nubel & Ricquier, 2006).

Can we fight cancer by inducing uncoupling?

1. *Dietary fatty acids* are natural uncouplers. Fatty acids can go to the inner mitochondrial membrane and make it permeable (more leaky). The change in the membrane allows the inner chamber (matrix) to swell up (edema) and rupture the outer membrane to release pro-death proteins (Samartsev, 2000).

2. *High-temperature situations (hyperthermia)*, such as after exercise or saunas, can trigger uncoupling in skeletal muscles. Mitochondrial uncoupling will increase oxidative stress. Could this be useful when the goal is to kill cancers? We do not know much about skeletal muscle UCP3 except that it might affect fat metabolism in some way.

   I must caution against using high temperatures to 'trigger' uncoupling. Scientists tested heart function in mice under conditions of high heat. At 37-40 degrees °F, proton leaks were not seen, but beyond 43 degrees °F, the uncoupling of the heart's mitochondria led to loss of ATP energy and death from heart failure (McAnulty, *et al.*, 2005).

   In addition, caution must be taken to ensure high temperatures do not cause tissue damage. We know that heat can damage tissues, and repeated exposure followed by faulty repair can be carcinogenic (Dewhirst, *et al.*, 2003).

3. *Fasting* can also increase UPC. So does strenuous exercise. We have evidence that fasting and caloric restriction prolong life. Aside from UPC, many other benefits of fasting are probably in motion (Klug, *et al.*, 1984).

4. *Cold stress* can activate uncoupling. The evidence is seen in hibernating squirrels and increased UPC after prolonged cold exposure (Brustovetskyi, *et al.*, 1990).

5. *CoQ10* induces mitochondrial uncoupling and potentially prevents dopamine loss in Parkinsons' disease (Horvath, *et al.*, 2016).

6. *Spices* such as turmeric can increase UCP1 to promote mitochondrial uncoupling, similar to brown fat tissue (Lone, *et al.*, 2016).

7. *Ginger* also has a similar effect. It can 'reprogram' our fat cells to make them release heat and promote weight loss. Again, UPCs are possibly involved (Seo, *et al.*, 2001).

8. *Omega 6 fatty acids* can activate and increase UCP2 through the nuclear receptor PPAR beta pathways. Many processed bakery goods use Omega 6 fats (Chevillotte, *et al.*, 2016).

9. *Genipin* is a UCP2 inhibitor that comes from the *Gardenia jasminoides fruit*. Genipin also has significant antioxidant and anticancer benefits. Chinese herbalists use Genipin to treat inflammation and jaundice and also use it as a food colorant (Kreiter, *et al.*, 2019).

10. *Bo-Mt-Ge* is the fruit extract of Gardenia jasminoides fruit, is a molecule channel blocker that can inhibit UCP2, limit the leaking of protons, and kill cancer stem cells by causing self-destruction or apoptotic cell death (Park, *et al.,* 2023).

Chapter Summary/Key Takeaways:

I gave you a glimpse into the emerging research on uncoupling proteins. Suffice it to say you know that uncoupling (proton leaking) is a natural, protective process. We find uncoupling proteins in our mitochondria, which help release built-up proton pressure to protect cells against stress and prolong lifespans. uncoupling proteins appear to prevent cancers by controlling our insulin-linked pathways and reducing reactive oxygen species stress. There is also conflicting evidence that uncoupling proteins are elevated in many cancers. Though it is tempting to think that UCPs can also encourage cancer growth via metabolic reprogramming, it is possible that these observed uncoupling protein overexpressions might be an after-effect rather than a cause of cancer.

We have very limited knowledge about uncoupling proteins, which I suspect has great potential as a future tool in fighting cancers.

In the next chapter, we will examine cancer stem cells closely.

FAQs

From the Facebook group "Keto For Cancer"

QUESTION:

Are there dangers of high-heat cooking? Is meat cooked on a grill dangerous?

ANSWER:

Foods cooked on a grill can cause carcinogens like heterocyclic amines (HCAs) and polycyclic aromatic hydrocarbons (PAHs) to develop. Marinating the meats for 30 minutes before cooking can help prevent these carcinogens from forming by creating a barrier between the meat and the heat.

End Notes

Brustovetsky NN, Amerkanov ZG, Yegorova ME, Mokhova EN, Skulachev VP. Carboxyatractylate-sensitive uncoupling in liver mitochondria from ground squirrels during hibernation and arousal. *FEBS Lett.* 1990 Oct 15;272(1-2): pp. 190-2. doi: 10.1016/0014-5793(90)80481-w. PMID: 2226831.

Chevillotte E, Rieusset J, Roques M, Desage M, Vidal H. The regulation of uncoupling protein-2 gene expression by omega-6 polyunsaturated fatty acids in human skeletal muscle cells involves multiple pathways, including the nuclear receptor peroxisome proliferator-activated receptor beta. *J Biol Chem.* 2001 Apr 6;276(14): e10853-60. doi: 10.1074/jbc.M008010200. Epub 2001 Jan 12. PMID: 11278377.

Deng S, Yang Y, Han Y, Li X, Wang X, Li X, et al. (2012) UCP2 Inhibits ROS-Mediated Apoptosis in A549 under Hypoxic Conditions. *PLoS ONE.* 7(1): e30714. https://doi.org/10.1371/journal.pone.0030714

Dewhirst MW, Lora-Michiels M, Viglianti BL, Dewey WC, Repacholi M. Carcinogenic effects of hyperthermia. *Int J Hyperthermia.* 2003 May-Jun;19(3): pp. 236-51. doi: 10.1080/0265673031000070811. PMID: 12745970.

Erlanson-Albertsson C. Uncoupling proteins—a new family of proteins with unknown function. *Nutr Neurosci.* 2002 Feb;5(1): pp.1-11. doi: 10.1080/10284150290007038. PMID: 11929192.

Esteves P, Pecqueur C, Alves-Guerra MC. UCP2 induces metabolic reprogramming to inhibit proliferation of cancer cells. *Mol Cell Oncol.* 2014 Dec 1;2(1): e975024. doi: 10.4161/23723556.2014.975024. PMID: 27308391; PMCID: PMC4905249.

Hirose M, Schilf P, Lange F, Mayer J, Reichart G, Maity P, Jöhren O, Schwaninger M, Scharffetter-Kochanek K, Sina C, Sadik CD, Köhling R, Miroux B, Ibrahim SM. Uncoupling protein 2 protects mice from aging. *Mitochondrion.* 2016 Sep;30: pp. 42-50. doi: 10.1016/j.mito.2016.06.004. Epub 2016 Jun 27. PMID: 27364833.

Horvath TL, Diano S, Leranth C, Garcia-Segura LM, Cowley MA, Shanabrough M, Elsworth JD, Sotonyi P, Roth RH, Dietrich EH, *et al.* Coenzyme Q induces nigral mitochondrial uncoupling and prevents dopamine cell loss in a primate model of Parkinson's disease. *Endocrinology.* 2003;144: e2757–60.

Jacobsson, A., Stadler, U., Glotzer, M. A., and Kozak, L. P. (1985). Mitochondrial Uncoupling Protein from Mouse Brown Fat. Molecular Cloning, Genetic Mapping, and mRNA Expression. *J Biol Chem.* 260(30): e16250–54. doi:10.1016/s0021-9258(17)36228-2

Klug GA, Krause J, Ostlund AK, Knoll G, Brdiczka D. Alterations in liver mitochondrial function as a result of fasting and exhaustive exercise. *Biochim Biophys Acta.* 1984 Mar 30;764(3): pp. 272-82. doi: 10.1016/0005-2728(84)90097-5. PMID: 6704385.

Kreiter J, Rupprecht A, Zimmermann L, Moschinger M, Rokitskaya TI, Antonenko YN, Gille L, Fedorova M, Pohl EE. Molecular Mechanisms Responsible for Pharmacological Effects of Genipin on Mitochondrial Proteins. *Biophys J.* 2019 Nov 19;117(10): e1845-57. doi: 10.1016/j.bpj.2019.10.021. Epub 2019 Oct 24. PMID: 31706565; PMCID: PMC7031773.

Kuai XY, Ji ZY, Zhang HJ. Mitochondrial uncoupling protein 2 expression in colon cancer and its clinical significance. *World J Gastroenterol.* 2010 Dec 7;16(45): e5773-8. doi: 10.3748/wjg.v16.i45.5773. PMID: 21128330; PMCID: PMC2997996. Colon cancer can be either with high UCP or low UCP levels.

Li W, Nichols K, Nathan CA, Zhao Y. Mitochondrial uncoupling protein 2 is up-regulated in human head and neck, skin, pancreatic, and prostate tumors. *Cancer Biomark.* 2013;13(5): pp. 377-83. doi: 10.3233/CBM-130369. PMID: 24440978.

Lone J, Choi JH, Kim SW, Yun JW. Curcumin induces brown fat-like phenotype in 3T3-L1 and primary white adipocytes. *J Nutr Biochem.* 2016 Jan;27: pp. 193-202. doi: 10.1016/j.jnutbio.2015.09.006. Epub 2015 Sep 21. PMID: 26456563.

McAnulty SR, McAnulty L, Pascoe DD, Gropper SS, Keith RE, Morrow JD, Gladden LB. Hyperthermia increases exercise-induced oxidative stress. *Int J Sports Med.* 2005 Apr;26(3): pp. 188-92. doi: 10.1055/s-2004-820990. PMID: 15776334.

Nübel T, Ricquier D. Respiration under control of uncoupling proteins: Clinical perspective. *Horm Res.* 2006;65(6): pp. 300-10. doi: 10.1159/000092847. PMID: 16641553.

Park M, Sunwoo K, Kim YJ, Won M, Xu Y, Kim J, Pu Z, Li M, Kim JY, Seo JH, Kim JS. Cutting Off H+ Leaks on the Inner Mitochondrial Membrane: A Proton Modulation Approach to Selectively Eradicate Cancer Stem Cells. *J Am Chem Soc.* 2023 Mar 1;145(8): e4647-58. doi: 10.1021/jacs.2c12587. Epub 2023 Feb 6. PMID: 36745678.

Pecqueur C, Bui T, Gelly C, Hauchard J, Barbot C, Bouillaud F, Ricquier D, Miroux B, Thompson CB. Uncoupling protein-2 controls proliferation by promoting fatty acid oxidation and limiting glycolysis-derived pyruvate utilization. *FASEB J.* 2008 Jan;22(1): pp. 9-18. doi: 10.1096/fj.07-8945com. Epub 2007 Sep 13. PMID: 17855623.

Pierelli G, Stanzione R, Forte M, Migliarino S, Perelli M, Volpe M, Rubattu S. Uncoupling Protein 2: A Key Player and a Potential Therapeutic Target in Vascular Diseases. *Oxid Med Cell Longev.* 2017: e7348372. doi: 10.1155/2017/7348372. Epub 2017 Oct 15. PMID: 29163755; PMCID: PMC5661070.

Robbins D, Zhao Y. New aspects of mitochondrial Uncoupling Proteins (UCPs) and their roles in tumorigenesis. *Int J Mol Sci.* 2011;12(8): e5285-93. doi: 10.3390/ijms12085285. Epub 2011 Aug 17. PMID: 21954358; PMCID: PMC3179165.

Samudio I, Fiegl M, Andreeff M. Mitochondrial uncoupling and the Warburg effect: molecular basis for the reprogramming of cancer cell metabolism. *Cancer Res.* 2009 Mar 15;69(6): e2163-6. doi: 10.1158/0008-5472.CAN-08-3722. Epub 2009 Mar 3. PMID: 19258498; PMCID: PMC3822436.

Samartsev VN. Fatty acids as uncouplers of oxidative phosphorylation. *Biochemistry (Mosc).* 2000 Sep;65(9): e991-1005. PMID: 11042489.

Schrauwen P, Hesselink M. UCP2 and UCP3 in muscle controlling body metabolism. *J Exp Biol.* 2002 Aug;205(Pt 15): e2275-85. doi: 10.1242/jeb.205.15.2275. PMID: 12110661.

Seo SH, Fang F, Kang I. Ginger (Zingiber officinale) Attenuates Obesity and Adipose Tissue Remodeling in High-Fat Diet-Fed C57BL/6 Mice. *Int J Environ Res Public Health.* 2021 Jan 13;18(2): e631. doi: 10.3390/ijerph18020631. PMID: 33451038; PMCID: PMC7828532.

Vozza A, Parisi G, De Leonardis F, Lasorsa FM, Castegna A, Amorese D, Marmo R, Calcagnile VM, Palmieri L, Ricquier D, Paradies E, Scarcia P, Palmieri F, Bouillaud F, Fiermonte G. UCP2 transports C4 metabolites out of mitochondria, regulating glucose and glutamine oxidation. *Proc Natl Acad Sci USA*. 2014 Jan 21;111(3): e960-5. doi: 10.1073/pnas.1317400111. Epub 2014 Jan 6. PMID: 24395786; PMCID: PMC3903233.

Yu X, Shi M, Wu Q, Wei W, Sun S and Zhu S (2022) Identification of UCP1 and UCP2 as Potential Prognostic Markers in Breast Cancer: A Study Based on Immunohistochemical Analysis and Bioinformatics. *Front Cell Dev Biol.* 10:891731. doi: 10.3389/fcell.2022.891731

Chapter Eighteen

Cancer Stem Cell Theory

Emerging evidence shows that there are also *cancer stem cells* (CSCs) when normal cells transform into cancer. CSCs are very early versions of the cancer cell, and we can identify them by their surface markers, such as CD44, CD90, and CD133.

Genetic mutations wake up CSCs, dividing and entering established tumors. The resulting cancer will contain some stem cells mixed with mature cancer cells (Ning, *et al.*, 2016). This coexistence of CSCs with more mature cancer cells may partly explain why we relapse after aggressive chemotherapy. Some leftover stem cells may survive chemotherapy or radiation and return to life after treatment ends.

How to fight cancer stem cells:

Radiation treats early-stage cancers, hopefully to cure. We add chemotherapy to help 'mop up' any remaining cancer cells that survived the radiation. Many original cancer cells die, but a small portion will survive radiation and mutate into a more resistant form. These mutated cells are often CSCs (Li, *et al.*, 2016).

Glioma (brain cancer), for example, is known to be treatment-resistant. Gliomas contain mature cancer cells and *glioma stem cells* (GSCs). Compared to mature glioma cells, the stem cells are less active. They use less glucose, make less lactate, and are less acidic than mature glioma cells. GSCs also store higher ATP energy levels and are more likely to survive radiation therapy.

Higher ATP energy levels mean a higher mitochondrial reserve and intact oxidation. Therefore, attempting to block glucose (glycolysis) in glioma may also be futile because these GSCs have the backup energy from intact mitochondria (Vlashi & Pajonk, 2015; Vlashi, *et al.*, 2011).

How, then, can we fight stem cells?

Repurposing non-chemotherapy drugs:

The following information reflects areas of research.

1. *Antibiotics* inhibit stem cells' OXPHOS. Small-cell lung cancer is challenging to treat and often relapses after chemotherapy or radiation. Small-cell lung CSCs produce less lactic acid than non-stem cancer cells. Like gliomas, their CSCs prefer to make more ATP energy through mitochondrial substrate-level phosphorylation (mitochondrial OXPHOS) instead of glucose (glycolysis). As a result, limiting glucose isn't as effective as targeting

the mitochondrial OXPHOS directly.

2. *Oligomycin* is an antibiotic that can block OXPHOS in small-cell CSCs (Gao, *et al.*, 2016). Oligomycin, however, is only available for laboratory use.

3. *Doxycycline,* another antibiotic, may suppress small-cell lung CSCs from multiplying and prevent invasiveness. In the lab, doxycycline had enough anti-mitochondrial activity to eradicate CSCs in six cancer cell lines: breast, ovarian, lung, melanoma, prostate, and pancreatic cancers (Lamb, *et al.*, 2015). Unlike oligomycin, doxycycline is available to consumers but needs a prescription if you live in the United States (Wang, *et al.*, 2016).

4. *Pantoprazole,* an over-the-counter stomach acid reducer, can inhibit gastric (stomach) CSCs by blocking the *EMT/β-catenin* pathway (Feng, *et al.*, 2016). Exercise caution if one is also on immunotherapy (i.e., immune checkpoint inhibitors such as *nivolumab* and *pembrolizumab*). Some studies show that using proton pump inhibitor acid reducers can lead to significantly worse survival (Lopes, *et al.*, 2023).

5. *EGFR inhibitors* are special chemotherapy drugs added to *5-fluorouracil* (5-FU) chemotherapy, which can be a very effective combination instead of 5FU alone. The combination can promote cancer cell self-destruction (autophagy) and spontaneous stem cell death (apoptosis)

(Feng, *et al.*, 2016). We are already practicing this in the clinic. The combination of 5FU plus *cetuximab* is widely used for treating colorectal cancer.

Using 'nanomedicine versions' of drugs can help improve penetrance into CSCs to improve efficacy.

When combined with *Docetaxel chemotherapy*, sulforaphane-loaded (sulforaphane is a substance seen in broccoli) nanoparticles can effectively target differentiated breast cancer and stem-cell-like breast cancer cells in *in vivo* experiments (Burnett, *et al.*, 2017).

6. *Metformin and Curcumin:* The anti-diabetic drug *metformin* and the culinary spice *curcumin* can prevent CSC conversion in oral cancer mouse models and pancreatic cancer cell lines (Siddappa, *et al.*, 2017; Ning, *et al.*, 2016).

7. *Extra virgin olive oil (EVOO).* CSC can help cancers metastasize by 'softening' the EMT zone. EVOO can nutritionally stop cancer stem cells and prevent EMT changes. EVOO contains *decarboxymethyl oleuropein aglycone* (DOA), which can bind to mTOR's ATP binding domains and to the *S-adenosyl-l-methionine* (SAM) co-factor binding pocket, which affects *methylation* of *DNA methyltransferase* (DNMT3A). Since EVOO contains DOA, this is a potential, naturally occurring, dual mTOR/DNMT inhibitor that could synergize with the effects of targeted therapies such as *everolimus* (mTOR inhibitors) and *azacytidine* (DNA methyltransferase inhibitor) (Corominas-Faja, *et al.*, 2018).

Chapter Summary/Key Takeaways:

The environment surrounding the cancer is just as important as fighting the cancer itself. Mutations—stem cell transformation—and changes in the epithelial-mesenchymal transition zones help cancers resist treatment and increase relapse.

We explored several areas of promising treatment options that need attention in future cancer research (Ning, *et al.*, 2016).

You now have a good background of knowledge on how cancer metabolism works. The next half of this book deals with the ketogenic diet, its history, variations, and potential uses in clinical medicine.

End Notes

Burnett JP, Lim G, Li Y, Shah RB, Lim R, Paholak HJ, McDermott SP, Sun L, Tsume Y, Bai S, Wicha MS, Sun D, Zhang T. Sulforaphane enhances the anticancer activity of taxanes against triple negative breast cancer by killing cancer stem cells. *Cancer Lett.* 2017 May 28;394: pp. 52-64. doi: 10.1016/j.canlet.2017.02.023. Epub 2017 Feb 27. PMID: 28254410; PMCID: PMC8892390.

Corominas-Faja B, Cuyàs E, Lozano-Sánchez J, Cufí S, Verdura S, Fernández-Arroyo S, Borrás-Linares I, Martin-Castillo B, Martin ÁG, Lupu R, Nonell-Canals A, Sanchez-Martinez M, Micol V, Joven J, Segura-Carretero A, Menendez JA. Extra-virgin olive oil contains a metabolo-epigenetic inhibitor of cancer stem cells. *Carcinogenesis.* 2018 Apr 5;39(4): e601-13. doi: 10.1093/carcin/bgy023. PMID: 29452350; PMCID: PMC5888987.

Feng S, Zheng Z, Feng L, Yang L, Chen Z, Lin Y, Gao Y, Chen Y. Proton pump inhibitor pantoprazole inhibits the proliferation, self-renewal and chemoresistance of gastric cancer stem cells via the EMT/β-catenin pathways. *Oncol Rep.* 2016 Dec;36(6): e3207-14. doi: 10.3892/or.2016.5154. Epub 2016 Oct 7. PMID: 27748935.

Feng Y, Gao S, Gao Y, Wang X, Chen Z. Anti-EGFR antibody sensitizes colorectal cancer stem-like cells to Fluorouracil-induced apoptosis by affecting autophagy. *Oncotarget.* 2016 Dec 6;7(49): e81402-9. doi: 10.18632/oncotarget.13233. PMID: 27833077; PMCID: PMC5348401.

Gao C, Shen Y, Jin F, Miao Y, Qiu X. Cancer Stem Cells in Small Cell Lung Cancer Cell Line H446: Higher Dependency on Oxidative Phosphorylation and Mitochondrial Substrate-Level Phosphorylation than Non-Stem Cancer Cells. *PLoS One.* 2016 May 11;11(5): e0154576. doi: 10.1371/journal.pone.0154576. PMID: 27167619; PMCID: PMC4863974.

Ning X, Du Y, Ben Q, Huang L, He X, Gong Y, Gao J, Wu H, Man X, Jin J, Xu M, Li Z. Bulk pancreatic cancer cells can convert into cancer stem cells (CSCs) in vitro and 2 compounds can target these CSCs. *Cell Cycle.* 2016;15(3): pp. 403-12. doi: 10.1080/15384101.2015.1127471. PMID: 26709750; PMCID: PMC4943690.

Lamb R, Ozsvari B, Lisanti CL, Tanowitz HB, Howell A, Martinez-Outschoorn UE, Sotgia F, Lisanti MP. Antibiotics that target mitochondria effectively eradicate cancer stem cells, across multiple tumor types: treating cancer like an infectious disease. *Oncotarget.* 2015 Mar 10;6(7): e4569-84. doi: 10.18632/oncotarget.3174. PMID: 25625193; PMCID: PMC4467100.

Li F, Zhou K, Gao L, Zhang B, Li W, Yan W, Song X, Yu H, Wang S, Yu N, Jiang Q. Radiation induces the generation of cancer stem cells: A novel mechanism for cancer radioresistance. *Oncol Lett.* 2016 Nov;12(5): e3059-65. doi: 10.3892/ol.2016.5124. Epub 2016 Sep 12. PMID: 27899964; PMCID: PMC5103903.

Lopes S, Pabst L, Dory A, Klotz M, Gourieux B, Michel B, Mascaux C. Do proton pump inhibitors alter the response to immune checkpoint inhibitors in cancer patients? A meta-analysis. *Front Immunol.* 2023 Jan 26;14: e1070076. doi: 10.3389/fimmu.2023.1070076. PMID: 36776847; PMCID: PMC9910608.

Ning X, Du Y, Ben Q, Huang L, He X, Gong Y, Gao J, Wu H, Man X, Jin J, Xu M, Li Z. Bulk pancreatic cancer cells can convert into cancer stem cells(CSCs) in vitro and 2 compounds can target these CSCs. *Cell Cycle.* 2016;15(3): pp. 403-12. doi: 10.1080/15384101.2015.1127471. PMID: 26709750; PMCID: PMC4943690.

Siddappa G, Kulsum S, Ravindra DR, Kumar VV, Raju N, Raghavan N, Sudheendra HV, Sharma A, Sunny SP, Jacob T, Kuruvilla BT, Benny M, Antony B, Seshadri M, Lakshminarayan P, Hicks W Jr, Suresh A, Kuriakose MA. Curcumin and metformin-mediated chemoprevention of oral cancer is associated with inhibition of cancer stem cells. *Mol Carcinog.* 2017 Nov;56(11): e2446-60. doi: 10.1002/mc.22692. Epub 2017 Jul 13. PMID: 28618017.

Vlashi E, Lagadec C, Vergnes L, Matsutani T, Masui K, Poulou M, Popescu R, Della Donna L, Evers P, Dekmezian C, Reue K, Christofk H, Mischel PS, Pajonk F. Metabolic state of glioma stem cells and nontumorigenic cells. *Proc Natl Acad Sci USA.* 2011 Sep 20;108(38): e16062-7. doi: 10.1073pnas.1106704108. Epub 2011 Sep 7. PMID: 21900605; PMCID: PMC3179043.

Vlashi E, Pajonk F. The metabolic state of cancer stem cells-a valid target for cancer therapy? *Free Radic Biol Med.* 2015 Feb;79: pp. 264-8. doi: 10.1016/j.freeradbiomed.2014.10.732. Epub 2014 Nov 10. PMID: 25450330; PMCID: PMC4339632.

Wang SQ, Zhao BX, Liu Y, Wang YT, Liang QY, Cai Y, Zhang YQ, Yang JH, Song ZH, Li GF. New application of an old drug: Antitumor activity and mechanisms of doxycycline in small cell lung cancer. *Int J Oncol.* 2016 Apr;48(4): e1353-60. doi: 10.3892/ijo.2016.3375. Epub 2016 Feb 4. PMID: 26846275.

PART II:

The Ketogenic Diet

Chapter Nineteen

The History of the Ketogenic Diet

With contributions by Apurva Pandey, M.D.

Fasting and diet were used as early as 500 BC to treat various diseases, including seizures (Wheless, 2008). In the Hippocratic collections of ancient Greece, fasting is mentioned as a therapy for epileptic seizures (Adams, 1849). Another influential figure in medicine, Galen (129-216 AD), built upon Hippocrates' theories and continued to treat seizures with fasting (Galen, *et al.*, 1976).

In 1911, Guelpa and Marie reported fasting as a treatment for French epileptic patients (Höhn, *et al.,* 2019). In 1921, Dr. R.M. Wilder, a doctor from the Mayo Clinic in Minnesota, coined the term ketogenic diet (KD) (p. 307). It describes a diet that produces elevated levels of ketones in the blood, an alternative treatment that mimics the biochemical and metabolic changes (i.e., ketosis, acidosis, and dehydration) seen during fasting (Wilder, 1921).

The KD limits dietary carbohydrates and increases the amount of dietary fats.

The first use of the KD was for seizures (epilepsy). Dr. M.G. Peterman (1925) at the Mayo Clinic studied seizure patients and found that the KD improved their control of seizures and the ability to recognize things by over 50% (e1979-83).

He built the diet to consist of 1 gram of protein per kilogram of body weight in children and 10-15 grams of carbohydrates daily, with the rest to be filled in with fat. The KD became an effective seizure treatment and appeared in many pediatric epilepsy textbooks.

In 1938, Merritt and Putnam discovered the anti-seizure drug *diphenylhydantoin* (Dilantin), and soon after that, similar drugs became commonly used (Wheless, 2008). The KD lost popularity, and scientific publications between 1970 and 2000 numbered less than ten. This dismal trend continued until 1994, when it became popular, with a rising number of studies published until 2017 (Wheless, 2008; Sinha & Kossoff, 2005).

In the early 1990s, public and media interest in the KD grew as news emerged on Charlie, a 2-year-old boy with difficult-to-treat seizures. Charlie became seizure-free while on the KD. His father formed the Charlie Foundation to promote awareness of the KD's role in epilepsy control (Freeman & Kossoff, 2010). Although not as popular as before, the KD remains quite effective in managing seizures that have not responded to medications.

From the 1970s to now, the KD has also become famous for

weight loss. In 1972, the Atkins diet was in vogue (Atkins, 1972). Although the Atkins diet follows a low carbohydrate approach, it does not limit or track protein or fats consumed.

Ketogenic diets: an overview

The standard American diet has a ratio of fat to carbohydrate of 0.3:1 (Kao, 2017). In contrast, a KD is high in fat, low in carbohydrates, and moderate in protein. This combination favors mitochondrial respiration over glycolysis for energy (Saks, *et. al.*, 2009; Branco, *et. al.*, 2016).

The KD mimics starvation. When glucose is low, the liver breaks down fats to make ketones, providing calories for energy and growth. KDs vary in composition, as carbohydrate intakes can be as low as 4%, while other KDs go up to 40%, or roughly < 20g to 50 grams a day (Yancy, *et. al.*, 2005; Saks, *et. al.*, 2009; Holloway, *et. al.*, 2011; Paoli, *et. al.*, 2011), with fats making up 60-70% and protein ~20%.

During adequate carbohydrate intake, acetoacetate levels are negligible (Paoli, *et al.*, 2011). During fasting or starvation, we make ketone bodies—such as acetoacetate and *β-hydroxybutyrate*—and send them into the blood to vital organs such as the brain and nervous system. The mitochondria change ketones into energy for cells to use. Acetone, the third ketone body, is made from the decarboxylation of acetoacetate. Acetone is then passed out in our breath and urine.

Modified KDs use ratios of 3:1, 2:1, or 1:1, depending on the desired level of ketosis and protein requirement. The classical KD underwent modifications to reduce restrictions and improve palatability and compliance. We now have the modified Atkins diet, the low glycemic, and the MCT diet.

Metabolically, when glucose is low, oxaloacetate (Krebs cycle acid) leaves the citric acid cycle (Krebs) towards gluconeogenesis to maintain glucose levels. Instead of sending the acetyl-CoA (produced from fatty acid metabolism) to be metabolized in the Krebs cycle, this is used to make ketone bodies, which then cross the blood-brain barrier to be used instead of glucose for energy. See Figure 13.

Figure 13 (for reference only; identical to Figure 1):

Krebs Cycle

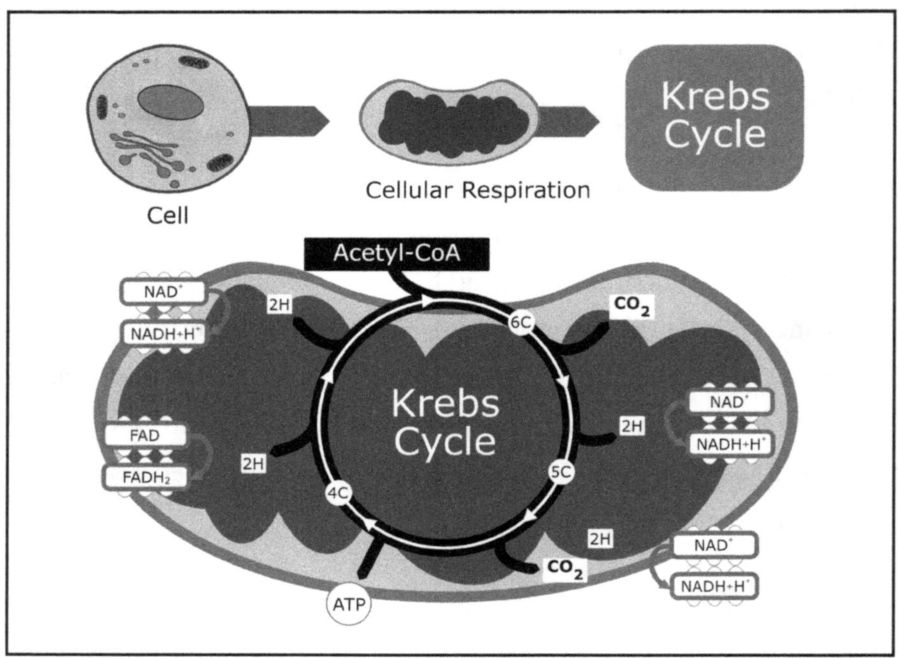

What are the common side effects?

Reported side effects of KDs in epileptic children included constipation, high cholesterol, drowsiness, low protein in the blood, excess uric acid and gout, kidney stones, and vitamin and mineral deficiency. Serious side effects such as respiratory failure and pancreatitis were seen in 0.5% or less. Over 50% discontinued the diet due to a lack of early results rather than side effects (Cai, *et al.*, 2017).

Common challenges for the beginner:

There are many perceived challenges with a KD. The basic KD is not tasty and is hard to follow in the long term. It requires close monitoring of kidney function and electrolytes (Cai, *et al.*, 2017). Patients with diabetes may suffer severe *hypoglycemia* (low blood sugar) while on the diet. However, when the KD is done correctly, reaching ketosis should be easy, and this would fuel the glucose-deprived brain. See this book's Appendices for the acceptable and unacceptable foods while on Keto, and a sample diet.

When do we NOT advise the ketogenic diet?

This diet is not advised for patients with liver failure, pancreatitis, disorders of fat metabolism, and deficiencies in the following: primary carnitine, carnitine palmitoyl transferase, carnitine translocase, porphyria or pyruvate kinase.

Emerging human safety trials suggest it is safe, but trace element deficiency is a significant problem for those who diet beyond three months (Tan-Shalaby, *et al.*, 2016). Intake of a multivitamin could make up for any subclinical deficiencies (Cai, *et al.*, 2017; Bergqvist, *et al.*, 2003). Side effects are covered in more detail in Chapter 7.

Chapter Summary/Key Takeaways:

We reviewed the beginnings of the classical ketogenic diet and how it evolved through the years.

We have an idea of what makes a diet ketogenic and reviewed some common side effects that have been seen in the past.

Remember that the ketogenic diet was the 'classical' form in the past. Many versions have evolved after that, as you will soon see in the next chapter.

End Notes

Adams F. (1849). On Regimen in Acute Diseases. *The Genuine Works of Hippocrates: Translated from the Greek with a preliminary discourse and annotations* (Vol. 1). The Sydenham Society.

Branco AF, Ferreira A, Simões RF, Magalhães-Novais S, Zehowski C, Cope E, Silva AM, Pereira D, Sardão VA, Cunha-Oliveira T. Ketogenic diets: from cancer to mitochondrial diseases and beyond. *Eur J Clin Invest.* 2016 Mar;46(3): pp. 285-98. doi: 10.1111/eci.12591. PMID: 26782788.

Bergqvist AG, Chee CM, Lutchka L, Rychik J, Stallings VA. Selenium deficiency associated with cardiomyopathy: a complication of the ketogenic diet. *Epilepsia.* 2003 Apr;44(4): e618-20. doi: 10.1046/j.1528-1157.2003.26102.x. PMID: 12681013.

Cai QY, Zhou ZJ, Luo R, Gan J, Li SP, Mu DZ, Wan CM. Safety and tolerability of the ketogenic diet used for the treatment of refractory childhood epilepsy: a systematic review of published prospective studies. *World J Pediatr.* 2017 Dec;13(6): pp. 528-36. doi: 10.1007/s12519-017-0053-2. Epub 2017 Jul 12. PMID: 28702868.

Freeman JM, Kossoff EH. Ketosis and the ketogenic diet, 2010: advances in treating epilepsy and other disorders. *Adv Pediatr.* 2010;57(1): pp. 315-29. doi: 10.1016/j.yapd.2010.08.003. PMID: 21056745.

Galen, C., Green, J. S., & Brock, A. J. (1976). Book 3, Chapter 10. In *On The Natural Faculties.* Leiden, Netherlands: Brill Academic Publishers.

Holloway CJ, Cochlin LE, Emmanuel Y, Murray A, Codreanu I, Edwards LM, Szmigielski C, Tyler DJ, Knight NS, Saxby BK, Lambert B, Thompson C, Neubauer S, Clarke K. A high-fat diet impairs cardiac high-energy phosphate metabolism and cognitive function in healthy human subjects. *Am J Clin Nutr.* 2011 Apr;93(4): e748-55. doi: 10.3945/ajcn.110.002758. Epub 2011 Jan 26. PMID: 21270386.

Höhn, S., Dozières-Puyravel, B., & Auvin, S. (2019). History of dietary treatment: Guelpa & Marie First Report of intermittent fasting for epilepsy in 1911. *Epilepsy & amp; Behavior*, 94, pp. 277–80. https://doi.org/10.1016/j.yebeh.2019.03.018

Kao, A., The Ketogenic Diet: Overcoming Challenges for Optimal Utilization in Epilepsy Treatment. *Practical Neurology*, 2017: pp. 29-31.

Paoli A, Rubini A, Volek JS, Grimaldi KA. Beyond weight loss: a review of the therapeutic uses of very-low-carbohydrate (ketogenic) diets. *Eur J Clin Nutr.* 2013 Aug;67(8): e789-96. doi: 10.1038/ejcn.2013.116. Epub 2013 Jun 26. Erratum in: *Eur J Clin Nutr.* 2014 May;68(5): e641. PMID: 23801097; PMCID: PMC3826507.

Peterman, MG., The Ketogenic Diet in Epilepsy. *JAMA,* 1925. 84(26): e979-83. doi:10.1001/jama.1925.02660520007003.

Atkins RC,, *Dr. Atkins' Diet Revolution: The High Calorie Way to Stay Thin Forever.* D McKay Co, New York, NY USA, 1972.

Sacks FM, Bray GA, Carey VJ, Smith SR, Ryan DH, Anton SD, McManus K, Champagne CM, Bishop LM, Laranjo N, Leboff MS, Rood JC, de Jonge L, Greenway FL, Loria CM, Obarzanek E, Williamson DA. Comparison of weight-loss diets with different compositions of fat, protein, and carbohydrates. *N Engl J Med.* 2009 Feb 26;360(9): e859-73. doi: 10.1056/NEJMoa0804748. PMID: 19246357; PMCID: PMC2763382.

Sinha SR, Kossoff EH. The ketogenic diet. *Neurologist.* 2005 May;11(3): pp. 161-70. doi:10.1097/01.nrl.0000160818.58821.d2. PMID:15860138.

Tan-Shalaby JL, Carrick J, Edinger K, Genovese D, Liman AD, Passero VA, Shah RB. Modified Atkins diet in advanced malignancies - final results of a safety and feasibility trial within the Veterans Affairs Pittsburgh Healthcare System. Nutr Metab (Lond). 2016 Aug 12;13:52. doi: 10.1186/s12986-016-0113-y. Erratum in: *Nutr Metab (Lond).* 2016;13(1): p. 61. PMID: 27525031; PMCID: PMC4983076.

Wheless JW. History of the ketogenic diet. *Epilepsia.* 2008 Nov;49 Suppl 8: pp. 3-5. doi: 10.1111/j.1528-1167.2008.01821.x. PMID: 19049574.

Wilder, R.J. The effects of ketonemia on the course of epilepsy. *Mayo Clinic Proceedings,* 2, pp. 307-308.

Yancy WS Jr, Foy M, Chalecki AM, Vernon MC, Westman EC. A low-carbohydrate, ketogenic diet to treat type 2 diabetes. *Nutr Metab (Lond).* 2005 Dec 1;2: p. 34. doi: 10.1186/1743-7075-2-34. PMID: 16318637; PMCID: PMC1325029.

Chapter Twenty

Beyond the Ketogenic Diet: Variations of the Diet

The classical ketogenic diet:

The classical diet began with a period of fasting followed by limited fluids and calories and strict ketone monitoring (Wirrell, 2008). Later data shows that children can reach ketosis without an initial fast (Wirrell, *et al.*, 2002; Miranda, *et al.*, 2012). A classical ketogenic diet (KD) can be divided into approximately 55% to 60% fat, 30% to 35% protein, and 5% to 10% carbohydrates. A typical KD comprises a macronutrient ratio of 4:1 (4g of fat to every 1g of protein, plus carbohydrates combined). Instead of carbohydrates, the primary source of calories shifts to fat. The diet is adjusted to maintain urinary ketones in the moderate to high range (80-160 mg/dl). Higher ratios (4:1) were felt to be less palatable (tasty). Lower proportions of 3:1, 2:1, or 1:1 are allowed based on individual and gastrointestinal tolerability, level of ketosis, and protein requirements (Wirrell, 2008).

The Mayo Clinic's KD has 1g/kg protein, 10 to 15g/day of carbohydrates, and the rest of the calories are fat. The carbohydrate content of medications also must be included. The ratio of weighed fat to non-fat (protein plus carbohydrates) ranges from 2:1 to 4:1. The higher the ratio, the more restrictive the KD is. This is the *long-chain triglyceride* (LCT) based diet (Wirrell, 2008).

Sticking to the strict KD can be a problem. Palatability issues and poor compliance are common. Cancer patients with significant weight loss might not benefit. With that, several alternatives come to mind.

Ketogenic diet alternatives:

Over the years, many variations of a KD have evolved. Confusion remains regarding suitable alternatives to the KD. From my clinical experience, several patients could not follow a strict KD or reach ketosis. They modified their diet, lost some unwanted weight, and felt good. Despite the absence of significant ketosis, they did better than I expected.

Try to learn as much as you can, then follow what you are best able to do.

The following is an overview. Among the existing liberal alternatives, there are:

- The medium-chain triglyceride-Ketogenic diet (MCT-KD).
- The modified Atkins diet (MAD).
- The low-glycemic index treatment (LGIT).

In treating refractory epilepsy, the efficacy of these alternative diets appears to be close to that of the classical KD (Miranda, *et al.*, 2012).

Medium-chain triglyceride (MCT) ketogenic diet:

The *medium-chain triglyceride* (MCT) diet was created in 1971 by Dr. Peter Huttenlocher at the University of Chicago (e1097-103). Medium-chain diets avoid the restrictions seen in the long-chain type. The MCT diet does not use ratios but instead uses a percentage of calories from MCT oils to get into ketosis. It bypasses the biochemical step where long-chain oils must be broken down into medium-chain fats. The long way uses LCTs mixed into chylomicrons (fat droplets) and transferred to the thoracic (chest) duct. They pass into blood mitochondria and enter the beta-oxidation (fat breakdown) process.

Triglycerides are 'three fats.' The MCT diet is a hack. Coconut oil, for example, is already medium in length. Choosing MCTs instead of LCTs uses less energy and is more efficient. MCTs are, therefore, more ketogenic.

Unlike LCTs (=/> 14 carbons), the gut absorbs MCTs (6-12 carbon atoms) more efficiently, and MCTs travel quickly to the liver. The liver is where medium-chain fatty acids beta-oxidize (break down), turn into acetyl-CoA, and become ketones, which are released into the blood. Because ketones quickly form from MCT, this diet is less restrictive, tastier, and allows more protein and carbohydrates. However, it causes diarrhea. Even so, this might be useful in patients who develop constipation with the classic KD.

Modified Atkins Diet (MAD):

The Modified Atkins Diet was created as a less restrictive diet at the Johns Hopkins Hospital. Protein and calories are unlimited. It begins by taking the standard Atkins diet and using it as an induction (introductory) phase. This phase lasts one month, and carbohydrates are restricted to 10-15 grams daily to expect ketosis. After the induction phase, carbohydrates are increased to 20 to 30 grams daily. Food does not need to be weighed, but carbohydrates do have to be counted. Everything is done as an outpatient. The ratio is 0.9:1 (fat: carbohydrate plus protein).

Low-glycemic index (low-GI) diet:

A fourth type is the low-GI diet, which is the least restrictive. Food does not need to be measured, and induction does not require hospitalization. It is done at the outpatient level. Total carbohydrate limits range from 40 to 60 grams per day. Fat is 60% calories, while 20-30% is protein and carbohydrates. It allows moderate carbohydrate intake with a glycemic index < 50, but this diet will not increase ketone levels.

How to control diarrhea from MCT oil:

Diarrhea can be lessened by adjusting the fat: protein + carbohydrate ratio. Lower ratios of 3:1, 2:1, or 1:1 can be used and titrated to individual tolerability, level of ketosis, and protein requirements (Wirrell, 2008).

Cutting the MCT doses to smaller portions and limiting total quantities to no more than 50-100 grams daily can control symptoms. Each tablespoon contains around 14 grams of fat. A maximum daily limit of seven tablespoons, divided into the number of meals, could be one strategy to lessen diarrhea.

Emulsification of the MCT is done by adding oil to a non-oily liquid, then shaking it until creamy, like mayonnaise. A recent human study involving ten healthy adults showed that MCT emulsification may reduce side effects and increase the ketogenic impact of MCTs (Courchesne-Loyer, *et al.*, 2017). Emulsification of the MCT creates smaller lipid droplets, which, therefore, will increase gut absorption and the bioavailability of MCT in humans by at least 2-3x. In turn, it may increase the acute ketogenic effect. (Courchesne-Loyer, *et al.*, 2013 & 2017). It also will decrease bloating and diarrhea by 50%. This is because the gastric and pancreatic enzymes (lipases) can easily reach the smaller fat droplets and free the medium-chain fatty acids, allowing the gut to absorb them.

Nutritional ketosis vs. Diabetic ketoacidosis:

Carbohydrates provide our primary energy source. However, when carbohydrates are scarce (less than 50 grams per day), we can find and release energy from muscle protein and fats (Cornejo, *et al.*, 2007). There is also less insulin secretion and less fat and glucose storage.

Gluconeogenesis means our body makes glucose by itself; with ketogenesis, we make ketones for energy. Ketones come from the breakdown of fats. We metabolize fatty acids to make the acetoacetate (first ketone), which produces two other ketones, β-*hydroxybutyrate* (BOHB) and *acetone*. The mitochondria of our heart, brain, muscle tissues, and kidneys use acetoacetate and BOHB to make energy. The third ketone is the fruity-smelling acetone, which we do not use as energy and eliminate through our breath and urine.

1. *Nutritional ketosis* is safe because ketone bodies are produced in minimal quantities without any acidity (blood pH) change when we go on a KD.

2. *Diabetic ketoacidosis* (DKA) is very different. DKA is a dangerous state of uncontrolled ketone production and life-threatening acidosis. People with diabetes with ketoacidosis cannot make enough insulin to fight excess blood glucose. The lack of insulin means glucose cannot enter the organs (liver, muscle, and fatty tissue), which need it for energy. The body senses this failure. Because insulin becomes 'incompetent,' the organs are starving for glucose even though plenty of glucose is hanging around. Glycogen (stored carbs) are broken down to release glucose for fuel to survive. Proteins and lipids also rescue and make glucose through their pathways. Blood sugars rise. Fats start breaking into fatty acids (lipolysis) to become alternative fuels. This rapid breakdown results in catastrophic blood ketone quantities, which quickly develop into life-threatening *metabolic acidosis*.

Other uses of the ketogenic diet:

1. *Glucose transporter type 1 deficiency syndrome* (GLUT1 deficiency) is an inborn metabolic defect where glucose can no longer

transport itself from the blood to the brain (Cornejo, *et al.*, 2007). We know glucose is the brain's leading food. Children with this defect will not have enough glucose to feed their brains and, therefore, will have seizures, low muscle tone, small skulls, and developmental delay. They also develop *hypoglycorrhachia* (low glucose levels in cerebrospinal fluid). A KD will be a very effective treatment for this disease and controls seizures well. Long-term, 5-year follow-ups of these GLUT-1 deficient patients show no significant effects of the KD on body composition, bone mineral content, or bone mineral density (Bertoli, *et al.*, 2014). Cardiovascular follow-up shows patients' abnormal cholesterol profiles resolve over time, with standard profiles maintained at ten years and carotid artery lining thickness stable years later (Spalice & Guido, 2018).

2. *Pyruvate dehydrogenase* (PDH) deficiency. PDH, sometimes known as *pyruvate dehydrogenase complex* (PDC), comprises three enzymes that change pyruvate to acetyl-CoA, which feeds into the citric acid cycle. A mutation of the mitochondrial PDC will result in a 'traffic jam' because pyruvate cannot transform into acetyl-CoA. As a result, the reaction shifts back to making lactate in glycolysis, developing severe congenital *lactic acidosis*. KDs will rescue the body from this crisis by replenishing acetyl-CoA. When our dietary carb content is low, our body turns to fat. We begin oxidizing (breaking down) fatty acids to produce the missing acetyl-CoA. Replenishing acetyl-CoA can keep the citric acid cycle and respiratory chain running to prevent lactate over-production (Weber, *et al.*, 2001).

3. *Acne and diabetes.* IGF-1 is a well-established effector of acne. The KD and its IGF-1 lowering effect could potentially treat acne and diabetes-related conditions (Burris, *et al.*, 2018; Paoli, *et al.*, 2012).

4. *Abnormal gut bacteria* (microbiota) can contribute to drug-refractory seizures. KDs can dramatically decrease *proteobacteria* and reshape gut microbiota to improve seizure control (Xie, *et al.*, 2017; Zhang, *et al.*, 2018).

5. *Improved neurobehavioral development* (gross and fine motor skills) was seen when a KD treated children with refractory seizures (Zhu, *et al.*, 2016).

Recommended monitoring:

During the first few months, it is reasonable to monitor *complete blood counts* (CBC), serum chemistries, lipid (fat and cholesterol), and liver tests, as well as monitor for *hyperuricemia* (high uric acid levels) (Tan-Shalaby, *et al.*, 2016). Weight gain or weight loss and compliance should be supervised. Monitoring for ketosis should include testing for hypoglycemia (low blood glucose) and ketosis. Serum BOHB levels can be calculated and compared to simultaneous glucose levels to achieve a value for the Glucose Ketone Index (GKI) (Tan-Shalaby, *et al.*, 2016; Meidenbauer, *et al.*, 2015). Preferably, there should be a dietician and social worker available. Supplemental education via pamphlets, videos, handouts, recipe books, shopping lists, and online support groups can help improve compliance. (Psst! Check out my group, Keto for Cancer, on FaceBook.)

Other supplements:

1. *Caffeine* can increase the ketogenic effect due to its actions on lipolysis and lipid oxidation (fat breakdown followed by ketone production) (Vandenberghe, *et al.*, 2017). Alzheimer's patients have decreased glucose uptake; hence, ketones could provide the needed brain energy in the event of brain glucose depletion. Caffeine given at breakfast in a dose-dependent manner raised plasma-free fatty acids and ketone levels in humans. It remains unknown whether this ketogenic effect of caffeine can add to the ketogenic influence of MCT, nor is it known if this effect will be long-term (Vandenberghe, *et al.*, 2016).

2. *Bezafibrate* (BEZA) is a cholesterol-lowering drug that boosts our good cholesterol called *high-density lipoproteins* (HDL). When added to MCTs in healthy adults, BEZA increased the ketogenic efficiency of MCT by 2.5-fold. However, it did not increase ketone levels (Courchesne-Loyer, *et al.*, 2015).

3. *KetoCal supplements.* In a 2011 study, adding a ketone shake supplement (KetoCal) to a modified Atkins diet (MAD) increased daily fat intake (Kossoff, *et al.*, 2011). It improved the ketogenic ratio (1.8:1 versus 1:1 in the MAD alone, P = .0002) but did not change levels of urinary or serum ketones (Kossoff, *et al.*, 2011).

4. *Raspberry ketones.* These supplemental ketones occur naturally in raspberries and are used as a flavoring agent. However, many over-the-counter supplements have doses that range

widely—between 100 and 1400 mg per day. There is concern that even with the lowest amount of 100 mg, it still exceeds minimum toxicology thresholds and could affect cardiac health and reproductive development (Bredsdorff, *et al.*, 2015).

Other popular dietary approaches:

Intermittent fasting (IF), therapeutic fasting (TF), timed meals, timed exercise, and caloric restriction (CR) have become popular. Although not necessarily ketogenic, these dietary approaches potentially benefit cancer management (Lv, *et al.*, 2014).

1. *Intermittent fasting* (IF), or *intermittent energy restriction* (IER), consists of periods of total fasting or marked energy restriction mixed with spells of normal eating. IF can improve insulin sensitivity and reduce inflammatory markers, *adipokines*, and IGFs. Compared to *continuous energy restriction* (CER), IF was superior in reducing tumor rates in mouse cancer models (Harvie & Howell, *et al.*, 2016). However, other IF studies in mouse prostate cancer tumors without weight loss failed to show survival benefits. Nor did we see improvement in survival or serum insulin, IGFBP-3 (insulin growth factor binding protein), or tumor phospho-Akt levels (pAKT) (Buschemeyer *et al.*, 2010).

2. *Therapeutic fasting* (TF) hopes to treat disease by triggering *autophagy* (self-renewal). By cleaning up chemotherapy-damaged cellular components, TF protects from

chemotherapy side effects (Davidson, *et al.*, 2006).

3. *Timed meals.* Tumors respond differently to chemotherapy based on circadian clocks. Studies show that rats with disrupted sleep will develop faulty central circadian rhythms that increase their cancer rates (Davidson, *et al.*, 2006). One way to fix this is by timing our meals. By restricting food intake to either day or night, we may readjust the disrupted circadian rhythms and improve the effectiveness of chemotherapy (van Niekerk, *et al.*, 2016).

4. *Timing our exercise* can also readjust disabled circadian clocks and help treat circadian rhythm-related disorders (Flôres, *et al.*, 2016).

Which is better? Intermittent or continuous fasting?

Is *continuous fasting* (CF) better than intermittent fasting (IF)? Fasting is also known as *continuous energy restriction* (CER), compared to *intermittent energy restriction* (IER). Both had similar effects on weight loss, heart disease, and glucose control even a year later (Carter, *et al.*, 2016; Sundfør, *et al.*, 2018; Harvie & Howell, *et al.*, 2016); however, found IF and IER to be superior to CER in improving insulin sensitivity (Harvie & Howell, *et al.*, 2016; Thomas *et al.*, 2010). That sounds like good news since it means we can take a break from fasting and still benefit.

Chapter Summary/Key Takeaways:

There is indeed more than one way to follow a ketogenic lifestyle. We learned about the different ketogenic diets and medium-chain triglycerides (MCT). We discussed how to deal with MCT oil issues and other medical conditions that could benefit from a ketogenic lifestyle. A few ketogenic supporting supplements were mentioned, and we discussed fasting as an additional tool to fight cancer.

The next chapter will examine the Glucose Ketone Index, another valuable tool for your ketogenic lifestyle.

(See this book's Appendices for the acceptable and unacceptable foods while on a true Keto diet, and sample diet for a day.)

FAQs

From the Facebook group "Keto For Cancer"

QUESTION:

What should my blood sugar be during ketosis? Mine was at 64 mg/dl.

ANSWER:

If you are in ketosis, the ketones will fuel your brain instead of glucose, and despite the low blood glucose, you should not feel weak or lightheaded. The glucose ketone index is a good ratio to aim for, not just the glucose level alone.

QUESTION:

When I'm testing with keto urine strips, the results are the darkest color on the strip. Is that a good thing?

ANSWER:

Ketones measure excess ketones that spill out into the urine. Once you see that the urine strip turns pink, it usually means that your serum should also have ketones.

End Notes

Bertoli S, Trentani C, Ferraris C, De Giorgis V, Veggiotti P, Tagliabue A. Long-term effects of a ketogenic diet on body composition and bone mineralization in GLUT-1 deficiency syndrome: a case series. *Nutrition.* 2014 Jun;30(6): e726-8. doi: 10.1016/j.nut.2014.01.005. Epub 2014 Jan 29. PMID: 24800673.

Bredsdorff L, Wedebye EB, Nikolov NG, Hallas-Møller T, Pilegaard K. Raspberry ketone in food supplements--High intake, few toxicity data--A cause for safety concern? *Regul Toxicol Pharmacol.* 2015 Oct;73(1): pp. 196-200. doi: 10.1016/j.yrtph.2015.06.022. Epub 2015 Jul 6. PMID: 26160596.

Burris J, Shikany JM, Rietkerk W, Woolf K. A Low Glycemic Index and Glycemic Load Diet Decreases Insulin-like Growth Factor-1 among Adults with Moderate and Severe Acne: A Short-Duration, 2-Week Randomized Controlled Trial. *J Acad Nutr Diet.* 2018 Oct;118(10): e1874-85. doi: 10.1016/j.jand.2018.02.009. Epub 2018 Apr 22. PMID: 29691143.

Buschemeyer WC 3rd, Klink JC, Mavropoulos JC, Poulton SH, Demark-Wahnefried W, Hursting SD, Cohen P, Hwang D, Johnson TL, Freedland SJ. Effect of intermittent fasting with or without caloric restriction on prostate cancer growth and survival in SCID mice. *Prostate.* 2010 Jul 1;70(10): e1037-43. doi: 10.1002/pros.21136. PMID: 20166128.

Carter S, Clifton PM, Keogh JB. The effects of intermittent compared to continuous energy restriction on glycaemic control in type 2 diabetes; a pragmatic pilot trial. *Diabetes Res Clin Pract.* 2016 Dec;122: pp. 106-12. doi: 10.1016/j.diabres.2016.10.010. Epub 2016 Oct 19. PMID: 27833048.

Cornejo VE, Cabello JF, Colombo MC, Raimann EB. Síndrome de deficiencia del transportador de glucosa tipo 1 (SDGLUT-1) tratado con dieta cetogénica. Caso clínico [Glucose transponer type 1 deficiency síndrome (GLUT-1 SD) treated with ketogenic diet. Report of one case]. *Rev Med Chil.* 2007 May;135(5): e631-5. Spanish. doi: 10.4067s0034-98872007000500011. Epub 2007 Jul 9. PMID: 17657332.

Courchesne-Loyer A, Fortier M, Tremblay-Mercier J, Chouinard-Watkins R, Roy M, Nugent S, Castellano CA, Cunnane SC. Stimulation of mild, sustained ketonemia by medium-chain triacylglycerols in healthy humans: estimated potential contribution to brain energy metabolism. *Nutrition.* 2013 Apr;29(4): pp. 635-40. doi: 10.1016/j.nut.2012.09.009. Epub 2012 Dec 28. PMID: 23274095.

Courchesne-Loyer A, Lowry CM, St-Pierre V, Vandenberghe C, Fortier M, Castellano CA, Wagner JR, Cunnane SC. Emulsification Increases the Acute Ketogenic Effect and Bioavailability of Medium-Chain Triglycerides in Humans: Protein, Carbohydrate, and Fat Metabolism. *Curr Dev Nutr.* 2017 Jun 21;1(7): e000851. doi: 10.3945/cdn.117.000851. PMID: 29955713; PMCID: PMC5998361.

Courchesne-Loyer A, St-Pierre V, Hennebelle M, Castellano CA, Fortier M, Tessier D, Cunnane SC. Ketogenic response to cotreatment with bezafibrate and medium chain triacylglycerols in healthy humans. *Nutrition.* 2015 Oct;31(10): e1255-9. doi: 10.1016/j.nut.2015.05.015. Epub 2015 Jun 6. PMID: 26333891.

Davidson AJ, Straume M, Block GD, Menaker M. Daily timed meals dissociate circadian rhythms in hepatoma and healthy host liver. *Int J Cancer.* 2006 Apr 1;118(7): e1623-7. doi: 10.1002/ijc.21591. PMID: 16231323; PMCID: PMC1464797.

Flôres DE, Bettilyon CN, Yamazaki S. Period-independent novel circadian oscillators revealed by timed exercise and palatable meals. *Sci Rep.* 2016 Feb 24;6: e21945. doi: 10.1038/srep21945. PMID: 26904978; PMCID: PMC4764932.

Harvie MN, Howell T. Could Intermittent Energy Restriction and Intermittent Fasting Reduce Rates of Cancer in Obese, Overweight, and Normal-Weight Subjects? A Summary of Evidence. *Adv Nutr.* 2016 Jul 15;7(4): e690-705. doi: 10.3945/an.115.011767. PMID: 27422504; PMCID: PMC4942870.

Huttenlocher PR, Wilbourn AJ, Signore JM. Medium-chain triglycerides as a therapy for intractable childhood epilepsy. *Neurology.* 1971 Nov;21(11): e1097-103. doi: 10.1212/wnl.21.11.1097. PMID: 5166216.

Kossoff EH, Dorward JL, Turner Z, Pyzik PL. Prospective study of the modified atkins diet in combination with a ketogenic liquid supplement during the initial month. *J Child Neurol.* 2011 Feb;26(2): pp. 147-51. doi: 10.1177/0883073810375718. Epub 2010 Sep 10. PMID: 20833798.

Lv M, Zhu X, Wang H, Wang F, Guan W. Roles of caloric restriction, ketogenic diet and intermittent fasting during initiation, progression and metastasis of cancer in animal models: a systematic review and meta-analysis. *PLoS One.* 2014 Dec 11;9(12): e115147. doi: 10.1371/journal.pone.0115147. PMID: 25502434; PMCID: PMC4263749.

Meidenbauer JJ, Mukherjee P, Seyfried TN. The glucose ketone index calculator: a simple tool to monitor therapeutic efficacy for metabolic management of brain cancer. *Nutr Metab (Lond).* 2015 Mar 11;12: p. 12. doi: 10.1186/s12986-015-0009-2. PMID: 25798181; PMCID: PMC4367849.

Miranda MJ, Turner Z, Magrath G. Alternative diets to the classical ketogenic diet--can we be more liberal? *Epilepsy Res.* 2012 Jul;100(3): pp. 278-85. doi: 10.1016/j.eplepsyres.2012.06.007. Epub 2012 Jul 6. PMID: 22771252.

Paoli A, Grimaldi K, Toniolo L, Canato M, Bianco A, Fratter A. Nutrition and acne: therapeutic potential of ketogenic diets. *Skin Pharmacol Physiol.* 2012;25(3): pp. 111-7. doi: 10.1159/000336404. Epub 2012 Feb 11. PMID: 22327146.

Spalice A, Guido CA. Cardiovascular Risks of Ketogenic Diet for Glut-1 Deficiency. *Pediatr Neurol Briefs.* 2018 Sep 5;32: p. 8. doi: 10.15844/pedneurbriefs-32-8. PMID: 30210142; PMCID: PMC6123241.

Sundfør TM, Svendsen M, Tonstad S. Effect of intermittent versus continuous energy restriction on weight loss, maintenance and cardiometabolic risk: A randomized 1-year trial. *Nutr Metab Cardiovasc Dis.* 2018 Jul;28(7): e698-706. doi: 10.1016/j.numecd.2018.03.009. Epub 2018 Mar 29. PMID: 29778565.

Tan-Shalaby JL, Carrick J, Edinger K, Genovese D, Liman AD, Passero VA, Shah RB. Modified Atkins diet in advanced malignancies - final results of a safety and feasibility trial within the Veterans Affairs Pittsburgh Healthcare System. *Nutr Metab (Lond).* 2016 Aug 12;13: p. 52. doi: 10.1186/s12986-016-0113-y. Erratum in: *Nutr Metab (Lond).* 2016;13(1): p. 61. PMID: 27525031; PMCID: PMC4983076.

Thomas JA 2nd, Antonelli JA, Lloyd JC, Masko EM, Poulton SH, Phillips TE, Pollak M, Freedland SJ. Effect of intermittent fasting on prostate cancer tumor growth in a mouse model. *Prostate Cancer Prostatic Dis.* 2010 Dec;13(4): pp. 350-5. doi: 10.1038/pcan.2010.24. Epub 2010 Aug 24. PMID: 20733612.

Vandenberghe C, St-Pierre V, Courchesne-Loyer A, Hennebelle M, Castellano CA, Cunnane SC. Caffeine intake increases plasma ketones: an acute metabolic study in humans. *Can J Physiol Pharmacol.* 2017 Apr;95(4): pp. 455-58. doi: 10.1139/cjpp-2016-0338. Epub 2016 Nov 25. PMID: 28177691.

Weber TA, Antognetti MR, Stacpoole PW. Caveats when considering ketogenic diets for the treatment of pyruvate dehydrogenase complex deficiency. *J Pediatr.* 2001 Mar;138(3): pp. 390-5. doi: 10.1067/mpd.2001.111817. PMID: 11241048.

Wirrell EC, Darwish HZ, Williams-Dyjur C, Blackman M, Lange V. Is a fast necessary when initiating the ketogenic diet? *J Child Neurol.* 2002 Mar;17(3): pp. 179-82. doi: 10.1177/08830 7380201700305. PMID: 12026232.

Wirrell EC. Ketogenic ratio, calories, and fluids: do they matter? *Epilepsia.* 2008 Nov;49 (Suppl 8): pp. 17-9. doi: 10.1111/j.1528-1167.2008.01825.x. PMID: 19049578; PMCID: PMC2656445.

Xie G, Zhou Q, Qiu CZ, Dai WK, Wang HP, Li YH, Liao JX, Lu XG, Lin SF, Ye JH, Ma ZY, Wang WJ. Ketogenic diet poses a significant effect on imbalanced gut microbiota in infants with refractory epilepsy. *World J Gastroenterol.* 2017 Sep 7;23(33): e6164-71. doi: 10.3748/wjg.v23.i33.6164. PMID: 28970732; PMCID: PMC5597508.

Zhang Y, Zhou S, Zhou Y, Yu L, Zhang L, Wang Y. Altered gut microbiome composition in children with refractory epilepsy after ketogenic diet. *Epilepsy Res.* 2018 Sep;145: p. 163-8. doi: 10.1016/j.eplepsyres.2018.06.015. Epub 2018 Jun 28. PMID: 30007242.

Zhu D, Wang M, Wang J, Yuan J, Niu G, Zhang G, Sun L, Xiong H, Xie M, Zhao Y. Ketogenic diet effects on neurobehavioral development of children with intractable epilepsy: A prospective study. *Epilepsy Behav.* 2016 Feb;55: pp. 87-91. doi: 10.1016/j.yebeh.2015.12.011. Epub 2016 Jan 13. PMID: 26773676.

Chapter Twenty-One

The Glucose Ketone Index (GKI)

The Glucose Ketone Index (GKI) is a calculated number using the molar ratio of blood glucose to blood ketone bodies, specifically the β-hydroxybutyrate (BOHB) (Meidenbauer, *et al.*, 2015).

GKI is a mathematical tool designed to help us reach our target blood glucose and ketone levels by comparing the quantities of the primary fermentable tumor fuel (glucose) to the non-fermentable fuel (ketones).

An example of how to calculate GKI is as follows:

<u>Divide</u> glucose level in millimoles (mmol) <u>by</u>

ketone (*β-hydroxybutyrate* [BHB]) in millimoles (mmol)

= Glucose Ketone Index (GKI)

Note: If glucose is in mg/dl, dividing it by 18 will convert it to millimoles.

A GKI of 3 means that one has reached a high level of ketosis (and a low level of glucose).

A GKI of 3-6 means one has achieved moderate ketosis, while 6-9 means a low level of ketosis. Remember, the lower the number, the better (normally) (Meidenbauer, *et al.*, 2015).

Based on preclinical and clinical data, the best results are predicted with values approaching 1.0 (Meidenbauer, *et. al.*, 2015).

Blood glucose and ketone values should be measured 2–3 hours after eating (Meidenbauer, *et al.*, 2015).

The GKI Calculator was first used in two pediatric patients with brain cancer: one with *anaplastic astrocytoma* and the other with *cerebellar astrocytoma* (Nebeling, & Lerner, 1995). Both patients had eight weeks of diet treatment. GKI dropped from about 27.5 to about 0.7–1.1. The anaplastic astrocytoma patient followed the diet without chemotherapy, and on a PET scan, the tumor had a 21.7% reduction in *fluoro-deoxyglucose* (FDG) uptake. The cerebellar astrocytoma patient received standard chemotherapy along with the ketogenic diet. Tumor FDG uptake was reduced by 21.8% (Nebeling & Lerner, 1995; Nebeling, 1995). Both are excellent responses!

Another case report was of a 65-year-old woman with *glioblastoma multiforme* (GBM). She followed a *calorie-restricted ketogenic diet* (KD-R) (600 kcal/day), standard chemotherapy, and radiation without steroids for eight weeks. GKI decreased from 37.5 to 1.4 in the first three weeks. At eight weeks, brain scans were tumor-free, and she was symptom-free. She decided to stop the ketogenic diet.

Unfortunately, her tumor returned ten weeks later (Zuccoli, *et al.*, 2010).

There were studies involving brain cancer cells implanted in mice (Zhou, *et al.*, 2007). Scientists ordered lab-grown CT-2A cancer cells (mouse brain cancer) and U87-MG (human glioma brain cancer) and injected both into adult mice. The mice were divided into three groups. They were assigned an unlimited standard diet, unrestricted calorie ketogenic diet, or KD-R separately. After eight days of therapy, mice with both calorie restriction and a ketogenic diet were the only ones that shrank their tumor weight. They also lived longer than the mice in the other two groups. Their GKIs ranged from 1.8 to 4.4. This success could be explained by the ketones' ability to shrink the *microvessels* that fed the cancer, and while starving the cancer of glucose, the ketones could still provide food for the brain. The brain tumors also had less active mitochondrial enzymes—low β-hydroxybutyrate dehydrogenase (β-OHBDH) and *succinyl-CoA:3-ketoacid CoA transferase* (SCOT). These enzymes normally metabolize or 'chew up and discard' the ketones. Less β-OHBDH and less SCOT activity mean ketones can 'hang out in the blood' longer to do their job, battling inflammation and cancer growth, since they are not quickly metabolized.

Chapter Summary/Key Takeaways:

The Glucose Ketone Index tool can help guide ketogenic diet therapy. Based on limited studies, the Glucose Ketone Index is a helpful tool to monitor the success of a shifting metabolism. Before using the Glucose Ketone Index in clinical practice, more clinical studies are needed.

The next chapter deals with ketogenic diet side effects in more detail.

End Notes

Meidenbauer JJ, Mukherjee P, Seyfried TN. The glucose ketone index calculator: a simple tool to monitor therapeutic efficacy for metabolic management of brain cancer. *Nutr Metab (Lond)*. 2015 Mar 11;12: p. 12. doi: 10.1186/s12986-015-0009-2. PMID: 25798181; PMCID: PMC4367849.

Nebeling LC, Lerner E. Implementing a ketogenic diet based on medium-chain triglyceride oil in pediatric patients with cancer. *J Am Diet Assoc.* 1995 Jun;95(6): e693-7. doi: 10.1016/S0002-8223(95)00189-1. PMID: 7759747.

Nebeling LC, Miraldi F, Shurin SB, Lerner E. Effects of a ketogenic diet on tumor metabolism and nutritional status in pediatric oncology patients: two case reports. *J Am Coll Nutr.* 1995 Apr;14(2): pp. 202-8. doi: 10.1080/07315724.1995.10718495. PMID: 7790697.

Zuccoli G, Marcello N, Pisanello A, Servadei F, Vaccaro S, Mukherjee P, Seyfried TN. Metabolic management of glioblastoma multiforme using standard therapy together with a restricted ketogenic diet: Case Report. *Nutr Metab (Lond)*. 2010 Apr 22;7: p. 33. doi: 10.1186/1743-7075-7-33. PMID: 20412570; PMCID: PMC2874558.

Zhou W, Mukherjee P, Kiebish MA, Markis WT, Mantis JG, Seyfried TN. The calorically restricted ketogenic diet, an effective alternative therapy for malignant brain cancer. *Nutr Metab (Lond)*. 2007 Feb 21;4: p. 5. doi: 10.1186/1743-7075-4-5. PMID: 17313687; PMCID: PMC1819381.

Chapter Twenty-Two

Ketogenic Diet Side Effects

With contributions by Hema Rai, M.D.

The ketogenic diet (KD) was first used more than eighty years ago to treat children suffering from seizures. The KD was commonly used in the early 1920s and was a very effective treatment (Wheless, 2008; Allen, *et al.*, 2014).

Other diseases also benefit from a KD. Obesity, migraines, infertility, psychiatric illness, and cancers were just a few. (Allen, *et al.*, 2014; Maggioni, *et al.*, 2011; Margoni, *et al.*, 2017). Although many reports had positive results, there were also side effects. Imbalances of macronutrients and micronutrients, deficits in protein, vitamins, and minerals, calories, and increased cholesterol (hyperlipidemia) are common concerns.

Disturbances of the digestive system commonly saw constipation. Changes in blood counts and thyroid, cardiac, bone, and electrolyte imbalances were added to the list (Doksöz, *et al.*, 2015).

With the mounting list of side effects, many wondered if the KD could be sustained long-term. Unfortunately, publications regarding the KD were few. Information and guidance on what to expect is only now reemerging.

Weight loss:

Ketogenic low-carbohydrate diets, if done correctly, will likely cause weight loss due to the initial loss of fat and water. Weight loss was pronounced in a safety and feasibility trial of advanced cancer patients, where the modified Atkins diet (MAD) resulted in a 13% median weight loss among all participants (Wheless, 2008; Abbasi, 2018; Paoli, *et al.*, 2008, Perez-Guisado, 2008; Taus, *et al.*, 2017).

Less hunger:

An interesting side effect of KDs is less hunger (Nymo, *et al.*, 2017). There will be a drop in blood levels of *ghrelin*, the hunger hormone. This is why many on the KD will actually eat less because their appetites are satisfied more efficiently, thanks to ghrelin (Nymo, *et al.*, 2017).

Cardiac complications:

Selenium levels are usually low when cardiac abnormalities are seen during a KD, which brings some concern.

In a case series of twenty children (without selenium deficiency) on a KD, three patients (15%) had electrocardiogram (EKG) changes (prolonged QT interval). The KD resulted in high ketone BOHB levels and low serum bicarbonate, which affected the beat-to-beat contractions (prolonged QTc). Three patients (15%) had cardiac chamber enlargement (Best, *et al.*, 2000).

A few reports show that selenium deficiency might cause *acquired cardiomyopathy* (abnormal heart muscle function). Most of our experience comes from individual case studies. Fortunately, each report showed that cardiomyopathy was reversed with selenium supplementation (Munguti, *et al.*, 2017; Constans, *et al.*, 1997).

Doksöz (2015) observed epileptic children on a KD for six months, and their heart muscles remained healthy (pp. 233-37). There were no disturbances in rhythm. There was some right-sided heart chamber enlargement (ventricular diastolic dysfunction), but in this case series, the children had normal selenium levels (Doksöz, *et al.*, 2015; Özdemir, *et al.*, 2016).

Ketogenic dieters should, therefore, monitor selenium levels and EKGs regularly (Bank, *et al.*, 2008).

Selenium:

Selenium is a micronutrient that regulates bodily functions, protects us from free radical damage and cancer, controls inflammation, maintains fertility and thyroid health, and is vital to cardiac health. There are no reported cardiac complications from the KD without selenium deficiency (Allen, *et al.*, 2014).

Meat, eggs, dairy, seafood, and grains are high in selenium. The *recommended daily allowance* (RDA) is between 55 and 70 mcg, not exceeding 400 mcg/day. Deficiency causes fatigue, hair loss, muscle weakness, weakened immunity, and infertility. Studies of otherwise healthy teenage children with anemia and poor memory revealed selenium deficiency (Ashu, 2016)

Seizure patients placed on a KD for twelve months had no serious side effects on their hearts. The study demonstrated no link to selenium levels, but they felt this was because the patients received trace element supplements during the KD (Guzel, *et al.*, 2016; Özdemir, *et al.*, 2016).

Another study of three hundred twenty children with intractable seizures on an olive oil based KD had low selenium levels between six and twelve months. Still, it showed no detectable cardiac findings (Guzel, *et al.*, 2016).

In another study, fifty-four KD patients had normal selenium levels at three months and were symptom-free with normal EKGs. Serum selenium changes were only seen after six and twelve months of the KD. We therefore recommend close monitoring of this trace element, especially around the six-month time frame (Arslan, *et al.*, 2017).

Hyperuricemia—too much uric acid:

Diets carrying protein-rich foods like meat, seafood, nuts, eggs, and poultry are rich in *purines*, which can break down into *uric acid*. Ketones can also raise uric acid levels.

How about carbohydrates? Whether carbohydrates can significantly increase blood uric acid levels is still being determined (Maggioni, *et al.*, 2011). Aldersberg and Umeda found that when one consumes a high-fat, low-carbohydrate diet, uric acid excretion will slow down, and blood uric acid levels rise (Doksöz, *et al.*, 2015; Abbasi, 2018).

Surprisingly, in a safety and feasibility trial of advanced cancer patients, blood uric acid levels remained steady while on the modified Atkins diet (MAD) (Wheless, 2008).

Bone mineral content and renal stones, vitamin D:

There is little data on KD's long-term effects on bone health. It is feared that a long-term KD will change the rate of bone mineralization and cause weak bones, especially in children and teens.

Bergqvist (2008) studied twenty-five children following a KD for intractable epilepsy (e1678-84). After fifteen months of dieting, *bone mineral content* (BMC) and blood levels of 25 hydroxy vitamin D and calcium fell. This was seen in inactive children (who did not exercise or walk) (Simm, *et al.*, 2017). The reason needed to be clarified.

Simm (2017) studied twenty-nine patients on the KD for six months (range 0.5–6.5 years old, mean 2.1 years) (pp. 62-66). He measured vitamin D levels and BMD using special blood tests using *dual-energy X-ray absorptiometry* (DEXA scans) and bone turnover (osteocalcin). Of twenty-nine patients, twenty (68%) developed low bone density, but only two developed fractures (Simm, *et al.*, 2017).

There was a similar study in animal models: Thirty-two albino rats were divided into two groups. One group was fed a KD, and the other a standard diet. The KD group received 4 grams of fat for every 1 gram of carbohydrates. They measured blood ketone, calcium, phosphorus, and IGF-1. The speed of bone fusion, bone mass, and minerals were also measured. The measurements were performed at four weeks and again at eight weeks. No differences in serum calcium or phosphorus levels were seen between the two groups. Still, the KD group did see higher blood ketones and lower serum IGF-1 compared to the standard diet group. Rats on KD also had delayed spinal fusion and decreased bone mass (Liu, *et al.*, 2018; Wu, *et al.*, 2017).

Vitamin A, E, zinc, magnesium, and selenium:

We see a difference in vitamin A levels depending on whether one follows a classical KD versus an MCT diet. One year of a KD decreased children's average blood vitamin A levels but increased in the MCT group (P<0.001) (Christodoulides, *et al.*, 2012). The mean plasma vitamin E increased in the classical KD and MCT groups. Plasma zinc levels remained stable at twelve months, but selenium levels decreased. No significant change in plasma zinc was seen at twelve months. However, the mean plasma selenium decreased (P<0.05), and the mean plasma magnesium decreased in the classical group (Christodoulides, *et al.*, 2012).

In a study, six Japanese patients with epilepsy on the ketone formula showed lower copper levels after six months of the KD

(Hayashi, *et al.*, 2013). After twelve months, we can expect changes in selenium, vitamins A and E, zinc, copper, and magnesium (Christodoulides, *et al.*, 2012; Bergqvist, *et al.*, 2003).

Dyslipidemia: cholesterol issues

Olive oil is rich in *monounsaturated fatty acids* (MUFAs) and anti-oxidant molecules; it helps improve cholesterol profiles, curbs inflammation, and acts as an antioxidant (Guzel *et al.*, 2016).

There were significant increases in their total and LDL-cholesterol (bad cholesterol) and triglyceride levels in 121 epileptic children who ate an olive oil-enriched, high-fat KD. Their total and LDL cholesterol and triglyceride levels rose after dietary treatment at one, three, six, and twelve months. No changes in cholesterol were seen during treatment. The HDL-cholesterol (good cholesterol) levels and the mean *body mass index* (BMI) did not change between start and finish (Guzel, *et al.*, 2016). You may review the issues of cholesterol by revisiting Chapter 8.

Thyroid function:

Fasting may lower levels of thyroid hormones—decrease conversion of *triiodothyronine* (T3) from *thyroxine* (T4).

Kose (2017) reported what he felt was the first study on thyroid function while on the KD (pp. 411-16). One hundred twenty children (mean age 7.3+/-4.3 years) with difficult-to-treat seizures resistant to medications were studied for one year while on the KD. They measured thyroid tests before and after the diet at months one, three, and six. Measurements of T3, free T4, and *thyroid-stimulating hormone* (TSH) levels were tallied. Sixteen percent of patients (20 pts total, 16.7%) developed hypothyroidism as early as one month after KD therapy. Females appeared to have a higher risk of low thyroid function. Thyroid function should be monitored, and given L-thyroxine replacement therapy if hypothyroidism develops (Kose, *et al.*, 2017).

Bone marrow issues:

Blood disorders rarely see copper deficiency as a cause. There was a case report of a child on a KD who later developed copper deficiency, followed by *neutropenia* (low white blood cell counts) plus anemia (low hemoglobin—oxygen carrier in the blood). This formed after the child's formula-based KD was changed to a pureed ketogenic food (Chin, 2018; Kose, *et al.*, 2018). We can't make any conclusions based on just one case, but it is worth mentioning for future reference.

Liver toxicities:

Liver side effects are rare (2% or less) but do happen. In a study, one hundred forty-one children were on the KD for multiple medical conditions, which included tuberous sclerosis, epilepsy, Doose syndrome, Landau Kleffner syndrome, and GLUT-1 deficiency (Arslan, *et al.*, 2016).

After six, twelve, and fifteen months of the KD, 2% (3 patients) developed fatty liver, 2% developed gallstones, and 2% had high liver transaminase enzymes.

Low white blood cell counts and anemia were even rarer, at 1.4% (2 patients) (Arslan, *et al.*, 2016).

Potential Benefits:

A. Improved behavior and mental awareness (cognition)

The KD improves behavior and memory in infants and older children treated for refractory seizures. They had better moods, increased social interaction, and longer attention spans (Nordli, *et al.*, 2001).

Other studies documented the same benefits. However, some scientists feel that perhaps it was not the KD per se but rather the "clarity that comes from diminishing seizures" that could have been responsible for the improved mental awareness. (For further study on improved mood, attention, etc., with the KD read: Brietzke, *et al.*, 2018; DM, *et al.*, 2016; Garcia-Penas 2018; Bergqvist, *et al.*, 2003.)

B. Anti-seizure activity

The anti-seizure benefits of a KD are well known to be as effective as traditional anti-seizure drugs in improving seizure severity and frequency (Li, *et al.*, 2013).

The KD has been used for seizure therapy since 1921. After the discovery of effective drugs (i.e., phenytoin, valproic acid, etc.), the diet lost popularity. Recently, it has made a comeback, particularly helping control seizures that didn't respond to drug therapy. In these complex cases, the diet was highly successful (Wijnen, *et al.*, 2017). In a 2008 randomized trial that enrolled one hundred forty-five children and teens with difficult-to-treat epilepsy, over 50% reduced seizures after only three months of dieting (Neal, *et al.*, 2008).

C. Cravings, sleep, sexual function

In a 2018 study, the very low-calorie variant of the KD (VLCKD) also improved the psychological well-being of obese patients (Castro, *et al.*, 2018). A good psyche helped them with long-term weight loss and allowed them to exercise outdoors. The study also found that loss of visceral (organ fat) and lower BMI had led to lowered food cravings, better sleep quality, and improved female sexual function (Castro, *et al.*, 2018).

Chapter Summary/Key Takeaways:

Many side effects do come from following a ketogenic diet. Fortunately, many side effects are helpful, and the unwelcome side effects are not too serious and manageable. Knowing what to expect when following a ketogenic diet can help prevent problems before they arise.

In the next chapter, we will dive deeper into the effects of the ketogenic diet on lipids (fats) and cholesterol.

End Notes

Abbasi J. Interest in the Ketogenic Diet Grows for Weight Loss and Type 2 Diabetes. *JAMA*. 2018 Jan 16;319(3): pp. 215-17. doi: 10.1001/jama.2017.20639. PMID: 29340675.

Allen BG, Bhatia SK, Anderson CM, Eichenberger-Gilmore JM, Sibenaller ZA, Mapuskar KA, Schoenfeld JD, Buatti JM, Spitz DR, Fath MA. Ketogenic diets as an adjuvant cancer therapy: History and potential mechanism. *Redox Biol.* 2014;2: e963-70. doi: 10.1016/j.redox.2014.08.002. Epub 2014 Aug 7. PMID: 25460731; PMCID: PMC4215472.

Arslan N, Guzel O, Kose E, Yılmaz U, Kuyum P, Aksoy B, Çalık T. Is ketogenic diet treatment hepatotoxic for children with intractable epilepsy? *Seizure.* 2016 Dec;43: pp. 32-38. doi: 10.1016/j.seizure.2016.10.024. Epub 2016 Nov 13. PMID: 27866088.

Arslan N, Kose E, Guzel O. The Effect of Ketogenic Diet on Serum Selenium Levels in Patients with Intractable Epilepsy. *Biol Trace Elem Res.* 2017 Jul;178(1): pp. 1-6. doi: 10.1007/s12011-016-0897-7. Epub 2016 Nov 21. PMID: 27873289.

Bank IM, Shemie SD, Rosenblatt B, Bernard C, Mackie AS. Sudden cardiac death in association with the ketogenic diet. *Pediatr Neurol.* 2008 Dec;39(6): pp. 429-31. doi: 10.1016/j.pediatrneurol.2008.08.013. PMID: 19027591.

Bergqvist AG, Chee CM, Lutchka L, Rychik J, Stallings VA. Selenium deficiency associated with cardiomyopathy: a complication of the ketogenic diet. *Epilepsia.* 2003 Apr;44(4): e618-20. doi: 10.1046/j.1528-1157.2003.26102.x. PMID: 12681013.

Bergqvist AG, Schall JI, Stallings VA, Zemel BS. Progressive bone mineral content loss in children with intractable epilepsy treated with the ketogenic diet. *Am J Clin Nutr.* 2008 Dec;88(6): e1678-84. doi: 10.3945/ajcn.2008.26099. PMID: 19064531.

Best TH, Franz DN, Gilbert DL, Nelson DP, Epstein MR. Cardiac complications in pediatric patients on the ketogenic diet. *Neurology.* 2000 Jun 27;54(12): e2328-30. doi: 10.1212/wnl.54.12.2328. PMID: 10881264.

Brietzke E, Mansur RB, Subramaniapillai M, Balanzá-Martínez V, Vinberg M, González-Pinto A, Rosenblat JD, Ho R, McIntyre RS. Ketogenic diet as a metabolic therapy for mood disorders: Evidence and developments. *Neurosci Biobehav Rev.* 2018 Nov;94: pp. 11-16. doi: 10.1016/j.neubiorev.2018.07.020. Epub 2018 Jul 31. PMID: 30075165.

Constans J, Sire S, Sergeant C, Simonoff M, Ragnaud JM. Cardiomyopathie dilatée et déficit en sélénium au cours du SIDA. A propos d'un cas [Dilated cardiomyopathy and selenium deficiency in AIDS. Apropos of a case]. *Rev Med Interne.* 1997;18(8): e642-5. French. doi: 10.1016/s0248-8663(97)82466-6. PMID: 9365739.

Castro AI, Gomez-Arbelaez D, Crujeiras AB, Granero R, Aguera Z, Jimenez-Murcia S, Sajoux I, Lopez-Jaramillo P, Fernandez-Aranda F, Casanueva FF. Effect of A Very Low-Calorie Ketogenic Diet on Food and Alcohol Cravings, Physical and Sexual Activity, Sleep Disturbances, and Quality of Life in Obese Patients. *Nutrients.* 2018 Sep 21;10(10): e1348. doi: 10.3390/nu10101348. PMID: 30241426; PMCID: PMC6213862.

Chin A. Copper Deficiency Anemia and Neutropenia Due to Ketogenic Diet. *Pediatrics.* 2018 May;141(5): e20173286. doi: 10.1542/peds.2017-3286. PMID: 29695584.

Christodoulides SS, Neal EG, Fitzsimmons G, Chaffe HM, Jeanes YM, Aitkenhead H, Cross JH. The effect of the classical and medium chain triglyceride ketogenic diet on vitamin and mineral levels. *J Hum Nutr Diet.* 2012 Feb;25(1): pp. 16-26. doi: 10.1111/j.1365-277X.2011.01172.x. Epub 2011 May 27. PMID: 21615805.

Doksöz Ö, Çeleğen K, Güzel O, Yılmaz Ü, Uysal U, İşgüder R, Çeleğen M, Meşe T. The Short-Term Effects of Ketogenic Diet on Cardiac Ventricular Functions in Epileptic Children. *Pediatr Neurol.* 2015 Sep;53(3): pp. 233-37. e1. doi: 10.1016/j.pediatrneurol.2015.06.009. Epub 2015 Jun 18. PMID: 26302701.

Garcia-Penas JJ. Epilepsia, cognicion y dieta cetogenica [Epilepsy, cognition and ketogenic diet]. *Rev Neurol.* 2018 Mar 1;66(S01): S71-S75. Spanish. PMID: 29516456.

Gashu D, Stoecker BJ, Bougma K, Adish A, Haki GD, Marquis GS. Stunting, selenium deficiency, and anemia are associated with poor cognitive performance in preschool children from rural Ethiopia. *Nutr J.* 2016 Apr 12;15: p. 38. doi: 10.1186/s12937-016-0155-z. PMID: 27067274; PMCID: PMC4828825.

Güzel O, Yılmaz U, Uysal U, Arslan N. The effect of olive oil-based ketogenic diet on serum lipid levels in epileptic children. *Neurol Sci.* 2016 Mar;37(3): pp. 465-70. doi: 10.1007/s10072-015-2436-2. Epub 2015 Dec 23. PMID: 26700799.

Hayashi A, Kumada T, Nozaki F, *et al.* [Changes in serum levels of selenium, zinc, and copper in patients on a ketogenic diet using Ketonformula]. *No to Hattatsu = Brain and Development.* 2013 Jul;45(4): pp. 288-93. PMID: 23951940.

IJff DM, Postulart D, Lambrechts DAJE, Majoie MHJM, de Kinderen RJA, Hendriksen JGM, Evers SMAA, Aldenkamp AP. Cognitive and behavioral impact of the ketogenic diet in children and adolescents with refractory epilepsy: A randomized controlled trial. *Epilepsy Behav.* 2016 Jul;60: pp. 153-57. doi: 10.1016/j.yebeh.2016.04.033. Epub 2016 May 18. PMID: 27206235.

Kose E, Guzel O, Arslan N. Analysis of hematological parameters in patients treated with ketogenic diet due to drug-resistant epilepsy. *Neurol Sci.* 2018 Jan;39(1): pp. 85-89. doi: 10.1007/s10072-017-3152-x. Epub 2017 Oct 16. PMID: 29038947.

Kose E, Guzel O, Demir K, Arslan N. Changes of thyroid hormonal status in patients receiving ketogenic diet due to intractable epilepsy. *J Pediatr Endocrinol Metab.* 2017 Apr 1;30(4): pp. 411-16. doi: 10.1515/jpem-2016-0281. PMID: 28076316.

Li HF, Zou Y, Ding G. Therapeutic Success of the Ketogenic Diet as a Treatment Option for Epilepsy: a Meta-analysis. *Iran J Pediatr.* 2013 Dec;23(6): e613-20. PMID: 24910737; PMCID: PMC4025116.

Liu Q, Wang X, Huang Z, Liu J, Ding J, Xu X, Kong G, Wu X, Yang Z, Zhu Q. Ketogenic diet delays spinal fusion and decreases bone mass in posterolateral lumbar spinal fusion: an in vivo rat model. *Acta Neurochir (Wien)*. 2018 Oct;160(10): e1909-16. doi: 10.1007/s00701-018-3616-7. Epub 2018 Jul 7. PMID: 29982887.

Maggioni F, Margoni M, Zanchin G. Ketogenic diet in migraine treatment: a brief but ancient history. *Cephalalgia.* 2011 Jul;31(10): e1150-1. doi: 10.1177/0333102411412089. Epub 2011 Jul 4. PMID: 21727144.

Munguti CM, Al Rifai M, Shaheen W. A Rare Cause of Cardiomyopathy: A Case of Selenium Deficiency Causing Severe Cardiomyopathy that Improved on Supplementation. *Cureus.* 2017 Aug 29;9(8): e1627. doi: 10.7759/cureus.1627. PMID: 29098137; PMCID: PMC5659335.

Neal EG, Chaffe H, Schwartz RH, Lawson MS, Edwards N, Fitzsimmons G, Whitney A, Cross JH. The ketogenic diet for the treatment of childhood epilepsy: a randomised controlled trial. *Lancet Neurol.* 2008 Jun;7(6): pp. 500-6. doi: 10.1016/S1474-4422(08)70092-9. Epub 2008 May 2. PMID: 18456557.

Nordli, D. R., Kuroda, M. M., Carroll, J., Koenigsberger, D. Y., Hirsch, L. J., Bruner, H. J., Seidel, W. T., & De Vivo, D. C. (2001). Experience With the Ketogenic Diet in Infants. *Pediatrics*, *108*(1), pp. 129–133. https://doi.org/10.1542/peds.108.1.129

Nymo S, Coutinho SR, Jørgensen J, Rehfeld JF, Truby H, Kulseng B, Martins C. Timeline of changes in appetite during weight loss with a ketogenic diet. *Int J Obes (Lond)*. 2017 Aug;41(8): e1224-31. doi: 10.1038/ijo.2017.96. Epub 2017 Apr 25. PMID: 28439092; PMCID: PMC5550564.

Özdemir R, Güzel O, Küçük M, Karadeniz C, Yılmaz Ü, Calik T, Meşe T. The Impact of 3:1 Ketogenic Diet on Cardiac Repolarization Changes in Children with Refractory Seizures: A Prospective Follow-Up Study. *Neuropediatrics.* 2016 Jun;47(3): pp. 157-61. doi: 10.1055/s-0036-1582139. Epub 2016 Apr 4. PMID: 27043293.

Paoli A, Bianco A, Grimaldi KA, Lodi A, Bosco G. Long term successful weight loss with a combination biphasic ketogenic Mediterranean diet and Mediterranean diet maintenance protocol. *Nutrients.* 2013 Dec 18;5(12): e5205-17. doi: 10.3390/nu5125205. PMID: 24352095; PMCID: PMC3875914.Perez-Guisado, J. 2008. "[Ketogenic diets and weight loss: basis and effectiveness]." *Arch Latinoam Nutr* 58 (2): pp. 126-31.

Taus M, Fumelli D, Busni D, et al. A very low calorie ketogenic diet improves weight loss and quality of life in patients with adjustable gastric banding. *Annali Italiani di Chirurgia.* 2017 ;88: S0003469X17026550. PMID: 28604374.

Simm PJ, Bicknell-Royle J, Lawrie J, Nation J, Draffin K, Stewart KG, Cameron FJ, Scheffer IE, Mackay MT. The effect of the ketogenic diet on the developing skeleton. *Epilepsy Res*. 2017 Oct;136: pp. 62-66. doi: 10.1016/j.eplepsyres.2017.07.014. Epub 2017 Jul 26. PMID: 28778055.

Wheless JW. History of the ketogenic diet. *Epilepsia.* 2008 Nov;49 Suppl 8: pp. 3-5. doi: 10.1111/j.1528-1167.2008.01821.x. PMID: 19049574.

Wijnen BFM, de Kinderen RJA, Lambrechts DAJE, Postulart D, Aldenkamp AP, Majoie MHJM, Evers SMAA. Long-term clinical outcomes and economic evaluation of the ketogenic diet versus care as usual in children and adolescents with intractable epilepsy. *Epilepsy Res.* 2017 May;132: pp. 91-99. doi: 10.1016/j.eplepsyres.2017.03.002. Epub 2017 Mar 21. PMID: 28364726.

Wu X, Huang Z, Wang X, Fu Z, Liu J, Huang Z, Kong G, Xu X, Ding J, Zhu Q. Ketogenic Diet Compromises Both Cancellous and Cortical Bone Mass in Mice. *Calcif Tissue Int.* 2017 Oct;101(4): pp. 412-421. doi: 10.1007/s00223-017-0292-1. Epub 2017 May 25. PMID: 28547346.

Chapter Twenty-Three

Cholesterol, Fats, and the Ketogenic Diet

With contributions by Arisha Patel, M.D., MBA

A high cholesterol blood level is a negative risk factor (warning signs) in cardiovascular (heart/blood vessel) disease.

Because the classical ketogenic diet (KD) has a high-fat content, we often blame it as the cause of high blood cholesterol. However, studies have shown that KD improves cardiovascular fitness. (See Sharman, *et al.*, 2002; Dashti, *et al.*, 2004; Sondike, *et al.*, 2003; Westman, *et al.*, 2006; Nordmann, *et al.*, 2006.)

The KD's low-carbohydrate and high-fat composition changes the dietary energy distribution, which is believed to be the reason behind the improved fat profile. Increased HDL—the good cholesterol—will improve overall cardiovascular health and foster weight loss. To understand the effects of the KD on lipid breakdown, realize that there are two classes of lipids (organic molecules that don't dissolve in water) within the circulatory system: triglycerides and cholesterol.

Triglycerides are fatty acids that serve as an energy source when broken into smaller parts. Elevated triglycerides increase the risk of chronic heart disease.

Cholesterol is the lipid type that serves as the backbone for hormones. Cholesterol also helps vitamin absorption and keeps cell membranes intact.

Fats attach themselves to proteins and become lipoproteins, which move freely in the blood.

You should be familiar with the different types of lipoproteins: *high-density lipoprotein* (HDL), *low-density lipoprotein* (LDL), and *very-low-density lipoprotein* (VLDL).

Why is HDL cholesterol good?

HDL cholesterol removes the cholesterol that is not used to make cell energy. It is known as good cholesterol because HDL has anti-inflammatory properties and blocks pro-inflammatory cytokines (proteins secreted by immune cells). Ultimately, HDL cholesterol is anti-inflammatory, keeps blood vessels healthy, and protects against heart disease (De Nardo, *et al.*, 2014).

On the extreme opposite is VLDL, which is responsible for transporting triglycerides to different body areas.

LDL is generally considered a bad cholesterol because of its ability to attach to the *vascular endothelium* (cells lining the blood vessels). LDL also oxidizes free radicals, which become highly inflammatory (Parthasarthy, *et al.*, 2008). We shouldn't fear LDL cholesterol as long as it's not oxidized.

High levels of both VLDL and LDL strongly predict future cardiovascular disease. Therefore, to protect our hearts, we need a diet to increase our good cholesterol (HDL) while lowering our bad cholesterol (VLDL and oxidized LDL) (Sharman, *et al.*, 2002; Dashti, *et al.*, 2006).

Can a loss of weight with the ketogenic diet be good for us?

Obesity is a risk factor for heart disease. There are several studies wherein KDs containing less than 20 grams of carbs daily effectively reduced weight in obese patients (Dashti, *et al.*, 2006; Sondike, *et al.*, 2003; Westman, *et al.*, 2005; Brinkworth, *et al.*, 2009). So, yes, KD-induced weight loss, especially in overweight patients, should be welcomed and encouraged.

What happens to our LDL cholesterol when on a ketogenic diet?

In a study, middle-aged men and women followed a low-carbohydrate KD for six weeks but did not lower total LDL cholesterol. However, they did shift from a small, dense LDL to a large, buoyant (fluffy) LDL. This positive change could lower the risk of heart disease (Westman, *et al.*, 2005).

Low-carbohydrate versus low-fat diets: What happens to our bad LDL cholesterol?

In a twenty-four-week study of one hundred twenty overweight volunteers with high cholesterol, they were randomly assigned to either a low-carbohydrate diet (LCD) or low-fat diet (LFD) group. The LC diet reduced the LDL and triglyceride levels more than the LFD (Yancy, *et al.*, 2004).

Here is another trial comparing the LCDs and LFDs. Bueno (2013) did a meta-analysis of thirteen *randomized control trials* (RCTs) with one thousand five hundred sixty-nine participants (e178-87). Patients were assigned to a VLKD and compared to LFDs (Beneno, *et al.*, 2013). Patients assigned to the VLKD had statistically significant greater weight loss, decreased triacylglycerol, decreased diastolic blood pressure, and increased HDL to LDL cholesterol ratio (Beneno, *et al.*, 2013).

Weight loss is faster with LCDs than with LFDs. A meta-analysis by Nordmann (2006) analyzed multiple published, high-quality studies (RCTs) that compared the effects of LCDs versus LFDs in overweight people (pp. 285-93). They all had a BMI greater than or equal to 25. They found five trials (447 people) that fit their strict criteria. The authors discovered that people who followed an LCD for at least six months lost more weight than those on an LFD (Nordmann, *et al.*, 2006).

The weighted difference was 3.3kg (95% confidence interval of 1.4 - 5.3 kgs). After twelve months, there was no longer any difference in weight or blood pressure between the two groups. After six months of an LCD, there was a noticeable decrease in triglyceride levels with an increase in HDL (good cholesterol) (Nordmann, *et al.*, 2006).

These studies show that because of its low-carbohydrate content, KD is more effective than LFDs in achieving weight loss and increasing total good HDL cholesterol (Sondike, *et al.*, 2003; Yancy, *et al.*, 2004; Dashti, *et al.*, 2006)

What does a ketogenic diet do to our cholesterol profile?

More of the good (HDL) and less of the bad (LDL, triglycerides).

In a six-week study of twelve normal-weight men, cardio-vascular disease *serum biomarkers* (blood tests that measure heart disease activity) were measured while on the KD (Sharman, *et al.*, 2002). The participants' diet comprised 8% carbohydrates (less than 50g/d), 61% fat, and 30% protein. This study similarly noted an increase in LDL even though there was no evidence of a change in *oxidative* LDL concentrations. Recall that the *oxidized* LDL form is responsible for heart disease and atherosclerosis. The participants' HDL levels were also elevated, leading the author to conclude that the KD is very beneficial. A good lipid biomarker profile did not have to depend on the amount of weight loss (Sharman, *et al.*, 2002).

Another 24-week observational study had eighty-three obese patients undergo a KD, which reduced LDL cholesterol and triglycerides but increased HDL levels (Dashti, *et al.*, 2006).

What happens when we follow the ketogenic diet for longer than a year?

The previous studies ran over a short period. Therefore, Brinkworth (2009) conducted similar research pitting the LFD against the LCD (pp. 23-32). This year-long study operated under strict energy-controlled conditions.

The findings were similar between both groups. Weight loss was nearly identical, but the LCD had fewer cases of insulin resistance. Interestingly, the LCD group had higher total LDL cholesterol levels (Brinkworth *et al.*, 2009).

Another long-term study using fifty-six weeks of the KD followed sixty-six obese patients (BMI> 30) with pre-existing hypercholesterolemia (above six mmol/L). They were compared to patients with normal cholesterol levels (Dashti, *et al.*, 2006). Both groups had significant (P<0.0001) body weight and BMI drops. They also decreased their total LDL triglycerides cholesterol and blood glucose levels and increased their HDL cholesterol (Dashti, *et al.*, 2006). The researchers concluded that the KD was safe to use in obese patients and improved the cholesterol profiles of those with pre-existing hypercholesterolemia (Dashti, *et al.*, 2006). The prolonged use of a KD is safe and can protect against heart disease.

A better test than LDL cholesterol: total-to-HDL cholesterol ratio

Studies have shown that the ratio of total-to-HDL cholesterol is a better test for the risk of coronary artery disease. The KD demonstrated that eating less carbohydrates will lead to more HDL cholesterol. Doing so can improve the total-to-HDL cholesterol ratio (Mensink, *et al.*, 2003). You can calculate this ratio by taking the total cholesterol value (mg/dl units) and dividing that by the HDL cholesterol. A ratio of 5 or more is considered harmful, but if your number is 3.5 or lower, that is ideal for heart health.

Which is better, the ketogenic diet or the Mediterranean diet?

This question remains unanswered because there is no head-to-head comparison of the ketogenic versus the Mediterranean diet.

A Spanish study tried incorporating the KD into the well-known healthy Mediterranean diet. To me, the researchers were not convinced of the heart benefits of the KD. Therefore, they wanted to see if they could improve upon it by incorporating some of the features of the Mediterranean diet to improve heart health. They studied thirty-one obese volunteers and created the Spanish Ketogenic Mediterranean Diet (SKMD). They mainly used virgin olive oil and allowed moderate red wine intake (200-400 ml/day). Carbohydrates were primarily salads and green vegetables. The diet was unlimited, and no calories were counted.

After twelve weeks, the researchers noted statistically significant weight loss, improved blood pressure, and a beautiful fat profile—lowered total LDL cholesterol and triacylglycerol, plus increased HDL-C. Potentially, the diet may improve cardiovascular outcomes and is seen as a benefit of future variations of the KD (Pérez-Guisado, *et al.*, 2008). Unfortunately, this study was small and enrolled only thirty-one volunteers. There was no control group for comparison, and the researchers could not tell if the benefits were due to the calorie restriction, the extra virgin olive oil, ketones, fish, salad, or red wine.

Chapter Summary/Key Takeaways:

Contrary to common misconceptions about fat, the ketogenic diet improves overall cardiovascular fitness by improving lipid (fat) subclasses despite the high-fat content of the diet. The ketogenic diet's low carbohydrate content helped increase the high-density lipoprotein cholesterol and created a healthier lipid profile. Combining the Mediterranean diet with a ketogenic diet showed benefits. However, to my knowledge, there is still no head-to-head comparison of the two diets to declare one better.

In the next chapter, we will explore some of the experiments that studied the effects of the ketogenic diet on animals and cancer cells in the lab.

End Notes

Brinkworth GD, Noakes M, Buckley JD, Keogh JB, Clifton PM. Long-term effects of a very-low-carbohydrate weight loss diet compared with an isocaloric low-fat diet after 12 mo. *Am J Clin Nutr.* 2009 Jul;90(1): pp. 23-32. doi: 10.3945/ajcn.2008.27326. Epub 2009 May 13. PMID: 19439458.

Bueno NB, de Melo IS, de Oliveira SL, da Rocha Ataide T. Very-low-carbohydrate ketogenic diet v. low-fat diet for long-term weight loss: a meta-analysis of randomised controlled trials. *Br J Nutr.* 2013 Oct;110(7): e1178-87. doi: 10.1017/S0007114513000548. Epub 2013 May 7. PMID: 23651522.

Dashti HM, Al-Zaid NS, Mathew TC, Al-Mousawi M, Talib H, Asfar SK, Behbahani AI. Long term effects of ketogenic diet in obese subjects with high cholesterol level. *Mol Cell Biochem.* 2006 Jun;286(1-2): pp. 1-9. doi: 10.1007/s11010-005-9001-x. Epub 2006 Apr 21. PMID: 16652223.

Dashti HM, Mathew TC, Hussein T, Asfar SK, Behbahani A, Khoursheed MA, Al-Sayer HM, Bo-Abbas YY, Al-Zaid NS. Long-term effects of a ketogenic diet in obese patients. *Exp Clin Cardiol.* 2004 Fall;9(3): pp. 200-5. PMID: 19641727; PMCID: PMC2716748.

De Nardo D, Labzin LI, Kono H, Seki R, Schmidt SV, Beyer M, Xu D, Zimmer S, Lahrmann C, Schildberg FA, Vogelhuber J, Kraut M, Ulas T, Kerksiek A, Krebs W, Bode N, Grebe A, Fitzgerald ML, Hernandez NJ, Williams BR, Knolle P, Kneilling M, Röcken M, Lütjohann D, Wright SD, Schultze JL, Latz E. High-density lipoprotein mediates anti-inflammatory reprogramming of macrophages via the transcriptional regulator ATF3. *Nat Immunol.* 2014 Feb;15(2): pp. 152-60. doi: 10.1038/ni.2784. Epub 2013 Dec 8. PMID: 24317040; PMCID: PMC4009731.

Mensink RP, Zock PL, Kester AD, Katan MB. Effects of dietary fatty acids and carbohydrates on the ratio of serum total to HDL cholesterol and on serum lipids and apolipoproteins: a meta-analysis of 60 controlled trials. *Am J Clin Nutr.* 2003 May;77(5): e146-55. doi: 10.1093/ajcn/77.5.1146. PMID: 12716665.

Nordmann, A.J., et al., Effects of low-carbohydrate vs low-fat diets on weight loss and cardiovascular risk factors: a metaanalysis of randomized controlled trials. *Arch Intern Med,* 2006. 166(3): pp. 285-93.

Parthasarathy S, Raghavamenon A, Garelnabi MO, Santanam N. Oxidized low-density lipoprotein. *Methods Mol Biol.* 2010;610: pp. 403-17. doi: 10.1007/978-1-60327-029-8_24. PMID: 20013192; PMCID: PMC3315351.

Pérez-Guisado J, Muñoz-Serrano A, Alonso-Moraga A. Spanish Ketogenic Mediterranean Diet: a healthy cardiovascular diet for weight loss. *Nutr J.* 2008 Oct 26;7: p. 30. doi: 10.1186/1475-2891-7-30. PMID: 18950537; PMCID: PMC2586625.

Sharman MJ, Kraemer WJ, Love DM, Avery NG, Gómez AL, Scheett TP, Volek JS. A ketogenic diet favorably affects serum biomarkers for cardiovascular disease in normal-weight men. *J Nutr.* 2002 Jul;132(7): e1879-85. doi: 10.1093/jn/132.7.1879. PMID: 12097663.

Sondike SB, Copperman N, Jacobson MS. Effects of a low-carbohydrate diet on weight loss and cardiovascular risk factor in overweight adolescents. *J Pediatr.* 2003 Mar;142(3): pp. 253-8. doi: 10.1067/mpd.2003.4. PMID: 12640371.

Westman EC, Yancy WS Jr, Olsen MK, Dudley T, Guyton JR. Effect of a low-carbohydrate, ketogenic diet program compared to a low-fat diet on fasting lipoprotein subclasses. *Int J Cardiol.* 2006 Jun 16;110(2): pp. 212-6. doi: 10.1016/j.ijcard.2005.08.034. Epub 2005 Nov 16. PMID: 16297472.

Yancy WS Jr, Olsen MK, Guyton JR, Bakst RP, Westman EC. A low-carbohydrate, ketogenic diet versus a low-fat diet to treat obesity and hyperlipidemia: a randomized, controlled trial. *Ann Intern Med.* 2004 May 18;140(10): e769-77. doi: 10.7326/0003-4819-140-10-200405180-00006. PMID: 15148063.

Chapter Twenty-Four

Animal Studies I: Effects of Ketogenic Diets on Cancer Growth

With contributions by Mariam Shalaby, M.D.

This chapter features and discusses several animal studies on the relationship between ketogenic diets (KDs) and cancer. The studies presented here include standard mouse studies concerning side effects and symptoms of cancer and the potential for KDs as complementary to chemotherapy. The studies vary by animal strain, tumor cell line type, diet, and time of diet initiation to tumor planting. As such, they exhibit a variety of results. However, diets with low-carbohydrate intake (0-20% energy) showed anti-tumor effects.

Several studies have used KDs in animal models with cancer. Some studies used KDs alone. Others were more sophisticated, combined KDs with other therapies, or measured the effect of the KDs on tumor growth, cachexia, and animal survival time.

These studies, included in this chapter, are presented under the subheading: "Normal Mouse Studies." In Chapters Twenty-Five and Twenty-Six, you will find "Combination Therapies," "Side Effects and Side Symptoms," and "Non-Conventional Therapies."

Normal Mouse Studies (van Alstyne and Beebe experiments)

The first experiment:

The first and most extensive animal study on the effects of a KD on tumor growth was performed in 1913 by Van Alstyne and Beebe (pp. 217-32). The researchers were inspired by the differences in cancer incidence in people of different groups. They surmised that diet or racial disparities may have had some influence on their cancer risk (Van Alstyne & Beebe, 1913). They conducted nine various experiments, back-to-back, on three hundred and three rats. They divided nine experiments into two broad groups. The first group tested the different diets for a set period before tumor implantation, while the second group began offering KDs simultaneously with the tumor implants (Van Alstyne & Beebe, 1913).

What you are about to see will probably not surprise you but might answer some commonly asked questions.

Did diet have any influence on cancer development?

In the first experiment, scientists injected buffalo sarcoma cells into experimental rats. The very first setup had two groups of seventeen rats each. One group received a carbohydrate-free KD consisting of casein (milk protein) and lard, while the other group ate only bread. After six weeks, all rats received implants of a buffalo sarcoma. The bread-eating group successfully implanted seven cancers and rejected ten. The carbohydrate-free group successfully implanted only four and rejected thirteen cancers. There were more live cancers in the group that ate the bread. It was tempting to conclude that the KD was better at rejecting tumors, but because of the tiny size of this trial, they could not make any solid conclusions.

The researchers continued with more experiments and used the same sample of sarcoma cells, which, with time, had become more aggressive.

We all feel disappointed when a planted seed fails to grow. We surmise that soil quality needs to be more conducive to plant development. Cancers, like plant seeds, need fertile soil to grow in.

The "poor soil quality" explains why some people develop many cancers while others remain cancer-free for most of their lives.

The second experiment:

The second experiment used twenty-seven rats. The carbohydrate-free diet group had fourteen, and the regular diet (RD) group had thirteen rats.

However, this time, the group that ate the RD successfully grew seven cancers, while the carbohydrate-free group grew only one. They found that the rats on the carb-free diet were healthier. They gained weight and had less tumor growth, with fewer deaths. The results show that the rodents on carb-free diets could resist the tumors and stay healthy. The researchers were so impressed that they continued with more experiments.

The third experiment:

A third experiment had both groups of rats dieting for two months before implantation (Van Alstyne & Beebe, 1913). Thirteen rats were ketogenic, and sixteen were on the RD. Both groups successfully implanted the cancers (100% rats per group). But, after the first and second weeks, the tumors in the RD group grew faster and tripled the size of the tumors in the KD group. By week three, the tumors were four times larger. One month passed, and six tumors shrank in the ketogenic group versus only three in the RD group.

By this time, the researchers did not doubt that the carbohydrate content of a diet was behind the astounding differences in tumor growth of the two groups. The low-carbohydrate diet (LCD) played a key role in limiting the size of the implanted cancers.

Despite the success of these experiments, they still need to be more prominent in scale to make conclusions.

More experiments:

The rest of the experiments saw similar results, but they also improved the experimental control in experiment five. You may recall that the early experiments used only bread as a control and compared it to casein and lard, which was not scientifically accurate. It could have been a better setup.

A new experiment had the KD comprised of casein and lard, compared to a control diet of casein, lard, and pure lactose (milk carb). After a month, the KD group again had significantly smaller tumors. They also noticed that the type of carbohydrate also mattered in cancer growth. The rats that received pure lactose (carbohydrate from milk) grew larger tumors than those fed with bread (Van Alstyne & Beebe, 1913).

A Second Class of Experiments

Did the timing of the KD matter? Should the KD begin before or after cancer shows up? A second class of experiments (experiments three to nine) was initiated to answer these questions. The researchers repeated the same setup, but the diet was timed to coincide with tumor implantation.

Dr. Van Alstyne and Beebe's (1913) team compared thirteen KD rats with sixteen RD rats, and in both groups, they implanted the tumors simultaneously with the start of feeding (pp. 217-32). The ketogenic rats developed ketosis. There were no differences in survival, tumor growth, and blood glucose between the KD and the RD groups.

The authors noted that starting the KD late (after the cancer appeared) was ineffective. Perhaps the body did not have enough time to build a metabolically healthy tissue environment, good enough to resist cancer. Starting the KD several weeks early gave the rats time to change the tumor microenvironment or "soil" into one that could fight cancer when it did arrive.

However, the scientists later had a pleasant surprise. After three weeks, the tumors of the rats on the RD were more than four times larger than those on the KD. After four weeks, there were six regressions on the KD versus three on the RD. By forty days post-implantation, seventeen rats had died while on the RD (fourteen tumor-related, three of unknown cause), compared to only three deaths in the KD group (two from the tumor and one from unknown cause). The results were so profound that they concluded that the diet played a key role in rejecting cancer even when the diet started after the onset of tumors.

Will ketogenic diet benefits persist after stopping the diet?

Experiment five had similar superior results as in experiments one to four. After five weeks, all the rats in both groups were returned to a non-ketogenic diet. After another twenty-five days, the KD group had twenty tumor regressions and two tumor-related deaths, plus four accidental deaths; all rats (100%) were cancer-free. Compare this to the control group, which had only two tumor regressions and eighteen tumor-related deaths, and in the remaining six living rats, there were large, ulcerated tumors. This suggests that the benefits of a KD can persist long after the rats resume an RD. Despite resuming the RD, the formerly ketogenic rats still benefitted and were cancer-free nearly one month later.

The researchers had several conclusions.

The rats fed on a carbohydrate-free diet for a few weeks before planting the tumor can largely resist cancer growth because "the period of preparation is vital to success" (Van Alstyne & Beebe, 1913, pp. 217-232). The team also concluded that it was possible to follow a KD and still see benefits intermittently. Tumor shrinkage and improved survival were seen in the rats that followed the KD but returned to a regular carbohydrate diet. The team noted, "Individual peculiarities are not eliminated by diet" (Van Alstyne & Beebe, 1913, pp. 217-32).

Are there any further high-quality experiments?

Lv (2014) published a meta-analysis (central review) of studies that used low-carbohydrate diets (LCD) containing a carbohydrate intake of zero to twenty percent. The tumors studied included prostate, brain, colonic, gastric, and metastatic cancers, all using transplanted models. "Eight of the nine studies supported that carbohydrate restriction is protective [against] cancer" (Lv, *et al.*, 2014, e115147). One negative study using the mouse model of colon cancer showed that the LCD could not slow down tumor growth (Lv, *et al.*, 2014).

In another review, Khodadadi (2017) and her team searched five large databases from inception to November 2015: PubMed, Scopus, Google Scholar, Science Direct, and Cochrane Library (p. 35). They looked at pancreatic, prostate, gastric, colon, brain, neuroblastoma, and lung tumor types and for the KD's effect on tumor growth and survival time in animal models. They used SYRCLE's RoB tool to screen for high-quality studies. They collected two hundred sixty-eight articles, but only thirteen studies passed the quality screening. Khodadadi (2017) and her colleagues found that nine out of thirteen reports showed the benefit of using the KD to slow tumor growth and improve survival time (p. 35).

This sounds like a trend towards benefit.

Are oils necessary for benefit? Does the type of oil matter?

Otto's (2008) research suggested that the KD was particularly effective with omega-3 fatty acids and MCTs (p. 122).

However, another researcher, Hao (2015), found the KD effective compared to RDs but found no benefit with MCT oil (e 2061-68). Hao (2015) injected thirty-five mice with colon cancer tumor cells, then randomly assigned the mice to three groups: a KD plus omega-3 fats and MCT oil, a ketogenic lard diet, or an RD (e 2061-68). The rats ate as much as they desired.

They ended the experiments when the tumors reached a target size, and they compared the growth and the time it took for the cancer to grow to the target size. The study found that the tumor growth in the KD (MCT-keto and lard-keto) groups was significantly slower than in the RD group. MCT and lard ketogenic groups also had considerably more tumor necrosis and less new blood vessel growth than the RD group (Hao, *et al.*, 2015).

KDs slowed cancer growth more than RDs, regardless of whether they included oils. We have yet to determine whether the type of oil makes the KD perform better because different researchers are finding different results.

Does the amount of calories matter?

The glucose levels of the mice in Hao's (2015) group did not differ between the KD and RD groups (e2061-8). The diets were all unrestricted in calories, which gave the ketogenic mice enough material to make glucose in response to the absence of carbohydrates (Hao, *et al.*, 2015).

Yes, calories do matter. Consuming excess calories might be the reason why some KDs fail.

Will adding MCT oil allow us to eat an unlimited ketogenic diet?

A previous experiment showed that unlimited calories can increase glucose blood levels even if the KD successfully produces ketones (Hao, *et al.*, 2015).

Would adding MCT oil help bring ketosis?

Let's refocus back on Otto's study. Otto (2008) studied mice with stomach cancer and found delayed tumor growth with an unrestricted KD supplemented with omega-3 fatty acids (i.e., fish oils) and MCTs (i.e., coconut oils) (p. 122). The mice were randomly assigned to two feeding groups. One group ate an unlimited KD (n=12), and the other ate an unlimited RD (n=12). The experiments ended once the tumors reached their target volume of 600 to 700 mm3. The KD mice had slower cancer growth compared to the RD group. There were fewer blood vessels in the KD group. Both groups had some left-over live cancer cells that contained glucose-loving cells and many GLUTs (transporters that allow glucose to pass into cells).

The researchers concluded that an unlimited KD plus omega-3 oils and MCT oil can delay stomach cancer growth in mice. The mice in this study, however, were not yet obese.

There are many angles to cancer. We cannot blame one thing. Instead, we should look at the entire picture and see which area of concern needs more attention.

Should we be focusing on making ketones? Or should we look at the quality and ingredients in our food?

Are we still overweight? Did we do the KD long enough?

Can the ketogenic diet boost our natural immunity to fight cancer?

The KD has been researched as a potential treatment for malignant glioma, a highly aggressive brain tumor with usually poor outcomes (Woolf & Scheck, 2014).

Gliomas are a type of aggressive brain cancer that is hard to cure because they are known to have depressed immune systems, sluggish CD8+ T cells, and *natural killer* (NK) cells. Yes, we fight infections with our immune system, but we can also prevent cancer from developing. Cancer risk rises when the immune system is depressed.

Each brain cell usually has an anti-cancer immune system. When there is a danger of turning into cancer, the immunity cells (CD8+ T cells and NK cells) can spew out unique anti-cancer proteins called *cytokines*. Cytokines activate the immune system to kill cancer. These cytokine proteins come in different fancy names. Well-known examples of cytokines in brain cancer are *interferon* (IFN), *interleukin-2* (IL-2), and *interleukin-10* (IL-10).

Lussier (2016) studied mice with implanted glioma cells (e115147). The mice were fed a KD, and their brains were examined using a *flow cytometry* technique. Flow cytometry goes down to the cellular level and can search for CD8+ & CD4+ T cells (anti-cancer immune cells) and NK cells.

Lussier concluded that the KD could help brain cancers by boosting their immunity.

Chapter Summary/Key Takeaways:

We had a glimpse into early ketogenic diet trials and cancer.

Ketogenic diets have benefits for fighting cancer. It slows down tumor growth, decreases blood glucose, boosts the immune system, prevents muscle wasting, increases survival, and blocks cancer signaling pathways.

The next chapter explores how and why the ketogenic diet is helpful when combined with current standard therapies.

End Notes

Hao GW, Chen YS, He DM, Wang HY, Wu GH, Zhang B. Growth of human colon cancer cells in nude mice is delayed by ketogenic diet with or without omega-3 fatty acids and medium-chain triglycerides. *Asian Pacific journal of cancer prevention*: *APJCP*. 2015;16(5): e2061-68.

Khodadadi S, Sobhani N, Mirshekar S, Ghiasvand R, Pourmasoumi M, Miraghajani M, Dehsoukhteh SS. Tumor Cells Growth and Survival Time with the Ketogenic Diet in Animal Models: A Systematic Review. *Int J Prev Med.* 2017 May 25;8: p. 35. doi: 10.4103/2008-7802.207035. PMID: 28584617; PMCID: PMC5450454.

Lussier DM, Woolf EC, Johnson JL, Brooks KS, Blattman JN, Scheck AC. Enhanced immunity in a mouse model of malignant glioma is mediated by a therapeutic ketogenic diet. *BMC Cancer.* 2016 May 13;16: p. 310. doi: 10.1186/s12885-016-2337-7. PMID: 27178315; PMCID: PMC4866042.

Lv M, Zhu X, Wang H, Wang F, Guan W. Roles of Caloric Restriction, Ketogenic Diet and Intermittent Fasting during Initiation, Progression and Metastasis of Cancer in Animal Models: A Systematic Review and Meta-Analysis. *PLOS ONE*. 2014;9(12): e115147.

Otto C, Kaemmerer U, Illert B, Muehling B, Pfetzer N, Wittig R, Voelker HU, Thiede A, Coy JF. Growth of human gastric cancer cells in nude mice is delayed by a ketogenic diet supplemented with omega-3 fatty acids and medium-chain triglycerides. *BMC Cancer*. 2008 Apr 30;8: p. 122. doi: 10.1186/1471-2407-8-122. PMID: 18447912; PMCID: PMC2408928.

Van Alstyne EV, Beebe SP. Diet Studies in Transplantable Tumors: I. The Effect of Non-carbohydrate Diet upon the Growth of Transplantable Sarcoma in Rats. *J Med Res.* 1913 Dec;29(2): pp. 217-32. PMID: 19972139; PMCID: PMC2099768.

Woolf EC, Scheck AC. The ketogenic diet for the treatment of malignant glioma. *J Lipid Res.* 2015 Jan;56(1): pp. 5-10. doi: 10.1194/jlr.R046797. Epub 2014 Feb 6. PMID: 24503133; PMCID: PMC4274070.

Chapter Twenty-Five

Animal Studies II: Ketogenic Diets Plus Standard Therapies

With contributions by Mariam Shalaby, M.D.

Can we safely use the ketogenic diet (KD) with immunotherapy? Will the KD enhance the standard of care for cancer therapies? Do KDs make immunotherapy more or less effective? These are natural questions, as we have probably heard of this newest anti-cancer treatment. Immunotherapy ads are in the news, on the radio, and even on billboards. It is an effective therapy that also promises to cure most cancers, but sadly, it still has not.

It is essential to know how immunotherapy works and, with this knowledge, why adding a KD to your armamentarium might help you beat your cancer.

Immune systems are great. They help us fight infections and fight cancer. Our immune system keeps us healthy, but an overactive immune system can also make us ill. We need something to keep the immune system in check so it doesn't overdo its job. For this reason, we have unique proteins that sit on the surface of our immune cells. Examples of these are *cytotoxic T-lymphocyte-associated protein 4* (CTLA -4) and *programmed death 1* (PD-1). We call them 'checkpoint proteins' or 'inhibitory proteins,' but they are officially known as *immune inhibitory receptors*. How do they work to fight cancer?

Cancer takes advantage of these proteins and cleverly uses them to blunt the immune system so that they can continue to do damage undisturbed. The FDA-approved drugs target these proteins. You've seen the commercials that advertise these drugs. Ipilimumab and Nivolumab are examples. The good news is that in Lussier's (2016) mouse model, KDs appeared to improve immunotherapy by increasing the cytokine proteins and decreasing the checkpoint inhibitory proteins (p. 310).

Did I lose you?

Let's review how immunotherapy works.

CTLA-4 and PD-1 receptors are proteins that sit and wait on the surface of T-cells, just like a security guard. They block their path of communication with other cells. In medical school, they call these proteins 'brakes.' I like to think of CTLA-4 and PD-1 as eye masks for sleeping that prevent T cells from recognizing other T-cells or even cancer cells.

Cancers overuse these checkpoints to their advantage. Too much CTLA-4 or PD-1 will dampen the immune system, making the immune system fail to recognize and kill cancers, which is not good because now the cancer can grow without fear of being attacked.

As a result, the immune system won't be able to jump into action when needed quickly. Anti-cancer drugs block CTLA-4 (i.e., Ipilimumab) and PD-1 (i.e., Nivolumab). The KD has a similar effect, so it makes sense to try the KD with immunotherapy.

Bottom line: The KD mice in Lussier's lab had higher levels of cytokine proteins. Adding the KD can potentially make immunotherapy more effective against brain cancer.

Do KDs have anti-cancer effects on mitochondrial metabolism?

Morscher (2016) investigated the effects of a KD and caloric restriction on neuroblastoma tumor growth (e0129802).

Neuroblastomas are malignant pediatric cancers from special brain cells called neural crest cells. These cells have defective, reduced respiration or mitochondrial oxidative phosphorylation (the defective cell energy 'factory').

In Morscher's study, they injected lab mice with small doses of neuroblastoma cancer cells and randomly separated them into four treatment groups. Each group received an RD, a calorie-restricted standard diet, a KD, or a calorie-restricted KD.

They measured blood glucose, tumor growth, and lifespan and examined the cancer tissue under the microscope to monitor for any effects or changes in the appearance of the cells. (Normal cells are aligned orderly, while cancer cells are in disarray.) They also measured the levels of the mitochondrial enzymes and DNA content.

He found that slow-growing neuroblastomas with low blood glucose had lower Ki-67 scores (higher scores mean actively dividing cells).

Neuroblastoma-carrying mice on the KD and calorie restriction had lower cancer mitochondrial OXPHOS energy, longer lifespans, and reduced tumor growth.

What is the effect of the KD on metabolism?

KDs and insulin growth factor (IGF):

We know insulin as an anti-diabetic drug. But did you know that insulin also regulates cell growth? Some of the early trials on cancer metabolism involved prostate cancer mice models.

Caso (2013) studied one hundred fifty mice, injected them with human prostate cancer cells, and randomly separated them into four groups (p. 449-54). The first group consumed an unrestricted Western diet, the second a *no-carbohydrate ketogenic diet* (NCKD), and the third and fourth groups consumed a 10% carbohydrate or 20% carbohydrate diet. Tumor growth was fastest in those fed the Western diet and the slowest among those fed the 20% carbohydrate diet (Caso, *et al.*, 2013).

Masko (2010) did similar trials but went a bit further by studying the effect of the KD on insulin and insulin signaling pathways (e1124-31).

One hundred sixty male laboratory mice were divided into three different diet groups and fed for four days, followed by injections of human prostate cancer cells. The diet groups comprised a KD, a low-fat diet (LFD), and a Western diet (Masko, *et al.*, 2010).

The NCKD had the following proportions: 84% fat, 0% carbohydrate, and 16% protein. The LFD allowed 12% fat, 72% carbohydrate, and 16% protein. Lastly, the Western diet contained 40% fat, 44% carbohydrate, and 16% protein.

The calories were equal in all three groups, and the mice stayed on their assigned diets for another twenty-four days before receiving prostate cancer cell injections. They euthanized the animals when the tumors reached a specific size (1000 cubic centimeters). Despite being fed equal calories in each group, the NCKD group lost more weight, survived longer, and had tumors that shrank 33% smaller than those from the other groups. The NCKD mice also had better insulin serum levels and lower IGF-1 levels than the Western or LFD groups (Masko, *et al.*, 2010).

Can KDs combined with signaling blockers help fight cancer?

Some breast cancer clinics are currently using Alpelisib (a phosphatidylinositol-3 kinase [PI3K] inhibitor) combined with Letrozole (a hormonal therapy) as a combination therapy to treat metastatic, hormone-positive breast cancers.

Unfortunately, patients develop resistance after some time and may no longer respond to anti-PI3K therapy. Why? The side effects of Apelisib include hyperinsulinemia (high blood insulin levels) and hyperglycemia (high blood glucose). Since glucose feeds cancers and insulin acts as a growth factor, the cancers will use this to their advantage, and before you know it, the drug no longer works (Mayer, *et al.*, 2017).

Hopkins (2018) investigated the reason behind this increase in insulin after exposure to PI3K inhibitors (pp. 499-503). He took mice-bearing implants of pancreatic cancer cells and treated them with PI3K inhibitors, while another group of mice did not receive any drug. After ninety minutes, all the mice went through a PET CT scanner. The mice treated with PI3K inhibitors had brighter-looking tumors (glucose-rich tumors) compared to the non-treated mice (Hopkins, *et al.*, 2018).

He concluded that a spike in blood insulin was the reason behind the higher levels of tumor glucose seen in the tumor. He then thought of a great solution.

Why not treat the insulin spike with a KD plus anti-diabetic drugs?

In a separate group of mice bearing pancreatic cancer grafts, Hopkins tried to add Metformin or an SGLT2 inhibitor to the KD.

He fed one group with a KD, another group with only the anti-diabetic drug Metformin, and a third group received a *sodium-glucose co-transporter* (SGLT2) inhibitor. This anti-diabetic medicine targets the SGLT2 and prevents glucose in the kidney from reabsorbing into the central bloodstream. After ten days, all the mice in all three groups received a PI3K inhibitor, and he compared their subsequent blood glucose levels.

Metformin-treated mice had minimal changes in their blood glucose or insulin levels.

Not surprisingly, the blood glucose and insulin levels were much lower in the KD-fed mice and those treated with SGLT2 inhibitors.

Of all the groups, the KD-fed group had the best response with the lowest glucose and insulin levels. This mouse study showed a positive benefit of using the KD and SGLT2 anti-diabetic drugs for cancer (Hopkins, *et al.*, 2018).

These are fascinating findings. But do these findings apply to humans? Perhaps.

Most of our human cancers do have defective PI3K and defective PTEN (phosphate tensin homolog) proteins.

PI3K is an enzyme protein necessary for maintaining normal cell cycle, growth, and proliferation. When you read scientific journals, you might come across PI3KCA and wonder if this is the same as PI3K protein. Yes, but PI3KCA is only a portion of the entire PI3K protein. PI3K contains the inhibitor (the brakes) and the catalytic subunit (the accelerator) called PI3KCA, standing for *phosphatidylinositol-4,5-bisphosphate 3-kinase catalytic subunit alpha.*

An excellent way to remember this is to think of a car. Cars have brakes and a gas pedal or accelerator. The inhibitor (the brake) and a PI3KCA catalytic subunit (the gas pedal) make up the PI3K protein, which helps move the cell growth cycle along. Defects often are seen in the PI3KCA portion.

The other protein, PTEN (Phosphatase and Tensin Homolog), is a tumor suppressor (anti-cancer). It is a long chain of 403 proteins and works closely with PI3K to control our cells' steady growth.

PTEN and PI3K proteins work together.

But, like a new car, proteins will eventually break down and have defects with time. Because PTEN and PI3K's jobs involve regulating cell growth, defects in PI3K or PTEN may result in uncontrolled growth and, eventually, cancer.

When that happens, cell growth goes out of control. There are now drugs that help block PI3K inhibitors, such as Alpelisib, which are very effective in slowing down cancer growth by blocking the underlying PI3K and PTEN signals.

We know that when we eat something sweet or starchy, our body will sense a rise in blood sugar and release insulin. Insulin helps our body transport that sugar to fuel other body parts.

Insulin connects to and activates PI3K to signal cell growth. The new anti-cancer drugs for blocking PI3K work by counteracting this signal.

Alpelisib is an oral medication that Novartis developed. This drug targets the PI3K cancer signaling pathways and effectively slows cancer growth.

Unfortunately, it has a troublesome side effect: hyperglycemia (high blood glucose). Soon, the doctor stops the drug because the high sugars fuel the cancer, and the treatment is declared a failure.

What is the reason behind the PI3K high sugar side effect?

When we block the insulin signaling pathway, we disrupt glucose metabolism. Glucose levels in the blood drop and cancer cells slow down.

The body senses this potential energy loss from glucose, so it makes up for this by breaking down some of its liver glycogen. Remember, glycogen is a branching network of smaller glucose molecules and serves as stored energy, as portrayed in Figure 9 on page 57. Break it down, and you have lots of smaller glucose molecules.

Insulin-resistant diabetics won't be able to use insulin to push glucose into skeletal muscles or fatty tissue. Their cells don't obey insulin, so glucose has difficulty getting to the cells anyway.

Hence, the glucose has no choice but to hang around in the bloodstream. Within hours of blocking PI3K, we see high blood glucose.

In non-diabetics, this is not a problem because the pancreas will recognize the insulin blockade and come to the rescue by releasing more insulin, which will restore the balance of glucose. People with diabetes, therefore, are more likely to have sustained high blood glucose and, therefore, are more likely to discontinue their cancer therapy.

Relapses occur, possibly because PI3K inhibitors can reactivate the mTOR pathway with time, another tumor signaling pathway.

Blocking mTOR can help make PI3K inhibitor therapies work better. You can block mTOR using Metformin or following a KD (Mayer, *et al.*, 2017). The mouse study, however, did not see any effect of Metformin when combined with PI3K inhibitors. This negative mouse study does not mean Metformin won't work in humans. We need more research.

Side Effects and Side Symptoms:

Can KDs improve cancer-related side effects?

A common negative symptom of cancer and other severe illnesses is cachexia (significant muscle and weight loss).

In a 2018 study, Nakamura studied the animal formula Keto Chow to see if it affected mouse tumor suppression and cachexia (p. 206). He divided a group of mice into three groups: normal diet-fed mice, tumor-bearing mice fed with standard chow, and tumor-bearing mice fed with Keto Chow. All mice ate without set limits on calories. Keto Chow fed tumor mice had smaller tumors but preserved their muscle weight (Nakamura, *et al.*, 2010).

The anti-inflammatory effect of blood ketones appeared to slow cancer growth and preserve muscle mass. As such, the KD may help to prevent cancer cachexia in humans by an anti-inflammatory mechanism.

The Keto Chow fed mice exhibited significantly lower tumor weight and plasma interleukin-6 (IL-6) (tumor-promoting protein) levels than the tumor-bearing normal-fed mice. Also, they preserved their body, muscle, and carcass weights. Keto Chow fed mice also had significantly elevated blood ketone body concentrations. The higher the blood ketones were, then the smaller the tumors became.

The study concluded that a KD may suppress cancer progression and lower the body's level of inflammation. In addition, it may prevent cancer cachexia by stopping cancer without worsening body weight or muscle mass (Nakamura, *et al.*, 2010).

Will KDs stunt growth, and if so, what can we do about it?

Not all studies are optimistic and rosy. One mouse study found growth stunting when animals consumed a commonly used ketogenic rodent chow. In Liskiewicz's 2018 study, young male mice consumed a modified food version, replacing the non-resorbable cellulose component with wheat bran (pp. 203-10). After a month of treatment with the modified wheat version, they measured their body weight and physical and mental performance. The modified chow corrected the emaciation, weakness, and brain undergrowth of the mice previously fed the unmodified chow version. Adding wheat bran helped restore IGF-1 and decreased corticosterone levels without causing ill side effects (Liskiewicz, *et. al.*, 2018).

Chapter Summary/Key Takeaways:

We discussed ways of combining the ketogenic diet with current standard-of-care therapies. In mice, this strategy has proven benefits.

The type of food, oil, anti-diabetic medications, caloric restriction, and timing can improve the ketogenic diet's effectiveness.

We reviewed animal research that combined the ketogenic diet with other therapies to improve cancer therapy efficacy—PI3K inhibitors, mTOR inhibitors, SGLT2 inhibitors, immunotherapies, 2-DG, and radiation.

The next step is to encourage human trials. The knowledge gained from animal research will become an acceptable medical practice backed up by human evidence-based trials.

End Notes

Caso J, Masko EM, Ii JA, Poulton SH, Dewhirst M, Pizzo SV, Freedland SJ. The effect of carbohydrate restriction on prostate cancer tumor growth in a castrate mouse xenograft model. *Prostate.* 2013 Apr;73(5): pp. 449-54. doi: 10.1002/pros.22586. Epub 2012 Oct 4. PMID: 23038057; PMCID: PMC3594433.

Hopkins BD, Pauli C, Du X, Wang DG, Li X, Wu D, Amadiume SC, Goncalves MD, Hodakoski C, Lundquist MR, Bareja R, Ma Y, Harris EM, Sboner A, Beltran H, Rubin MA, Mukherjee S, Cantley LC. Suppression of insulin feedback enhances the efficacy of PI3K inhibitors. *Nature.* 2018 Aug;560(7719): pp. 499-503. doi: 10.1038/s41586-018-0343-4. Epub 2018 Jul 4. Erratum in: Nature. 2018 Aug 29;: PMID: 30051890; PMCID: PMC6197057.

Liśkiewicz AD, Kasprowska-Liśkiewicz D, Sługocka A, Nowacka-Chmielewska MM, Wiaderkiewicz J, Jędrzejowska-Szypułka H, Barski JJ, Lewin-Kowalik J. The modification of the ketogenic diet mitigates its stunting effects in rodents. *Appl Physiol Nutr Metab.* 2018 Feb;43(2): pp. 203-10. doi: 10.1139/apnm-2017-0374. Epub 2017 Oct 18. PMID: 29045796.

Lussier DM, Woolf EC, Johnson JL, Brooks KS, Blattman JN, Scheck AC. Enhanced immunity in a mouse model of malignant glioma is mediated by a therapeutic ketogenic diet. *BMC Cancer.* 2016 May 13;16: p. 310. doi: 10.1186/s12885-016-2337-7. PMID: 27178315; PMCID: PMC4866042.

Masko EM, Thomas JA 2nd, Antonelli JA, Lloyd JC, Phillips TE, Poulton SH, Dewhirst MW, Pizzo SV, Freedland SJ. Low-carbohydrate diets and prostate cancer: how low is "low enough"? *Cancer Prev Res (Phila).* 2010 Sep;3(9): e1124-31. doi: 10.1158/1940-6207.CAPR-10-0071. Epub 2010 Aug 17. PMID: 20716631; PMCID: PMC3757152.

Mayer IA, Abramson VG, Formisano L, Balko JM, Estrada MV, Sanders ME, Juric D, Solit D, Berger MF, Won HH, Li Y, Cantley LC, Winer E, Arteaga CL. A Phase Ib Study of Alpelisib (BYL719), a PI3Kα-Specific Inhibitor, with Letrozole in ER+/HER2- Metastatic Breast Cancer. *Clin Cancer Res.* 2017 Jan 1;23(1): pp. 26-34. doi: 10.1158/1078-0432.CCR-16-0134. Epub 2016 Apr 28. PMID: 27126994; PMCID: PMC5085926.

Morscher RJ, Aminzadeh-Gohari S, Feichtinger RG, Mayr JA, Lang R, Neureiter D, Sperl W, Kofler B. Inhibition of Neuroblastoma Tumor Growth by Ketogenic Diet and/or Calorie Restriction in a CD1-Nu Mouse Model. *PLoS One.* 2015 Jun 8;10(6): e0129802. doi: 10.1371/journal.pone.0129802. PMID: 26053068; PMCID: PMC4459995.

Nakamura K, Tonouchi H, Sasayama A, Ashida K. A Ketogenic Formula Prevents Tumor Progression and Cancer Cachexia by Attenuating Systemic Inflammation in Colon 26 Tumor-Bearing Mice. *Nutrients.* 2018 Feb 14;10(2): p. 206. doi: 10.3390/nu10020206. PMID: 29443873; PMCID: PMC5852782.

Chapter Twenty-Six

Animal Studies III: Ketogenic Diets Plus Complementary Therapies

With contributions by Mariam Shalaby, M.D.

The ketogenic diet (KD) can potentially be a complementary cancer treatment. Animal studies showed that the KD can delay tumor growth when prescribed with other therapies, such as *hyperbaric oxygen therapy* (HBO2T).

Non-Drug Combination Therapies:

Ketogenic diet + Hyperbaric oxygen + Ketone supplements:

A 2013 mouse study investigated the combinatory effects of KD and HBO2T on long-term survival in mice with widespread metastatic cancer. Dr. Poff (2013) studied mice with stage 4 breast cancer and treated them with unlimited calorie KD plus hyperbaric oxygen (e65522). She treated a similar group with the KD only.

They used "firefly luciferase," a bioluminescent imaging substance tagged to cancer cells to measure tumor glucose uptake and growth. Mice received these labeled cancer cells and ate either a standard or an unlimited KD.

Dr. Poff (2013) found that the mice on the KD alone had significantly lowered blood glucose, "slowed tumor growth, and increased mean survival time by 56.7% in mice with systemic metastatic cancer" (e65522).

HBO2T given alone did not affect tumor growth. However, the KD alone improved blood glucose, delayed tumor growth, and improved survival by 56.7%.

With the KD and HBO2T combined, blood glucose dropped, and survival improved by 77.9%!

There was also a significant decrease in "blood glucose, tumor growth rate, and 77.9% increase in mean survival time compared to controls" (Poff, 2013, e65522).

Another study published in 2015 corroborated these findings. Dr. Poff (2015) again studied the KD and HBO2T, but this time around, they added dietary ketone supplements (e0127407).

Like the KD, ketone supplements significantly decreased the tumor cell population and growth. Additionally, this combination therapy increased the stress inside the cancer cells by increasing ROS production of HBO2.

Can calorie restriction and MCT oil improve the ketogenic diet?

Previous studies showed that a KD combined with calorie restriction can slow down tumor growth and enhance the effectiveness of low-dose, oral cyclophosphamide chemotherapy.

In 2017, Aminzadeh-Gohari tried to improve the KD by using additional oils to shrink cancer, hoping to improve the KD without calorie restriction (e64728-44).

Aminzadeh-Gohari studied mice bearing neuroblastoma (pediatric nerve cell cancer) treated with low-dose oral chemotherapy. The mice consumed calorie-restricted KDs containing different levels of MCT oil.

She and her team found that the MCT oil version with eight carbons, in addition to the KD, helped immensely in blocking tumor growth, and the cancer's blood vessel networks became thinner.

They also found increased levels of glutamine, serine, and glycine. This tiny observation of increased glutamine brings a bit of worry. Some cancers use glutamine, and perhaps it is cleverly trying to escape the tumor-starving effects of KDs by boosting glutamine. It might be a good idea then to try glutamine-targeted therapies in addition to KDs and chemotherapy. Doctors call this strategy *multimodal therapy*.

We use multimodality therapy often in oncology. Combining drugs that have different targets might bring a better clinical result.

For example, we might give chemotherapy to directly kill cancer and add an antibody-like *bevacizumab* to target the blood vessels, plus another targeting drug, such as *sorafenib*, to block a signaling pathway.

Can lactate blockade + ketogenic diets help fight cancer?

Dr. Kim (2012) knew lactate levels are high in some cancers, and calorie restriction could help slow tumor growth (e1062-9). Armed with this knowledge, he considered using both techniques in prostate cancer-bearing mice. Dr. Kim wanted to find out whether we can fight cancer better by limiting lactate and glucose, so he injected 120 male mice, six to eight weeks old, with lab-grown prostate cancer cells (Kim, *et al.*, 2012).

He then separated them into four groups. Group One received a Western diet only. Group Two had a Western diet plus a drug lactate blocker. Group Three received a zero-carb diet only. Group Four had a zero-carb diet plus a lactate blocker.

The Western diet was 35% fat, 16% protein, and 49% carbohydrate. The KD was 84% fat, 16% protein, and 0% carbohydrate.

Dr. Kim and his team fed and weighed the mice three times weekly, adjusting the feed to keep the weights steady. Tumor size measurements occurred twice a week.

On day 53, they euthanized all the mice and analyzed tumors and blood.

This experiment showed that simply blocking lactate without restricting carbohydrates (Western diet plus lactate inhibitor) did not shrink tumors but did make the tumors partially necrotic (disintegrate). All the groups on a zero-carb diet had smaller tumors.

Lactate inhibition (blocking) can help fight cancers by changing the arrangement of the tissue surrounding the tumor. Scientists like to call this microscopic tissue the tumor micro-environment.

This finding brings us hope that metabolic therapies targeted at lactate could someday be a part of standard prostate cancer therapy.

Can the ketogenic diet + chemoradiation improve outcomes?

Radiation therapy can increase the levels of stress inside cancers. They turn oxygen molecules into highly reactive chemicals, ROS. Soon, the pressure reaches a level that is enough to kill cancer cells.

KDs can fight cancers by lowering oxidative stress and inflammation. However, when combined with radiation, the KD enhances the radiation effect.

Allen (2013) and his team wanted to confirm this hypothesis, so they injected some mice with lung cancer cells (e3905-13). The mice that developed cancers after the injections received a KD (4:1 ratio of fats: proteins + carbohydrates) and then radiation combined with carboplatin chemotherapy, while another group received radiation only. They measured tumor size, oxidative stress proteins, and fat and searched for signs of DNA damage or abnormal cell proliferation. The mice on KDs and radiation had slower tumors than those on radiation alone (Allen, *et al.*, 2013).

The radiation plus KD-fed mice probably had increased internal oxidative stress, which KD helped enhance and delay their growth. The KD made the radiation more effective in killing tumors.

What is the data on the ketogenic diet + 2 deoxyglucose?

2-Deoxy-D-glucose (2-DG) is a potent anti-cancer research drug. It can fight glucose-hungry cancers by acting as a glucose analog (imposter) and cannot undergo normal glucose metabolism; therefore, it is useless as an energy source. 2-DG can imitate the effects of fasting by inhibiting glycolysis.

Marsh (2008) studied the effect of a KD in combination with the non-metabolizable glucose analog, 2-DG (p. 33). He separated adult mice injected with astrocytoma brain cancer into four groups. One group ate an unrestricted Western diet; the second group ate a Western diet plus the 2-DG drug for ten days. The third group followed a restricted KD only. The fourth followed a restricted KD plus the 2-DG medication for ten days. The most tumor shrinkage was in the mouse on the restricted KD plus the 2-DG, which was better than the KD alone. The restricted KD plus 2-DG is very potent (Marsh, *et al.*, 2008).

Are there any harmful effects of the ketogenic diet?

While many of the previously discussed articles exhibited positive KD results, some studies have shown adverse effects on cancer. Research results by Xia (2017) suggest that a KD might worsen cancer depending on a patient's particular oncogene mutation (pp. 358-73).

Xia (2017) also reported that acetoacetate, a ketone body, worsens cancers that possess the BRAF V600E mutation (pp. 358-73). This mutation activates the MET pro-cancer signaling pathway, and they found that the KD causes a rise in acetoacetate ketones, which resulted in an increased "tumor growth potential of" human melanoma cells that expressed BRAF V600E in mice (Xia, *et al.*, 2017).

After discovering the tumor growth, they treated one group of mice with fat-lowering medication to lower the circulating acetoacetate serum. This helped slow down the cancer (Xia, *et al.*, 2017).

In all, Xia (2017) concluded that ketones appeared to fuel cancer in these cancers with BRAF V600E tumors, but dietary fat also boosted melanoma cancer signals (pp. 358-73). Adding an anti-cholesterol-lowering drug helped limit growth.

When can the ketogenic diet be ineffective?

Sometimes, we don't see benefits even when following the KD correctly.

The KD might be ineffective with continued obesity.

Many studies examined the KD's role in obesity-associated tumor development.

In a study published in 2017, Allott studied obese mice with prostate cancer (pp. 165-71). Their research showed that carbohydrate and calorie restriction delayed tumor growth in earlier prostate cancer mouse models. They divided 5-week-old mice into two groups: 44 mice were assigned to the unlimited KD (1% carbohydrate, 82% fat) and 39 mice to the Western diet (42% carbohydrate and 40% fat). The mice were euthanized at age 3 or 6 months, and they examined the prostate's weights and microscopic features of malignancy (Allott, *et al.*, 2017).

Remember, all the mice ate unlimited amounts of their assigned diets.

The ketogenic mice ate a lot more calories and, as a result, were significantly heavier at six months compared to the Western diet mice (45g versus 38g). Too many calories can still increase weight, even on a KD.

Despite the heavier weights, the prostate tissue had fewer inflammation features and was smaller at 3 and 6 months. Tumor-related signaling protein levels were also lower in the ketogenic mice's prostates than in the Western diet mice. Sounds encouraging.

But, after six months, the KD mice had more cancers (100% vs. 80%, P=0.04) than the Western diet mice.

The study observed that mice fed KDs with unlimited calorie intake had higher body weights. The carbohydrate restriction decreased obesity-related inflammation and prostate weight, but persistent obesity might be a reason behind KD's failure to prevent cancer (Allott, *et al.*, 2017).

Liśkiewicz (2016) studied the effect of a 4, 6, and 8-month KD on renal tuberous sclerosis tumors in Eker rats (Tsc2+/-) (e 21807). They found prolonged KD feeding resulted in oleic acid accumulation, growth hormone overproduction, and increased mTOR and ERK ½ signaling (mTOR and ERK are pro-cancer signals), ultimately causing tumor growth. The KD also promoted a parallel increase in anti-tumor mechanisms, which, unfortunately, were overcome by the simultaneous pro-tumor effects. Despite the anti-tumor benefits of the KD in this rat study, the tumors failed, and the authors noted that the reason could be the observed parallel increase in mTOR signaling. Whether the KD caused this mTOR and ERK signaling is still subject to further research (Liśkiewicz, *et al.*, 2016).

While many studies show the benefits of KDs on cancers, there are some (melanoma BRAFV600, tuberous sclerosis—a type of kidney cancer—lung, and some prostate cancer studies) that show that cancers may grow while under a KD. Remember that these studies were done in cancer cell lines and animal studies. We need more repeated studies done and have human ones before we can draw any firm conclusions.

Chapter Summary/Key Takeaways:

We had a glimpse into early ketogenic diet trials and cancer.

Cancer patients benefit from the ketogenic diet by slowing down tumor growth, decreasing blood glucose, boosting the immune system, preventing muscle wasting, increasing survival, and blocking cancer signaling pathways.

The type of food, oil, anti-diabetic medications, caloric restriction, and timing can improve the ketogenic diet's effectiveness.

We discussed combining the ketogenic diet with other therapies to improve cancer therapy efficacy, such as PI3K inhibitors, mTOR inhibitors, SGLT2 inhibitors, immunotherapies, 2-DG, and radiation. We also discussed hyperbaric oxygen therapy and ketone supplements. The ketogenic diet alone is beneficial. There is some benefit to the combination of the ketogenic diet with hyperbaric oxygen and ketone supplements.

Ketogenic diets, taken liberally and without calorie restriction, improve inflammation but may lead to weight gain. Persistent obesity can influence the ketogenic diet's ability to enhance tumor outcomes.

Progress is painfully slow, and past research is often forgotten. However, interest in ketogenic diets and cancers is reemerging.

Animal studies are all preliminary, so we can only use the information presented to make real-life medical decisions once confirmed by high-quality human research.

End Notes

Allen BG, Bhatia SK, Buatti JM, Brandt KE, Lindholm KE, Button AM, Szweda LI, Smith BJ, Spitz DR, Fath MA. Ketogenic diets enhance oxidative stress and radio-chemo-therapy responses in lung cancer xenografts. *Clin Cancer Res.* 2013 Jul 15;19(14): e3905-13. doi: 10.1158/1078-0432.CCR-12-0287. Epub 2013 Jun 6. PMID: 23743570; PMCID: PMC3954599.

Allott EH, Macias E, Sanders S, Knudsen BS, Thomas GV, Hursting SD, Freedland SJ. Impact of carbohydrate restriction in the context of obesity on prostate tumor growth in the Hi-Myc transgenic mouse model. *Prostate Cancer Prostatic Dis.* 2017 Jun;20(2): pp. 165-171. doi: 10.1038/pcan.2016.73. Epub 2017 Feb 28. PMID: 28244492; PMCID: PMC5429178.

Aminzadeh-Gohari S, Feichtinger RG, Vidali S, Locker F, Rutherford T, O'Donnel M, Stöger-Kleiber A, Mayr JA, Sperl W, Kofler B. A ketogenic diet supplemented with medium-chain triglycerides enhances the anti-tumor and anti-angiogenic efficacy of chemotherapy on neuroblastoma xenografts in a CD1-nu mouse model. *Oncotarget.* 2017 Aug 8;8(39): e64728-44. doi: 10.18632/oncotarget.20041. PMID: 29029389; PMCID: PMC5630289.

Kim HS, Masko EM, Poulton SL, Kennedy KM, Pizzo SV, Dewhirst MW, Freedland SJ. Carbohydrate restriction and lactate transporter inhibition in a mouse xenograft model of human prostate cancer. *BJU Int.* 2012 Oct;110(7): e1062-9. doi: 10.1111/j.1464-410X.2012.10971.x. Epub 2012 Mar 6. PMID: 22394625; PMCID: PMC3371292.

Liśkiewicz AD, Kasprowska D, Wojakowska A, Polański K, Lewin-Kowalik J, Kotulska K, Jędrzejowska-Szypułka H. Long-term High Fat Ketogenic Diet Promotes Renal Tumor Growth in a Rat Model of Tuberous Sclerosis. *Sci Rep.* 2016 Feb 19;6: e21807. doi: 10.1038/srep21807. PMID: 26892894; PMCID: PMC4759602.

Marsh J, Mukherjee P, Seyfried TN. Drug/diet synergy for managing malignant astrocytoma in mice: 2-deoxy-D-glucose and the restricted ketogenic diet. *Nutr Metab (Lond).* 2008 Nov 25;5: p. 33. doi: 10.1186/1743-7075-5-33. PMID: 19032781; PMCID: PMC2607273.

Poff AM, Ari C, Seyfried TN, D'Agostino DP. The ketogenic diet and hyperbaric oxygen therapy prolong survival in mice with systemic metastatic cancer. *PLoS One.* 2013 Jun 5;8(6): e65522. doi: 10.1371/journal.pone.0065522. PMID: 23755243; PMCID: PMC3673985.

Poff AM, Ward N, Seyfried TN, Arnold P, D'Agostino DP. Non-Toxic Metabolic Management of Metastatic Cancer in VM Mice: Novel Combination of Ketogenic Diet, Ketone Supplementation, and Hyperbaric Oxygen Therapy. *PLoS One.* 2015 Jun 10;10(6): e0127407. doi: 10.1371/journal.pone.0127407. PMID: 26061868; PMCID: PMC4464523.

Xia S, Lin R, Jin L, Zhao L, Kang HB, Pan Y, Liu S, Qian G, Qian Z, Konstantakou E, Zhang B, Dong JT, Chung YR, Abdel-Wahab O, Merghoub T, Zhou L, Kudchadkar RR, Lawson DH, Khoury HJ, Khuri FR, Boise LH, Lonial S, Lee BH, Pollack BP, Arbiser JL, Fan J, Lei QY, Chen J. Prevention of Dietary-Fat-Fueled Ketogenesis Attenuates BRAF V600E Tumor Growth. *Cell Metab.* 2017 Feb 7;25(2): pp. 358-73. doi: 10.1016/j.cmet.2016.12.010. Epub 2017 Jan 12. PMID: 28089569; PMCID: PMC5299059.

Chapter Twenty-Seven

Ketogenic Diet Human Trials

With contributions by Christine A. Garcia, M.D., MPH

Only a handful of human trials have studied the role of ketogenic diets (KDs) in cancer. Between 1902 and 1957, only a few papers in the medical world adequately covered this subject. Most early studies and case reports involving the KD in human cancer focused on brain tumors (Schwartz, *et al.*, 2015; Winter, *et al.*, 2017; Van der Louw, *et al.*, 2019). Human studies using KDs in other types of cancers were limited to small, non-randomized, brief trials (4-12 weeks) or single case studies (Schwartz, *et al.*, 2015; Maroon, *et al.*, 2013) (see Table 1 on page 406). Many of these studies were small safety trials, partly due to poor patient accrual and lack of standardization. Some trials were based outside the United States. Earlier trials involved patients with different tumor types (Schmidt, *et al.*, 2011; Tan-Shalaby, *et al.*, 2016; Fine, *et al.*, 2012), whereas others have attempted only to study specific tumors (Rieger, *et al.*, 2014; Champ & Klement, 2015).

Table 1:

Low-Carbohydrate Pilot Safety and Tolerability Trials

Abbreviations: ERGO, ketogenic diet for recurrent glioblastoma; RECHARGE, Reduced Carbohydrates Against Resistant Growth Tumor.

Trial	Diet Duration	Patients Enrolled, n	Patients Tolerated Diet, n	Patients That Quit Early or Unable to Diet Due to Poor Health, n	Early Deaths, n	Stable Disease, n	Progressive Disease, n	Partial Response, n	Adverse Effects	Comments
RECHARGE: Fine and colleagues	4 wk	10 Breast Ovarian/ fallopian Colorectal Lung Esophageal	5	5	0	5 (4 wk)	4	1	Mean weight loss: 4.1% ($P = .45$) No adverse effects	Modified Atkins diet: 20 carbohydrate g/d Unlimited protein 2 cups of vegetables per day Ketosis correlated with standardized uptake value on positron emission tomography–computed tomography Stable disease correlated to 3-fold ketosis ($P = .018$)
ERGO: Rieger and colleagues	Until progression	20 Relapsed glioblastoma	17	3 Poor intake	0	0	17 1 minor response 2 patients with stable disease (6 wk)	Seen only after salvage chemotherapy with or without radiation 8 patients total received salvage 1 complete response 5 partial responses	Mean weight loss: 2.2% (statistically significant) 2 patients had grade 3 leucopenia No other grade 3 adverse effects	60 carbohydrate g/d Low-carbohydrate diet and plant oils Unlimited calories Primary endpoint: % discontinuation of diet Secondary endpoints: safety, % achieving ketosis, quality of life 8 of the 17 patients with progressive disease underwent salvage chemotherapy and dietary changes, which resulted in 5 partial responses and 1 complete response Median overall survival with diet: 32 wk Median progression-free survival: 5 wk
Wuerzburg study: Schmidt and colleagues	5–12 wk	16 Utero-ovarian Breast Parotid Sarcoma Pancreas Thyroid Colon Lung	5 (12 wk) 2 (6 wk) 2 (7 wk) 2 (8 wk) 1 (5 wk) 1 (4 wk) 3 (2 wk)	3	2	5	6	0	Mean weight loss: 2.9% ($P < .05$) No adverse effects	Stable lipid and cholesterol profile 70 carbohydrate g/d Low-carbohydrate diet Oil-protein shakes as snacks
VA Pittsburgh safety trial: Tan and colleagues	4–116 wk	17	12 (≥ 2 wk) 11 (≥ 4 wk) 6 (≥ 8 wk) 4 (≥ 16 wk)	6 Screen failures	0	6 (4 wk) 6 (8 wk) 4 (16 wk)	5 (4 wk) 1 voluntary withdrawal (8 wk)	2 mixed responses (16 wk) 1 no evidence of disease status postmetastectomy	Mean weight loss: 8% ($P < .0001$) 8 patients had grade 3 weight loss	Modified Atkins diet: 20–40 carbohydrate g/d Primary endpoints: safety and feasibility Quality of life unchanged Ketosis did not correlate with glucose or weight loss

Reproduced with Permission of Federal Practitioner. Modified Format. • Fed Pract. 2017 February; 34(supp 1):37S-42S | doi:10.12788/fp.0457, & Author: Jocelyn Tan-Shalaby, M. (2024, January 18). *Ketogenic diets and cancer: Emerging evidence*. Federal Practitioner. https://www.mdedge.com/fedprac/article/151962/oncology/ketogenic-diets-and-cancer-emerging-evidence

Only a handful of clinical trials ever reported on the effect of a KD on a cancer patient's tumor response and survival. These studies are summarized in the next section for each tumor type. Each trial may have an NCT identifier number to help you search for it within the clinical trials website.

Relapsed brain cancers – KD + chemotherapy + radiation:

The 2014 ERGO trial (NCT00575146) was an open-label, prospective, single-arm pilot feasibility study of twenty recurrent glioblastoma (brain cancer) patients. Rieger (2014) had recurrent glioblastoma patients treated with salvage chemotherapy and radiation, followed by an unrestricted KD (e2605). The diet was low in carbohydrates and supplemented with plant oils. They did not include patients with diabetes on insulin treatment or those with poor heart function (Rieger, *et al.*, 2014).

Three of twenty patients discontinued the diet early (2-3 weeks) because they felt their quality of life worsened. The remaining seventeen patients quickly followed the diet and had no severe side effects. Collectively, they lost 2.2% of their body weight, which was small but statistically significant. It was easy to reach ketosis. Of twelve urine ketone-positive patients, 73% had stable ketosis (Rieger, *et al.*, 2014).

After six weeks, three patients had stable disease, one patient had a minor response, and eight had worsening tumors and received more treatment—ACNU/teniposide (n=1), bevacizumab alone (n=4), or bevacizumab + irinotecan (n=3)—all while continuing the diet. The overall response rate was 85% (one complete response, five partial responses). On average, those on *bevacizumab* survived without disease for 20.1 weeks (12-124 weeks). At six months, 43% were still cancer-free. Rieger (2014) compared the *bevacizumab* + ketogenic diet group to a similar group of twenty-eight patients who were on *bevacizumab* only (no diet, six months PFS =16.1 weeks) and found no significant difference between the two (p=0.38) (e1843-52).

Newly diagnosed brain cancers – KD + chemotherapy + radiation:

Champ (2015) published the results of a retrospective cohort study of newly diagnosed glioblastoma multiforme (GBM) patients (pp. 281-2). He wanted to see if adding a KD to their radiation and chemotherapy would decrease serum glucose levels while raising ketones. Seven patients had an unrestricted regular diet (RD), while six underwent the KD during treatment. After 14 months, four of the KD patients were still alive. One patient had fatigue, but no serious adverse effects were seen, including hypoglycemia (low blood glucose). Patients on the KD had average glucose levels of 84 mg/dl, while those on the RD had 122 mg/dl. Despite being on high-dose steroids, the KD significantly reduced serum glucose levels in patients with GBM (Champ & Klement, 2015).

A single case of glioblastoma – KD + oral chemotherapy:

The case of a 65-year-old female with GBM demonstrated radiographic shrinkage after treatment with *temozolomide* oral chemotherapy along with the KD (Zuccoli, *et al.*, 2010). The patient tapered off her steroids before the KD + chemotherapy treatment. She discontinued the diet after a year and began *bevacizumab* therapy (anti-blood vessel targeted therapy). However, the disease worsened, resulting in the patient's death (Zuccoli, *et al.*, 2010).

Glioblastoma case – KD + fasting + surgery + chemotherapy + radiation:

Elsakka (2018) from the University of Alexandria in Egypt published a case report that described the 24-month follow-up of a 38-year-old male patient with glioblastoma (p. 33). Their patient complained of headaches, nausea, and vomiting. His left upper arm became weak, and he developed partial motor seizures. Treatment began with a 72-hour water-only fast, followed by surgical removal and chemotherapy. After the fast, he switched to a 900 kilocalorie KD. The calorie content gradually increased until he reached 1500 kilocalories in the following weeks.

In addition, he received the anti-diabetic drug *metformin* at 1,000 mg daily dose and *temozolomide* chemotherapy plus radiation. He took multiple supplements, including *chloroquine* (anti-malaria drug), *epigallocatechin* (green tea extract), and *methylfolate* (folic acid derivative drug). He also underwent weekly hour-long HBO2T sessions. When they surgically removed the remaining tumor, they found evidence of decreased tumor invasiveness and hyalinized blood vessels (degenerating blood vessels), suggesting tumor response (Elsakka, *et al.*, 2018). He was symptom-free 24 months later.

Ketogenic metabolic therapy, without chemo or radiation:

In 2014, a 32-year-old male with GBM and an IDH (isocitrate dehydrogenase) mutation followed a KD after he refused chemotherapy or radiation. His diet consisted mostly of saturated fats, some vegetables, and various meats. He maintained low *glucose ketone index* (GKI) values near 2.0 without much weight loss. His tumor grew slowly until it needed repeat surgery in 2017. He continued the KD and was in ketosis after the surgery. He maintained complete remission up to eighty months after 'debulking' and enjoyed a good quality of life, seizure-free. A therapeutic metabolic synergy between the IDH mutation and the KD was felt responsible for his medical success (Seyfried, *et al.*, 2021).

Review article – 32 gliomas – KD + standard therapies:

Schwartz and colleagues (2018) published a review of 32 glioma patients—5 from case reports, 19 from a clinical trial by Rieger (2014) and colleagues, and eight from Champ and Klemen (2012). All but one patient consumed energy-restricted KD combined with some standard therapy. Schwartz (2018) also reported on 2 of their glioma cases treated with the energy-restricted KD and studied tissues for expression of crucial ketolytic enzymes (p. 11). Unfortunately, these two glioma cases developed worsening tumors while on the energy-restricted diet, which they believe is related to the positive mitochondrial ketolytic enzyme expressions seen in their tissue samples.

Overall, they observed prolonged remission ranging from four months to more than five years amongst all observed patients (Rieger, *et al.*, 2014; Champ & Klement, 2015; Schwartz *et al.*, 2018; Chang, *et al.*, 2013).

Pediatric case series:

Van der Louw (2019) attempted to study the KD in pediatric patients with pontine glioma (p. e27561). They could only recruit three patients out of fourteen referred to them. Out of the three, two completed the study with minimal side effects. One died before completion. It was a small study, and conclusions regarding survival could not be made (Van der Louw, *et al.*, 2019).

Melanoma and female reproductive cancers – insulin therapy:

In 1962, Dr. S. Koroljow from the New York Department of Mental Hygiene published an article about two women admitted for depression, whose metastatic cancers disappeared after a series of daily treatments with insulin (pp. 261-70). These patients did not undergo conventional electric shock therapy due to safety concerns about their coexisting cancers. Instead, they received medically induced (insulin) psychotherapy.

The first patient was a 53-year-old female with cervical cancer metastasizing to her abdomen's lymph nodes. A biopsy confirmed her diagnosis. When doctors attempted surgery, they aborted the procedure when they opened her abdominal cavity and saw that the cancer had spread widely. She had no appetite, lost 24 pounds, and was sent to psychiatry for marked depression. Doctors began ambulatory insulin treatment, which put her into a sub-comatose state. Her depression cleared almost entirely after four weeks.

At that point, she regained her appetite, gained weight, and had improved energy. Several months later, her surgeon could not find any evidence of malignancy. She was alive and well a year after insulin therapy (Koroljow, 1962).

The second case was a 62-year-old woman with melanoma of the left leg that had metastasized to the inguinal region. She became depressed and suicidal over her diagnosis and was emaciated when referred to psychiatry for treatment. Her doctors started her on insulin therapy, and by the fourth week, her depression disappeared. Her tumor and symptoms were gone by the fifteenth week, and she returned to her regular employment a year later (Koroljow, 1962).

Her doctors felt that the hypoglycemic (extremely low blood sugar) coma caused a significant and unopposed increase in venous blood and tissue oxygen concentration, thereby increasing tissue fluid pH (alkaline). The resulting alkalosis and low blood glucose levels produced a particularly unfavorable environment for certain cellular enzymes. The malignant cells may be more sensitive to those biochemical changes than normal cells, thus suffering selective destruction (Koroljow, 1962).

Low blood glucose and acid-base imbalance caused by insulin therapy have a potent anticancer effect. Before attempting this in clinical practice, this observation deserves further investigation in clinical trials.

Randomized trial – female cancers – KD vs ACS diet:

More recently, Cohen (2018a) recruited 73 women with

endometrial (uterine) or ovarian cancers (e1253-60).

After randomly separating them into two groups, one group received a KD of 70% fat, 25% protein, and 5% carbohydrates. In contrast, the other received the American Cancer Society (ACS) diet (low fat, high fiber).

They measured baseline and 12-week values of serum glucose, insulin, C-peptide, IGF-1, IGFBP-1, and the ketone β-hydroxybutyrate. In both groups, the dropout rate was similar (32% KD vs 33% ACS diet).

Ketosis was easy to reach in the KD group. The trial measured urine ketones and set a goal of 0.5 mmol/L as their minimum target. Within three weeks, 80% of the participants (20 out of 25) achieved this 0.5 mmol/L urine ketone goal.

The KD group made more significant amounts of ketones and higher serum β-hydroxybutyrate (ketone) levels than the ACS group. Fat loss was also more significant in the KD group. After twelve weeks, the KD group lost 21.2% of their visceral (internal body) fat, a 21% loss compared to the ACS group, which only lost 4.6% of body fat. More fat breakdown led to lower insulin and higher ketones in the blood.

Higher β-hydroxybutyrate ketones also meant lower IGF-1 levels,.which is good for fighting cancer.

After 12 weeks, the KD patients had fewer food cravings, were less tired, and had a better quality of life (Cohen, *et al.*, 2018b).

Cancers of the digestive system:

Pancreatic cancer trial – KD + chemotherapy + radiation:

Zahra (2017) reported on the results of a Phase 1 clinical trial, KETOPAN (NCT01419483), run by researchers at the University of Iowa (pp. 743-54.). KETOPAN was a tiny trial where two pancreatic cancer patients consumed the KD while undergoing chemotherapy plus radiation over three years. All meals prepared in the metabolic kitchen provided a 4:1 ratio of fat grams to grams of protein + carbohydrate (90% of calories from fat, 8% from protein, and 2% from carbohydrates). The subjects used Nutricia's Ketocal 4:1 supplement. This study ended early due to poor recruitment. Only two patients joined the trial, one of whom completed the study with suboptimal compliance with the diet. At the same time, the other withdrew because of a dose-limiting toxicity. It certainly did not end well. We, therefore, cannot draw any conclusions based on such small numbers (Zahra, *et al.*, 2017).

High-fat formula vs high-dextrose

A tiny 27-patient study of patients with gastrointestinal cancers compared a high-fat (80% calories from fat) against a high-sugar (100% calories from dextrose) diet (Rossi-Fanelli, *et al.*, 1991). The patients received their food intravenously. After two weeks, there was decreased cell proliferation in the high-fat group, but the drop was insignificant. There were no differences in glucose levels between the two groups. Nice try. This negative study doesn't mean that the KD doesn't work. We need more trials.

Randomized trial of colon cancer – KD modified + chemotherapy

During the 2018 American Society of Clinical Oncology Conference, an abstract (e15709) by Furukawa and colleagues was presented. They reported on ten Stage IV recurrent colon cancer patients who received chemotherapy plus a modified MCT ketogenic diet (MCTKD). The comparison group included fourteen patients with Stage IV colon cancer on a standard diet plus chemotherapy. The body weights and serum albumin were not significantly different between the two groups. Still, the blood levels of ketones were considerably higher in the KD group. The group that received chemotherapy and the modified MCTKD had more tumor shrinkage than the group on the standard diet. Standard dieters had a 21% response rate compared to a 60% response rate in the ketogenic dieters (Furukawa, *et al.*, 2019).

Stage four colon cancers that relapse after first-line treatment usually respond poorly to a second attempt at chemotherapy. This trial showed that adding the KD to second-line chemotherapy dramatically resulted in more tumor shrinkage the second time around.

Hematologic malignancies (blood cancers):

Research on blood cancers and the KD are few, if any.

Dr. Tan (2018) recently reported on three lymphoma patients who limited their diets to a daily carbohydrate intake of 20-40 grams and gave up sweets and starches (e24222). The study included details of their history, dietary, and clinical outcomes. All patients tolerated the diet well and had varying degrees of weight loss. Two of the four patients remained disease-free after two years (Tan-Shalaby, *et al.*, 2018).

Breast Cancer – KD + HT + HBOT + insulin + surgery + chemotherapy:

The reasons behind the anticancer effects of hyperthermia and hyperbaric oxygen (HBO) are unclear. Hyperthermia can cause mitochondrial uncoupling, and hyperbaric oxygen (HBO) can help improve tumors' hypoxia. The KD plus insulin therapy can dramatically drop glucose levels to starve cancers of energy. The ketosis can feed and protect the brain against the effects of low blood glucose or hypoglycemia. This approach of using several metabolic therapies is considered aggressive but effective. It does need further attention and investigation.

Iyikesici (2017) reports a case from Turkey that describes an overweight 29-year-old female diagnosed with metastatic, triple-negative (estrogen receptor-negative, progesterone receptor-negative, and HER2-negative) invasive ductal carcinoma of the breast with liver and lymph node involvement (e1445). She received a combination of standard chemotherapy, KD, hyperthermia therapy (HT), and HBOT with subsequent mastectomy. She received chemotherapy after a 12-hour fast and 5 to 10 units of insulin. A year and a half after her initial diagnosis, she still enjoyed a complete remission (Lyikesici, *et al.*, 2017).

These results are very encouraging. More clinical trials are required to investigate the effect of combined metabolic treatments.

Non-small cell lung cancer + KD + Keto Cal:

Can supplemental ketogenic shakes help patients follow the KD successfully? Zahra (2017) from The University of Iowa recruited patients into a Phase 1 study of the KD using Nutricia KetoCal 4:1 as a supplement in NSCLC patients (KETOLUNG, NCT01419587) (pp. 743-54). Seven non-small cell lung cancer patients enrolled. Of the seven, four patients with locally advanced NSCLC could not comply with the diet and withdrew. Two completed the study. The two who conducted the study had suboptimal compliance. Due to the small sample size, no conclusions were drawn from this study (Zahra, *et al.*, 2017).

Miscellaneous metastatic tumors: pilot KD studies

Schmidt (2011) ran an early pilot study that looked at the safety of a KD by studying sixteen patients with advanced metastatic cancers who followed a KD (limited to 70 g carbs daily) for three months (p. 54). She included ovarian, breast, colon, granulosa, osteosarcoma, esophageal, parotid, pancreatic, thyroid, colon, endometrial, lung, and stomach cancers. Oil-protein shakes were allowed, and urine ketones were measured.

Five of 16 patients dieted for three months, and seven dieted for at least five weeks, while two died during the trial. There was significant weight loss but no severe side effects or events. Quality of life improved. LDL cholesterol (bad) dropped significantly while total cholesterol and white blood cell counts increased. An insulin-requiring diabetic required 75% less insulin while in the study. The quality-of-life questionnaire scores showed a slight improvement in emotional functioning and a slight worsening of physical functioning. There was fatigue, which was temporary, but insomnia improved (Schmidt, *et al.*, 2011).

This early study of a KD in advanced cancers showed mixed results. There was significant weight loss and increased premature fatigue. Still, there were also improvements in cholesterol, glucose blood levels, sleep quality, and emotional functioning. Overall, the patients tolerated the KD well.

Solid cancers and four weeks of modified Atkins diet:

Fine (2012) conducted a pioneering trial that placed advanced cancer patients on the modified Atkins diet (MAD) and measured responses via PET CT scans (e1028-35). This study offered MAD (≤ 20 g of carbohydrates daily) to advanced solid cancer patients with a PET scan. Positive means a PET scan that reveals tumors with high glucose uptake. When blood ketones reached 3-fold higher levels, the PET CT scans recorded stable disease. There was no correlation between caloric restriction and weight loss in patients with worsening illness (Fine, *et al.*, 2012).

The SUV scores of the PET scan were high (bright) with more elevated ketones, but the brightness of the scans did not follow any disease worsening. It's a very early study with small numbers of patients. Although the diet appeared safe in this group of patients, we cannot draw any conclusions based on such a small study.

Brain cancers – surgery + modified ketogenic diet +/– MCT oil:

The KEATING trial (clinicaltrials.gov reference number: NCT03075514) was a single-center pilot study that recruited twelve glioblastoma patients. This trial wanted to see how easy and safe it is for brain cancer patients to follow the diet successfully after surgery (Martin-McGill, *et al.*, 2020).

All patients previously underwent surgery to remove their tumors. They were randomly assigned 1:1 to a modified ketogenic diet (MKD) versus an MCTKD. Twelve weeks after starting the diet, the researchers measured ketone levels, glucose, and the number of dropouts. The primary outcome measured was the three-month retention rate. Recruitment was low at 28.6%, and retention needed improvement, with only 4 out of the 12 patients completing the trial at three months. Caretakers also influenced the participants' decision-making and retention.

Ongoing and terminated clinical trials:

The following trials are a compilation of current and past trials. We have listed them in no specific order. The NCT refers to the reference number, which you will need to locate the trial under www.clinicaltrials.gov.

1. **Central nervous system tumors:**

NCT01092247

Tel Aviv Sourasky Medical Center in Israel is

recruiting patients with high-grade glial tumors previously treated with chemoradiation to see whether the KD effectively prevents recurrence. This trial was posted in 2010 but needs its status updated.

NCT02046187

St. Joseph's Hospital and Medical Center (Phoenix, AZ) recruited newly diagnosed glioblastoma patients for a Phase 1/2 prospective trial involving upfront resection followed by KD with radiotherapy and concurrent *temozolomide*, followed by adjuvant *temozolomide* chemotherapy. The primary endpoint was the number of patients with adverse events, and the secondary endpoints were overall survival, time to progression, and quality of life. Unfortunately, this trial was terminated early due to excessive protocol deviations. The researchers felt the strict nature of the diet requirements was partly responsible for the poor compliance.

NCT03328858

Nicklaus Children's Hospital (Miami Children's Hospital) was recruiting patients for a Phase 2 study to evaluate the effect of KD on tumor size and quality of life in pediatric patients with malignant or recurrent/ refractory brain tumors. The trial was first posted on clinicaltrials.gov on November 1, 2017, but was terminated due to the loss of its principal investigator. The trial recruited two patients, both lost to follow-up.

The last update was in February 2020.

2. **Uterine/endometrial cancer (NCT03285152):**

Memorial Sloan Kettering, in collaboration with the Weill Medical College of Cornell University, is recruiting 30 patients for a prospective, multicenter, randomized, feasibility pilot study of the ketogenic diet (KD) vs. standard diet (SD) in treatment for naïve, newly diagnosed, overweight, or obese endometrial cancer patients. The timing of the diet will occur during the presurgical window period between diagnosis and surgical staging. Thirty patients are targeted for enrollment. The KD cohort will receive a rotating 7-day meal plan prepared by the Clinical Translational Science Center (CTSC) at Weill Cornell Medical Center (WCMC) with weekly food pick-up. The meal plan will provide a 3:1 fat-to-net carbohydrate ratio and calories for weight maintenance (30 kcals/kg for a BMI < 30kg/m2 and 25 kcal/kg for a BMI 30kg/m2). Investigators plan to measure markers of inflammation, glucose, insulin, and cholesterol in blood, urine, and endometrial tissue from the surgical sample. All will be examined for genetic and metabolic markers. As of October 1, 2023, the trial is still active but no longer recruiting.

3. **Breast cancer (NCT03962647):**

The Vanderbilt-Ingram Cancer Center recruited 30 patients with early-stage, ER-positive (estrogen receptor) breast cancer to test the feasibility of a 2-week KD combined with hormone therapy before surgery. Their secondary goal is to determine whether the KD and hormone therapy will reduce insulin pathway signaling and inhibit breast cancer cell proliferation. Ki-67 markers (a measure of cell division) will be recorded, in addition to weight, body composition, and changes in insulin resistance. Meal replacement shakes will be available. Hormonal therapy of *letrozole* 2.5 mg daily will be offered as standard care treatment. The study began in July 2019 and is active as of February 2023.

4. **KETO-CARE (NCT03535701):**

   Twenty women were enrolled in a six-month KD program. The women were closely supervised and provided with KD meals during the first three months. They then underwent nutritional coaching and transitioned to a self-administered KD for three months.

   Trial results were published in January of 2024. They showed that after three months, 15 out of 20 women achieved nutritional ketosis, a 10% body fat weight loss, and a significant decrease in insulin resistance, plasma insulin, and fasting plasma glucose. These benefits persisted as long as six months later.

5. **Comparison of healthy diets on breast cancer markers: KetoBreast (NCT02744079)**

Dr. Fine of the Albert Einstein College of Medicine recently completed this study, which recruited women with biopsy-proven breast cancer. The biopsies will have shown cancer that was either estrogen receptor-positive or negative. Forty-five women followed a ketogenic (insulin-inhibiting), low-carbohydrate diet (LCD), and twenty patients followed the low-fat diet (LFD) with whole grains, fruits, and vegetables. Before and after initiation of the diets, a biopsy will compare changes in proliferation (Ki-67) and apoptosis biomarkers (TUNEL). Results nor publications were not available at the time of this writing.

6. **Digestive tract cancers:**

NCT03510429 (Ketogenic Plus)

Yonsei University is recruiting for a clinical trial to validate nutritional supplements ("Ketogenic Plus") clinically developed for pancreaticobiliary cancer patients. These patients were chosen because pancreaticobiliary surgery can cause a profound decrease in bowel function and loss of appetite postoperatively. The drink "Ketogenic Plus" contains a "beefsteak mint" flavor. The goal is to see if the addition of a nutritional supplement will increase food intake and improve perioperative outcomes, including improvement of oncologic outcomes.

NCT04631445

In collaboration with the Translational Genomics Research Institute, a study sponsored by the Translational Drug Development group launched the "Study

Evaluating the Ketogenic Diet in Patients with Metastatic Pancreatic Cancer" on November 17, 2020.

This Phase 2 randomized trial will use two different nutritional approaches. Subjects with biopsy-proven metastatic pancreatic adenocarcinoma, not previously treated for their cancers, are eligible. They will randomly assign volunteers to one of two groups. One group will receive standard chemotherapy consisting of *nab-paclitaxel*, *cisplatin*, and *gemcitabine* given every 21 days, with a non-KD. The other arm will have the same chemotherapy plus a KD consisting of less than 30 grams of carbohydrates per day and a daily protein target of 1.5 grams/kg, the ideal body weight.

The primary outcome to be measured is progression-free survival (how long it will take to see a relapse). They will also count the number of patients who have improved their tumors as seen on imaging scans and as measured by serum cancer markers (such as CA19-9, CA125, and CEA). This trial posted no updates at the time of this writing.

7. **Lung cancer (NCT03785808):**

The R.I.G.H.T trial (Reducing Insulin, Growth Hormones, and Tumors) recruited lung cancer patients. They compared the effect of the KD versus a low-fat, high-carbohydrate, whole foods, plant-based diet versus the standard American diet (USDA control). They measured blood tests to see the effect of each diet on inflammation—Interleukin-6 (IL-6), C-reactive protein (CRP), adiponectin, IGF-1, and IGFBP-3. The study collected three patients and stopped due to a lack of enrollment.

8. Cancers with PI3K or PTEN mutation (lymphoma, uterine) (NCT04750941):

Study of Copanlisib and the KD. This multicenter, open-label, pilot Phase 2 study will recruit 23 patients with follicular Non-Hodgkin lymphoma (recurrent or refractory) and 19 patients with recurrent or refractory endometrial cancer and with a documented PI3KCA or PTEN mutation. Patients will receive the targeted therapy—PI3K inhibitor, copanlisib, plus KD.

They will record the number of patients with complete, partial, and overall response rates and observe compliance with the KD. The study was posted on clinicaltrials.gov in March 2021, with an expected completion date of December 2021. As of June 7, 2023, this study is still active but no longer recruiting.

9. Lymphoma (NCT04231734):

The Weill Medical College of Cornell University sponsored and first posted "The Ketogenic Diet in Patients with Untreated and Low Burden Mantle Cell Lymphoma" study on January 18, 2020. This single-arm Phase 1 feasibility study will recruit at least eight patients with low tumor burden, 'treatment naïve' mantle cell lymphoma, and have them follow a 12-week ketogenic diet followed by 28 days of observation. They will measure serum metabolic markers and changes in body composition and examine tumor specimens. The expected study completion date is June 2023. However, according to an online update on August 24, 2023, this study was withdrawn and is no longer active.

10. Prostate cancer:

NCT00932672

Duke University collaborated with the Greater Los Angeles Veteran Affairs Medical Center and the University of California, Los Angeles, to conduct a randomized study of the Atkins diet and androgen deprivation therapy for patients with prostate cancer. Androgen deprivation therapy, such as Leuprolide injections, often results in metabolic side effects such as insulin resistance, impaired glucose tolerance, and weight gain. Limiting carbohydrates might prevent these consequences. Unfortunately, the study was terminated early due to slow accrual, lack of funding, and relocation of the principal investigator.

NCT03194516

This study by The University of Maryland is still active but is currently not recruiting. This study observed overweight prostate cancer patients while on the eight-week KD. Blood tests before and after the diet period will measure levels of inflammation. There will be no randomization; all patients will receive the diet intervention.

NCT03679260

Carbohydrate Restricted Diet Intervention for Men on Prostate Cancer Active Surveillance is a Phase 2, waitlist-controlled, randomized trial for prostate cancer. This study (sponsored by Cedars Sinai Medical Center) aims to randomize 40 men to a carbohydrate-restricted diet versus no dietary intervention. They plan to compare the two groups' proliferative index (Ki67) differences over six months. This study is now complete, but results are not yet available.

11. Renal Cell Carcinoma (NCT04316520):

The University Hospital in Angers, France, sponsored this trial and posted it first on March 20, 2020. This pilot study will study the KD in combination with standard-of-care therapies for metastatic renal cell carcinoma (CETOREIN).

The trial started on July 22, 2020, and should be complete by May 2024. The medications involved in this study include the following: Nivolumab + Ipilimumab, Pembrolizumab + Axitinib, Sunitinib, or Pazopanib. These are combined immunotherapy and targeted therapies.

Chapter Summary/Key Takeaways:

Data from recent case reports and trials suggest that the ketogenic diet is safe and tolerable for patients with cancer.

Emerging data shows that combining a ketogenic diet with standard chemotherapy and radiotherapy may help improve tumor response and quality of life.

Examining gene expression patterns (how our genes are arranged) in mitochondria and mutations in ketolytic and glycolytic enzymes may help us predict which patients will likely benefit from ketogenic diets.

We should conduct a more extensive, randomized study. Making specific ketogenic dietary recommendations a part of our standard of care is still premature.

For now, investigators must work with existing sparse data. More research is desperately needed.

The ketogenic diet has come a long way. From being an anti-seizure diet, the ketogenic diet can potentially improve cancer outcomes and outcomes in other disease states (cardiology, endocrinology, immunology, and psychiatry).

End Notes

Buga A, Harper DG, Sapper TN, Hyde PN, Fell B, Dickerson R, Stoner JT, Kackley ML, Crabtree CD, Decker DD, Robinson BT, Krystal G, Binzel K, Lustberg MB, Volek JS. Feasibility and metabolic outcomes of a well-formulated ketogenic diet as an adjuvant therapeutic intervention for women with stage IV metastatic breast cancer: The Keto-CARE trial. *PLoS One.* 2024 Jan 2;19(1): e0296523. doi: 10.1371/journal.pone.0296523. PMID: 38166036; PMCID: PMC10760925.

Champ, C.E., and R.J. Klement, Commentary on "*Strong adverse prognostic impact of hyperglycemic episodes during adjuvant chemoradiotherapy of glioblastoma multiforme.*" Strahlenther Onkol, 2015. 191(3): pp. 281-2.

Chang, H.T., Olson, L.K. & Schwartz, K.A. Ketolytic and glycolytic enzymatic expression profiles in malignant gliomas: implication for ketogenic diet therapy. *Nutr Metab (Lond).* 10, p. 47 (2013). https://doi.org/10.1186/1743-7075-10-47.

Cohen CW, Fontaine KR, Arend RC, Alvarez RD, Leath CA III, Huh WK, Bevis KS, Kim KH, Straughn JM Jr, Gower BA. A Ketogenic Diet Reduces Central Obesity and Serum Insulin in Women with Ovarian or Endometrial Cancer. *J Nutr.* 2018 Aug 1;148(8): e1253-60. doi: 10.1093/jn/nxy119. PMID: 30137481; PMCID: PMC8496516.

Cohen CW, Fontaine KR, Arend RC, Soleymani T, Gower BA. Favorable Effects of a Ketogenic Diet on Physical Function, Perceived Energy, and Food Cravings in Women with Ovarian or Endometrial Cancer: A Randomized, Controlled Trial. *Nutrients.* 2018 Aug 30;10(9): e1187. doi: 10.3390/nu10091187. PMID: 30200193; PMCID: PMC6163837.

Elsakka AMA, Bary MA, Abdelzaher E, Elnaggar M, Kalamian M, Mukherjee P, Seyfried TN. Management of Glioblastoma Multiforme in a Patient Treated With Ketogenic Metabolic Therapy and Modified Standard of Care: A 24-Month Follow-Up. *Front Nutr.* 2018 Mar 29;5: p. 20. doi: 10.3389/fnut.2018.00020. PMID: 29651419; PMCID: PMC5884883.

Furukawa, K., Shigematsu, K., Katsuragawa, H., Tezuka, T., & Hataji, K. (2019). Investigating the effect of chemotherapy combined with ketogenic diet on stage IV colon cancer. *Journal of Clinical Oncology*, 37(15_suppl), e15182. https://doi.org/10.1200/JCO.2019.37.15_suppl.e15182.

Fine EJ, Segal-Isaacson CJ, Feinman RD, Herszkopf S, Romano MC, Tomuta N, Bontempo AF, Negassa A, Sparano JA. Targeting insulin inhibition as a metabolic therapy in advanced cancer: a pilot safety and feasibility dietary trial in 10 patients. *Nutrition.* 2012 Oct;28(10): e1028-35. doi: 10.1016/j.nut.2012.05.001. Epub 2012 Jul 26. PMID: 22840388.

İyikesici MS, Slocum AK, Slocum A, Berkarda FB, Kalamian M, Seyfried TN. Efficacy of Metabolically Supported Chemotherapy Combined with Ketogenic Diet, Hyperthermia, and Hyperbaric Oxygen Therapy for Stage IV Triple-Negative Breast Cancer. *Cureus.* 2017 Jul 7;9(7): e1445. doi: 10.7759/cureus.1445. PMID: 28924531; PMCID: PMC5589510.

Koroljow S. Two cases of malignant tumors with metastases apparently treated successfully with hypoglycemic coma. *Psychiatr Q.* 1962 Apr;36: pp. 261-70. doi: 10.1007/BF01586115. PMID: 14458502.

Maroon J, Bost J, Amos A, Zuccoli G. Restricted calorie ketogenic diet for the treatment of glioblastoma multiforme. *J Child Neurol.* 2013 Aug;28(8): e1002-8. doi: 10.1177/0883073813488670. Epub 2013 May 13. PMID: 23670248.

Martin-McGill KJ, Marson AG, Tudur Smith C, Young B, Mills SJ, Cherry MG, Jenkinson MD. Ketogenic diets as an adjuvant therapy for glioblastoma (KEATING): a randomized, mixed methods, feasibility study. *J Neurooncol.* 2020 Mar;147(1): pp. 213-27. doi: 10.1007/s11060-020-03417-8. Epub 2020 Feb 8. PMID: 32036576; PMCID: PMC7076054.

Rieger J, Bähr O, Maurer GD, Hattingen E, Franz K, Brucker D, Walenta S, Kämmerer U, Coy JF, Weller M, Steinbach JP. ERGO: a pilot study of ketogenic diet in recurrent glioblastoma. *Int J Oncol.* 2014 Jun;44(6): e1843-52. doi: 10.3892/ijo.2014.2382. Epub 2014 Apr 11. Erratum in: *Int J Oncol.* 2014 Dec;45(6): p. 2605. PMID: 24728273; PMCID: PMC4063533.

Rossi-Fanelli F, Franchi F, Mulieri M, Cangiano C, Cascino A, Ceci F, Muscaritoli M, Seminara P, Bonomo L. Effect of energy substrate manipulation on tumour cell proliferation in parenterally fed cancer patients. *Clin Nutr.* 1991 Aug;10(4): pp. 228-32. doi: 10.1016/0261-5614(91)90043-c. PMID: 16839923.

Schmidt M, Pfetzer N, Schwab M, Strauss I, Kämmerer U. Effects of a ketogenic diet on the quality of life in 16 patients with advanced cancer: A pilot trial. *Nutr Metab (Lond).* 2011 Jul 27;8(1): p. 54. doi: 10.1186/1743-7075-8-54. PMID: 21794124; PMCID: PMC3157418.

Schwartz KA, Chang HT, Nikolai M, Pernicone J, Rhee S, Olson K, Kurniali PC, Hord NG, Noel M. Treatment of glioma patients with ketogenic diets: report of two cases treated with an IRB-approved energy-restricted ketogenic diet protocol and review of the literature. *Cancer Metab.* 2015 Mar 25;3: p. 3. doi: 10.1186/s40170-015-0129-1. PMID: 25806103; PMCID: PMC4371612.

Schwartz KA, Noel M, Nikolai M, Chang HT. Investigating the Ketogenic Diet As Treatment for Primary Aggressive Brain Cancer: Challenges and Lessons Learned. *Front Nutr.* 2018 Feb 23;5: p. 11. doi: 10.3389/fnut.2018.00011. PMID: 29536011; PMCID: PMC5834833.

Seyfried TN, Shivane AG, Kalamian M, Maroon JC, Mukherjee P, Zuccoli G. Ketogenic Metabolic Therapy, Without Chemo or Radiation, for the Long-Term Management of IDH1-Mutant Glioblastoma: An 80-Month Follow-Up Case Report. *Front Nutr.* 2021 May 31;8: e682243. doi: 10.3389/fnut.2021.682243.

Tan-Shalaby JL, Carrick J, Edinger K, Genovese D, Liman AD, Passero VA, Shah RB. Modified Atkins diet in advanced malignancies - final results of a safety and feasibility trial within the Veterans Affairs Pittsburgh Healthcare System. *Nutr Metab (Lond).* 2016 Aug 12;13: p. 52. doi: 10.1186/s12986-016-0113-y. Erratum in: *Nutr Metab (Lond).* 2016;13(1): p. 61. PMID: 27525031; PMCID: PMC4983076.

Tan Shalaby, Jocelyn & Thomas, Roby & Carrick, Jennifer & Liman, Andrew & Passero, Vida & Patel, Arisha & Shields, Jenna. (2018). Modified ketogenic diet in lymphoma: A case series in the Veteran Affairs Pittsburgh Healthcare System. *Journal of Clinical Oncology.* 36. e24222. 10.1200/JCO.2018.36.15_suppl.e24222.

Van der Louw EJTM, Olieman JF, van den Bemt PMLA, Bromberg JEC, Oomen-de Hoop E, Neuteboom RF, Catsman-Berrevoets CE, Vincent AJPE. Ketogenic diet treatment as adjuvant to standard treatment of glioblastoma multiforme: a feasibility and safety study. *Ther Adv Med Oncol.* 2019 Jun 21;11: e1758835919853958. doi: 10.1177/1758835919853958. PMID: 31258628; PMCID: PMC6589986.

Van der Louw EJTM, Reddingius RE, Olieman JF, Neuteboom RF, Catsman-Berrevoets CE. Ketogenic diet treatment in recurrent diffuse intrinsic pontine glioma in children: A safety and feasibility study. *Pediatr Blood Cancer.* 2019 Mar;66(3): e27561. doi: 10.1002/pbc.27561. Epub 2018 Nov 28. PMID: 30484948.

Winter SF, Loebel F, Dietrich J. Role of ketogenic metabolic therapy in malignant glioma: A systematic review. *Crit Rev Oncol Hematol.* 2017 Apr;112: pp. 41-58. doi: 10.1016/j.critrevonc.2017.02.016. Epub 2017 Feb 20. PMID: 28325264.

Zahra A, Fath MA, Opat E, Mapuskar KA, Bhatia SK, Ma DC, Rodman SN III, Snyders TP, Chenard CA, Eichenberger-Gilmore JM, Bodeker KL, Ahmann L, Smith BJ, Vollstedt SA, Brown HA, Hejleh TA, Clamon GH, Berg DJ, Szweda LI, Spitz DR, Buatti JM, Allen BG. Consuming a Ketogenic Diet while Receiving Radiation and Chemotherapy for Locally Advanced Lung Cancer and Pancreatic Cancer: The University of Iowa Experience of Two Phase 1 Clinical Trials. *Radiat Res.* 2017 Jun;187(6): pp. 743-54. doi: 10.1667/RR14668.1. Epub 2017 Apr 24. PMID: 28437190; PMCID: PMC5510645.

Zuccoli G, Marcello N, Pisanello A, Servadei F, Vaccaro S, Mukherjee P, Seyfried TN. Metabolic management of glioblastoma multiforme using standard therapy together with a restricted ketogenic diet: Case Report. *Nutr Metab (Lond).* 2010 Apr 22;7: p. 33. doi: 10.1186/1743-7075-7-33. PMID: 20412570; PMCID: PMC2874558.

Chapter Twenty-Eight

Common Foods and Cancer Risk

High-fat, meat-heavy diets

Is there a relationship between fat intake and cancer risk?

How about red meat?

Many fear that overeating fat can worsen cancer outcomes. This book taught us that cancers prefer to make their fats versus directly using dietary fats.

Many published studies linking *high-fat diets* (HFDs) to cancers have, indeed, studied diets high in fat. Still, their carbohydrate contents were also much higher. These were not in the same category as ketogenic diets (KDs), which are high in fat but very low in carbohydrates (Tan-Shalaby, 2018).

It is well-accepted that colon cancer risk increases by consuming processed meats preserved with sodium nitrite (meat preservative). But does red meat increase cancer risk? Studies on diet are easily flawed because of confounding factors that are difficult to control. Many subjects who consume diets rich in red meat also consume high amounts of carbohydrates.

Let's look at some of the scientific studies.

Ovarian cancer:

Gurr (1999) found no evidence that HFD, high-meat diets increased the risk of ovarian cancer (pp. 187-8).

Breast cancer:

In breast cancer-induced models, there were more tumors when rats consumed HFDs (Magaki, *et al.*, 2017).

Colon cancer:

Mouse models of colon cancer were fed standard plus high-fat chow and likewise had higher cancer rates than the control (Rodriguez, *et al.*, 1988). Note that there was no effort to limit carbohydrates in the colon cancer model fed high-fat trials. The mice, therefore, ate a high fat + high carbohydrate diet. The mouse diet was not a KD. The high fat + non-low carbohydrate diet was more 'Akin' to today's standard American diet.

Liver cancer:

Mice with *non-alcoholic fatty liver disease* (NAFLD) fed low-fat/ high-carbohydrate diets had more hepatic (liver) damage and increased cancer risk compared to mice fed standard chow (control group) (Tessitore, *et al.*, 2017). Could it be that carbohydrates had a contributory role? Does the type of fat matter?

Prostate cancer:

Two separate trials of men with prostate cancer who were on low-fat, high-fiber, fruit, and vegetable diets showed no difference in serum *prostate-specific antigen* (PSA) levels compared to their baselines and controls (Shike, *et al.*, 2002; Walsh, 2003).

Fish oil supplements and breast cancer:

During the prenatal period, fish oil supplements diminished the detrimental effects of a HFD on carcinogen-induced rat mammary cancers (Su, *et al.*, 2010).

Soy, cancer growth factors, and signals:

IGF-1 and IGFBP-3 can boost cancer growth. There is concern that consuming more soy protein may promote cancer by increasing IGF-I and IGFBP-3 (McLaughlin, *et al.*, 2011). However, in the same trial, soy consumption led to decreased levels of *sex hormone-binding globulin* (SHBG), which might promote cancer growth. Chemotherapy can boost NF-κB activity in tumor cells, diminish cancer cell killing, and increase drug resistance. Therefore, NF-κB helps cancer cells survive! *Soy genistein* can counteract this and improve chemotherapy by inhibiting NF-κB activity (Li, *et al.*, 2005).

Soy and gastrointestinal cancers (colon, rectal, and stomach):

A meta-analysis of 17 studies on soy intake and colon cancer showed a protective effect of soy, significantly reducing the risk of colorectal cancer (CRC) (Yu, *et al.*, 2016). In a prospective study of 83,063 Japanese men and women ages 45 to 74, isoflavone, miso soup, and soy food intake had no connection to colorectal cancer. In the group with colon cancer, increased soy food intake lowered the risk of right-sided colon cancer (Akhter, *et al.*, 2008). Kim (2004) found that soy saponins (soy concentrates) reduced colon cancer growth, possibly inhibiting inflammation (pp. 1-6). Frequent soybean/tofu intake decreased the risk of stomach cancer (Ko, *et al.*, 2013). Finally, a 2017 soy intake meta-analysis found fewer stomach cancers in women than men (Lu, *et al.*, 2017).

Soy and breast cancers:

In a study of mice with breast cancer, soy processing influenced whether or not it encouraged cancer growth. Soy flour had no impact on development compared to soy molasses or pure soy (Allred, *et al.*, 2004).

Another study of breast cancer survivors showed that soy did not increase the risk of relapse (Harvard Women's Health Watch, 2011).

In the lab setup, breast cancer cell lines treated with the soy isoflavone genistein had an anti-cancer effect. There was a reversal of DNA *hypermethylation* and restoration of the expression of the oncosuppressor genes BRCA1 and BRCA2 (Bosviel, *et al.*, 2012). Genistein is a plant-based estrogen that has anti-cancer properties. It stops the formation of blood vessels that may supply tumors (Farina, *et al.*, 2006).

Fermented soymilk product (FSP) applied to various human breast cancer cell lines inhibited cancer growth (Chang, *et al.*, 2002).

More recently, Zhang (2009) from the Friedman School of Nutrition Science and Policy at Tufts University did an epidemiological study of 6,000 female American and Canadian breast cancer patients who consumed foods with soy-derived isoflavones (p. 501-7). Soy gave a 21% decrease in all-cause mortality. This benefit was seen only in women with hormone-receptor-negative tumors who never received hormone therapy (Zhang, *et al.*, 2009).

However, pro-tumor effects were seen in mice implanted with MCF-7 breast cancer cells and later fed with soy isoflavone extracts during adolescence or life. Both menopausal and post-menopausal models saw tumor growth (Wu, *et al.*, 2012).

Soy and prostate cancers:

A 2018 meta-analysis by the University of Illinois researchers on men who consumed soy products, which included genistein, *daidzein* (soy plant hormone counterparts), and unfermented soy food, found that they had a significantly lower risk of developing prostate cancer (Applegate, *et al.*, 2018; Adjakly, *et al.*, 2011).

There was another randomized, double-blind trial on 177 men at high risk of relapse after prostate cancer surgery. It ran for over 13 years at seven US centers. It compared daily soy protein supplementation vs. placebo and found that soy did not protect against relapse (Bosland, *et al.*, 2013).

Another recent meta-analysis of eight randomized controlled trial studies of soy and soy isoflavones in prostate cancer found no increased risk. There was a significant reduction in the diagnosis of prostate cancer in two studies after the intake of soy isoflavones (risk ratio = 0.49, 95% CI 0.26, 0.95). There were no significant differences in PSA levels or sex steroid endpoints (Van Die, *et al.*, 2014).

Soy's effect against lung and bladder cancers:

The Shanghai Women's Health Study (Shanghai, China) in 1997-2000 studied 71,550 women and found that soy intake may reduce aggressive lung cancer risk in nonsmoking menopausal women (Yang, *et al.*, 2011). Exogenous estrogens may contribute to lung cancer risk. In a subgroup study of never-smoker Asian women, soy consumption offered a statistically significant protective effect against lung cancer (Yang, *et al.*, 2011).

The Takayama study involved 14,233 men and 16,584 women aged 35 or older in September 1992. They found that over a follow-up of 13 years, higher soy intake protected against the development of bladder cancer in men (Wada, *et al.*, 2018).

Chapter Summary/Key Takeaways:

A single food item does not cause cancer—for example, meat. Frequently, it is a combination of foods that is the culprit. Often to blame for many diseases, meat does not, but it may increase risk in combination with other foods such as high carbohydrates. Conflicting results are seen with soy. The beneficial effects seem to outweigh the negatives.

We mentioned some data on plant-based diets and fish oils. I focused more on fats, meats, and soy because I often receive questions regarding the safety and benefits of consuming these when faced with a cancer diagnosis. There are indeed more foods to cover, but to discuss this topic extensively is beyond the purpose and scope of this book. Please be encouraged to read more about this topic.

FAQs

From the Facebook group "Keto For Cancer"

QUESTION 01:

Is a Mediterranean diet better as a hormone-based therapy? If high fats and animal protein can cause elevated levels of glutamine, can a ketogenic diet feed cancer?

ANSWER 01:

Mediterranean diets (MD) use plenty of olive oil, fruit, vegetables, legumes, cereals, nuts, eggs, and poultry. They also moderate the red wine, fish, seafood, yogurt, and cheese intake and discourage excess sweets and processed red meats. Sounds like a healthy diet. However, if our goal is to get into ketosis, not all Mediterranean diets are ketogenic. It all boils down to the total carbohydrate content. Too many carbs, even if on a healthy

Mediterranean diet, will not get you into ketosis. For purposes of cancer, a diet alone is an additional weapon, but should not be used as a stand-alone therapy to fight cancer. As for your question regarding high protein and a ketogenic diet. The high protein is not necessary to make a diet ketogenic. It is not a requirement to be meat or protein-heavy. Rather, the ABSENCE of high carbohydrates triggers the production of ketones. Glutamine is everywhere in your body and essential to your immune system, wound healing, and overall health. Cutting back on dietary glutamine in your diet is not possible or effective. Please review the glutamine chapters in this book to learn more.

QUESTION 02:

How much fat, protein, and carbs I am supposed to have daily? Doesn't fat also feed cancer?

ANSWER 02:

When we eat a high-fat keto diet, cancers do not grow; they die. Cancers cannot feed on fat. But they can make fat to use for creating a structure for themselves. Cancers cannot ferment fat to use as energy. Please review the chapters on fatty acid synthesis, to learn more.

QUESTION 03:

I was advised to do a plant-based diet, with the assertion that meat and dairy make breast cancer worse. I am a type 2 diabetic, and when I do the plant-based, it always spikes my blood sugar to 135 or higher.

ANSWER 03:

Plant-based diets are great for preventing cancer. However, it will be hard to get into ketosis while on a plant-based diet because to achieve ketosis, you will have to cut back on your food amounts. All vegetables are carbohydrates and will add to the daily total carbohydrate limit.

End Notes

Adjakly M, Bosviel R, Rabiau N, Boiteux JP, Bignon YJ, Guy L, Bernard-Gallon D. DNA methylation and soy phytoestrogens: quantitative study in DU-145 and PC-3 human prostate cancer cell lines. *Epigenomics*. 2011 Dec;3(6): e795-803. doi: 10.2217/epi.11.103. PMID: 22126297.

Akhter M, Inoue M, Kurahashi N, Iwasaki M, Sasazuki S, Tsugane S; Japan Public Health Center-Based Prospective Study Group. Dietary soy and isoflavone intake and risk of colorectal cancer in the Japan public health center-based prospective study. *Cancer Epidemiol Biomarkers Prev*. 2008 Aug;17(8): e2128-35. doi: 10.1158/1055-9965.EPI-08-0182. PMID: 18708407.

Allred CD, Allred KF, Ju YH, Goeppinger TS, Doerge DR, Helferich WG. Soy processing influences growth of estrogen-dependent breast cancer tumors. *Carcinogenesis.* 2004 Sep;25(9): e1649-57. doi: 10.1093/carcin/bgh178. Epub 2004 May 6. PMID: 15131010.

Applegate CC, Rowles JL, Ranard KM, Jeon S, Erdman JW. Soy Consumption and the Risk of Prostate Cancer: An Updated Systematic Review and Meta-Analysis. *Nutrients*. 2018 Jan 4;10(1): p. 40. doi: 10.3390/nu10010040. PMID: 29300347; PMCID: PMC5793268.

Bosland MC, Kato I, Zeleniuch-Jacquotte A, Schmoll J, Enk Rueter E, Melamed J, Kong MX, Macias V, Kajdacsy-Balla A, Lumey LH, Xie H, Gao W, Walden P, Lepor H, Taneja SS, Randolph C, Schlicht MJ, Meserve-Watanabe H, Deaton RJ, Davies JA. Effect of soy protein isolate supplementation on biochemical recurrence of prostate cancer after radical prostatectomy: a randomized trial. *JAMA*. 2013 Jul 10;310(2): pp. 170-8. doi: 10.1001/jama.2013.7842. PMID: 23839751; PMCID: PMC3921119.

Bosviel R, Dumollard E, Déchelotte P, Bignon YJ, Bernard-Gallon D. Can soy phytoestrogens decrease DNA methylation in BRCA1 and BRCA2 oncosuppressor genes in breast cancer? *OMICS*. 2012 May;16(5): pp. 235-44. doi: 10.1089/omi.2011.0105. Epub 2012 Feb 17. PMID: 22339411.

Chang WH, Liu JJ, Chen CH, Huang TS, Lu FJ. Growth inhibition and induction of apoptosis in MCF-7 breast cancer cells by fermented soy milk. *Nutr Cancer*. 2002;43(2): pp. 214-26. doi: 10.1207/S15327914NC432_12. PMID: 12588701.

Farina HG, Pomies M, Alonso DF, Gomez DE. Antitumor and antiangiogenic activity of soy isoflavone genistein in mouse models of melanoma and breast cancer. *Oncol Rep*. 2006 Oct;16(4): e885-91. PMID: 16969510.

Gurr MI. Diet and the prevention of cancer. No evidence has linked ovarian cancer with high intakes of fat and meat. *BMJ*. 1999 Jul 17;319(7203): pp. 187-8. PMID: 10498416.

Kim HY, Yu R, Kim JS, Kim YK, Sung MK. Antiproliferative crude soy saponin extract modulates the expression of IkappaBalpha, protein kinase C, and cyclooxygenase-2 in human colon cancer cells. *Cancer Lett.* 2004 Jul 8;210(1): pp. 1-6. doi: 10.1016/j.canlet.2004.01.009. PMID: 15172114.

Ko KP, Park SK, Yang JJ, Ma SH, Gwack J, Shin A, Kim Y, Kang D, Chang SH, Shin HR, Yoo KY. Intake of soy products and other foods and gastric cancer risk: a prospective study. *J Epidemiol.* 2013 Sep 5;23(5): pp. 337-43. doi: 10.2188/jea.je20120232. Epub 2013 Jun 29. PMID: 23812102; PMCID: PMC3775527.

Li Y, Ahmed F, Ali S, Philip PA, Kucuk O, Sarkar FH. Inactivation of nuclear factor kappaB by soy isoflavone genistein contributes to increased apoptosis induced by chemotherapeutic agents in human cancer cells. *Cancer Res.* 2005 Aug 1;65(15): e6934-42. doi: 10.1158/0008-5472.CAN-04-4604. Erratum in: Cancer Res. 2005 Dec 1;65(23):11228. PMID: 16061678.

Lu, D., Pan, C., Ye, C. *et al.* Meta-analysis of Soy Consumption and Gastrointestinal Cancer Risk. *Sci Rep.* 2017. 7(1): e4048. doi: https://doi.org/10.1038/s41598-017-03692-y.

Magaki M, Ishii H, Yamasaki A, Kitai Y, Kametani S, Nakai R, Dabid A, Tsuda H, Ohnishi T. A high-fat diet increases the incidence of mammary cancer inc-Ha-*ras* proto-oncogene transgenic rats. *J Toxicol Pathol.* 2017 Apr;30(2): pp. 145-52. doi: 10.1293/tox.2016-0052. Epub 2016 Dec 8. PMID: 28458452; PMCID: PMC5406593.

McLaughlin JM, Olivo-Marston S, Vitolins MZ, Bittoni M, Reeves KW, Degraffinreid CR, Schwartz SJ, Clinton SK, Paskett ED. Effects of tomato- and soy-rich diets on the IGF-I hormonal network: a crossover study of postmenopausal women at high risk for breast cancer. *Cancer Prev Res (Phila)*. 2011 May;4(5): e702-10. doi: 10.1158/1940-6207.CAPR-10-0329. Epub 2011 Mar 23. Erratum in: Cancer Prev Res (Phila). 2012 Mar;5(3): p. 498. Dosage error in article text. PMID: 21430071; PMCID: PMC3837570.

Rodriguez PM, Cruz NI, Gonzalez CI, Lopez R. The effect of a high fat diet on the incidence of colonic cancer after cholecystectomy in mice. *Cancer.* 1988 Aug 15;62(4): e727-9. doi: 10.1002/1097-0142(19880815)62:4<727::aid-cncr2820620414>3.0.co;2-f. PMID: 3395956.

Shike, M., Latkany, L., Riedel, E., Fleisher, M., Schatzkin, A., Lanza, E., Corle, D., & Begg, C. B. (2002). Lack of effect of a low-fat, high-fruit, -vegetable, and -fiber diet on serum prostate-specific antigen of men without prostate cancer: Results from a randomized trial. *Journal of Clinical Oncology*, 20(17): e3592–98. doi: 10.1200/jco.2002.02.040.

Soy may be okay for breast cancer survivors. Prospective studies show no increased risk of recurrence. *Harv Womens Health Watch.* 2011 Jun;18(10): pp. 1-2. PMID: 27024121.

Su HM, Hsieh PH, Chen HF. A maternal high n-6 fat diet with fish oil supplementation during pregnancy and lactation in rats decreases breast cancer risk in the female offspring. *J Nutr Biochem.* 2010 Nov; 21(11): e1033-7. doi: 10.1016/j.jnutbio.2009.08.007. Epub 2009 Dec 1. PMID: 19954943.

Tan-Shalaby JL. Dietary carbohydrate intake and mortality: reflections and reactions. *Lancet Public Health.* 2018 Nov;3(11): e517. doi: 10.1016/S2468-2667(18)30207-X. PMID: 30409400.

Tessitore A, Mastroiaco V, Vetuschi A, Sferra R, Pompili S, Cicciarelli G, Barnabei R, Capece D, Zazzeroni F, Capalbo C, Alesse E. Development of hepatocellular cancer induced by long term low fat-high carbohydrate diet in a NAFLD/ NASH mouse model. *Oncotarget.* 2017 Jun 21;8(32): e53482-94. doi: 10.18632/oncotarget.18585. PMID: 28881825; PMCID: PMC5581124.

Van Die MD, Bone KM, Williams SG, Pirotta MV. Soy and soy isoflavones in prostate cancer: a systematic review and meta-analysis of randomized controlled trials. *BJU Int.* 2014 May;113(5b): e119-30. doi: 10.1111/bju.12435. PMID: 24053483.

Wada K, Tsuji M, Tamura T, Konishi K, Goto Y, Mizuta F, Koda S, Uji T, Hori A, Tanabashi S, Matsushita S, Tokimitsu N, Nagata C. Soy Isoflavone Intake and Bladder Cancer Risk in Japan: From the Takayama Study. *Cancer Epidemiol Biomarkers Prev.* 2018 Nov;27(11): e1371-75. doi: 10.1158/1055 -9965.EPI-18-0283. Epub 2018 Aug 21. PMID: 30131436.

Walsh PC. Lack of effect of a low-fat, high-fruit, -vegetable, and -fiber diet on serum prostate-specific antigen of men without prostate cancer: results from a randomized trial. *J Urol.* 2003 Apr;169(4): e1592-3. PMID: 12641090.

Wu Q, Yang Y, Yu J, Jin N. Soy isoflavone extracts stimulate the growth of nude mouse xenografts bearing estrogen-dependent human breast cancer cells (MCF-7). *J Biomed Res.* 2012 Jan;26(1): pp. 44-52. doi: 10.1016/S1674-8301 (12)60006-2. PMID: 23554729; PMCID: PMC3596079.

Yang G, Shu XO, Chow WH, Zhang X, Li HL, Ji BT, Cai H, Wu S, Gao YT, Zheng W. Soy food intake and risk of lung cancer: evidence from the Shanghai Women's Health Study and a meta-analysis. *Am J Epidemiol.* 2012 Nov 15;176(10): e846-55. doi: 10.1093/aje/kws168. Epub 2012 Oct 24. PMID: 23097255; PMCID: PMC3626060.

Yang WS, Va P, Wong MY, Zhang HL, Xiang YB. Soy intake is associated with lower lung cancer risk: results from a meta-analysis of epidemiologic studies. *Am J Clin Nutr.* 2011 Dec;94(6): e1575-83. doi: 10.3945/ajcn.111.020966. Epub 2011 Nov 9. PMID: 22071712; PMCID: PMC3252551.

Yu Y, Jing X, Li H, Zhao X, Wang D. Soy isoflavone consumption and colorectal cancer risk: a systematic review and meta-analysis. *Sci Rep.* 2016 May 12;6: e25939. doi: 10.1038/srep25939. PMID: 27170217; PMCID: PMC4864327.

Zhang C, Ho SC, Lin F, Cheng S, Fu J, Chen Y. Soy product and isoflavone intake and breast cancer risk defined by hormone receptor status. *Cancer Sci.* 2010 Feb;101(2): e501-7. doi: 10.1111/j.1349-7006.2009.01376.x. Epub 2009 Sep 29. PMID: 19860847.

EPILOGUE

Final Thoughts

Congratulations on making it to the end of this book! We covered many topics: The ketogenic diet and the history and metabolic workings behind what makes a cancer tick.

Cancer was, and still is, largely incurable. However, we are entering exciting times. Standard therapies are getting more advanced. More doctors are using immune therapies in more cases. Targeted therapies are beginning to take over chemotherapies as the standard of care in some cancers (i.e., kidney and melanoma). Metabolic therapies are likewise emerging, but attention to this field must catch up in clinical practice and research.

You are at a good starting point. I hope this book helped you understand more about the basics of the metabolic basis of cancer. You've learned how cancers develop and manipulate their environment to survive. I reviewed some basic metabolic concepts to help you understand why a ketogenic diet is helpful against cancer.

We took a deep dive into a review of past and current clinical trials that study the ketogenic diet and its role in cancer care. Throughout this book, I also mentioned many compounds, drugs, and supplements that are relevant to each chapter. Some are investigational, while others are readily available as grocery or pharmacy food, prescription drugs, or over-the-counter. The comprehensive list is meant for information only (not medical advice). It is wise to consult your doctors before taking any medication or supplement to prevent harm from drug interactions or organ toxicity.

Take-home messages:

1. The cause of cancer is more than just one thing. We cannot blame it on a single food, mutation, or bad habit. Like a tree, many roots feed cancer and are all connected somehow.

2. Diet alone is not a cure but a powerful tool. Cancer feeds primarily on glucose but also glutamine. Lactate and fat metabolism is very active in cancers, but events come after the cancer has evolved. The sugar causes inflammation, which damages respiration in the mitochondria. This event, impaired respiration, is where cancer begins. The damaged mitochondria and upset glucose metabolism fuel and are the central origin of cancer. Once the tumor develops, it makes a lot of fat, but the role of fat is not for fuel but for building material. Lactate is high because it is a byproduct of glucose breakdown. Lactate is not a fuel, but it does help cancers metastasize, and the microenvironment can become more aggressive. We obviously cannot stop eating, but we can

prioritize what to eat and avoid what cancers love most. Glucose (sugar) is still a favorite food of cancers. Cancers that rewire to use glutamine will need novel strategies to fight them.

3. I believe that to fight cancer effectively, we need to pay more attention to cancer metabolism and examine our lifestyles. The cancer fight does not end upon achieving a first remission. To prevent relapse, a new lifestyle must replace the old. For this reason, integrative medicine is beginning to enter clinical oncology practice.

   Cancer patients often suffer from a lack of sleep, exercise, and many other things unrelated to food: excess stress, mutations, chemicals, and bad habits. To counteract these, we must learn to destress, sleep, and move more, eat less, and eat well.

4. Choose and cook your food the right way. It is better to boil, steam, or bake than deep fry, broil, or grill your food. Try to choose food that is as close to nature as possible (non-processed) and try to limit sugar. Be aware of the hidden forms of sugar like those in starches: pasta, bread, rice, and potatoes. Learn to love green vegetables and eat more seafood. Pay attention to your vitamins. More is not always better. Correct any vitamin deficiencies, but also avoid excesses. Lifestyle changes are needed to optimize an anticancer profile.

5. When cancer arrives, we try to remove, burn, and poison it with surgery, radiation, and chemotherapy. Aside from trying to kill the cancer, we should pay attention to the other things that keep it going. We now have targeted drugs that deal with oncogenes (pro-cancer genes). Still, there are different ways cancer can escape death. We need ways to target the loss of tumor suppressors, abnormal proteins, overactive cancer signaling pathways, uncoupling proteins that bring imbalance to our mitochondria, and disrupted immune systems, to name just a few. Cancer also thrives in low oxygen, stabilizing and activating hypoxia-inducible factors and, eventually, other signals. Walk more, stop smoking, and do breathing exercises daily. These are ways we can improve any low oxygen condition. The research behind hyperbaric oxygen is still emerging and seems promising. Mindful breathing helps us relax and lowers stress hormones such as cortisol.

6. Spread the word. We are already using integrative therapies in our clinical practice. Others are following and creating integrative approaches of their own. We hope to see the same happen with metabolic therapies.

About the Author

Dr. Jocelyn Tan is a Clinical Associate Professor at the University of Pittsburgh School of Medicine and the founding director of Integrative Oncology at the Veterans Affairs Pittsburgh Healthcare System. She is an internist with subspecialty board certifications in Medical Oncology and Lifestyle Medicine, trained in Integrative Oncology and Mind-Body Medicine. Dr. Tan can be found at her Facebook group, **"Keto for Cancer,"** and on the web at **www.ketoonc.com**.

Acknowledgments

I am fortunate to have worked with a group of energetic clinical and research staff who have shared my excitement about studying keto-oncology. I would like to personally thank my former clinical trainees and colleagues who supported my vision and contributed to the creation of this work:

Doctors Christine A. Garcia, M.D., MPH, Apurva Pandey, M.D., Arisha Patel, M.D., MBA, Chaoyuan Kuang, M.D., Ph.D., Hema Rai, M.D., Mariam Shalaby, M.D., Kevin A. Quann, M.D., Ph.D., Brittaney-Belle Gordon, M.D., and Jennifer Carrick, RN, MS.

Special mention goes to Dr. Thomas Seyfried and Dr. Tomas Duraj of Boston College, Dr. Nadia Shalaby of Ain Shams University, Mujahed Lateef, M.D., Zorica Kurtesevic, RN, Joseph Tan, M.D., and Sharif El Komi for their review and helpful comments.

Finally, this book would not have been possible without my family, my husband Alaa Shalaby, M.D., and children, Mariam, Yusuf, and Ramy. I am deeply grateful for their patience and endless support.

Index

Appendices

APPENDIX A: Sample Diet (a day's menu)

BREAKFAST

- Sausage
- Two eggs (any style)
- Shredded cheddar cheese (1/4 cup)
- Black coffee (1 cup)
- Optional stevia sweetener (1 tsp)
- Optional cream (1 tbsp heavy cream or almond milk)

LUNCH

- Stir-fried broccoli – 1 cup
- Fried mushrooms – 1/2 cup
- Chicken breast – 1 piece (baked or fried, non-breaded)
- Non-sweetened iced tea

DINNER

- Salmon steak (baked or broiled)
- Cauliflower rice (1 cup)
- Garden salad (½ cup)
- Seasoning (salt, garlic, butter to taste)
- A glass of unsweetened seltzer water

APPENDIX B: Acceptable Foods on Keto

Breads and Grains: None

Dairy

butter
cream cheese
heavy cream
plain coconut milk
cheeses—sliced, sticks, block, or cubed non-low-fat cheeses
sour cream

Drinks and Beverages

water (best choice)
broth
caffeine-free teas
caffeine-free coffees
club soda
liquor (Note: This should be consumed in moderation due to health risks.)
unsweetened seltzer water

Okay but not as good:
diet sodas
diet teas with a sugar substitute

Note: Try to avoid soda, and try to avoid sweeteners even if sugar-free. We want to keep the gut bacteria healthy and sweeteners might adversely change this.

Fats and Oils

canola oil
coconut oil
oil-based salad dressing
olive oil
olives (limit to 5 pieces a day)
pork rinds
real mayonnaise

Fruits

avocados

Note: Be careful to measure the amount; large avocados can easily exceed 20 grams daily.

Other Proteins

peanut butter (plain, without any added glucose, fructose, and/or sugar)
soy
tempeh
tofu

Meats

Beef:

- luncheon meats
- roast beef
- spareribs
- steaks
- veal cuts

Lamb

Pork:

- bacon
- chops
- ribs
- sausage

Poultry:

- chicken breasts
- chicken drumsticks
- chicken thighs
- duck
- eggs
- quail
- turkey
- un-breaded nuggets

Venison

Miscellaneous Items

fat bombs (homemade; be careful with the ingredients.)
fresh and dried herbs
nuts (in small amounts)
pickles
salt
pepper
spicy sauce
sugar-free jello
sugar-free sauces
sugar-free soy sauce
sugar substitutes—allulose, monk fruit, stevia
Worcestershire sauce (limit to 1 tsp a day)

Seafood

clams
cod
crab
halibut
lobster
scallops

sardines
shrimp
tuna
salmon

Vegetables

asparagus
bok choy
broccoli
Brussels sprouts
cabbage
cauliflower
celery
cucumber
eggplants
kale
lettuce
mushrooms
onions (daily limit of 2 tablespoons)
peppers
radishes
spinach
turnips
watercress
bitter melon

Note: Try to limit vegetables to 1 cup of raw serving per day or 1/2 cup of cooked serving per day. Organic food is nice but not required to achieve ketosis.

APPENDIX C: Unacceptable Foods on Keto

Breads and Grains

breads—whole wheat, rye, oat, sourdough, bagels, French toast, brioche, waffles, naan bread, breadcrumbs
cereal
chips
french fries
pasta
popcorn
potatoes
pretzels
rice
sweet potatoes
tortillas

Dairy

cottage cheese
ice cream
milk (both low-fat and skim)
ricotta
yogurt

Drinks and Beverages

beer
chocolate beverages sweetened with sugar
drinks with fructose or dextrose
fruit juices
milk
non-diet tonic water
regular soda
sugared coffee drinks
sweetened iced tea
wine

Fats and Oils

cream-based salad dressings
creamed soups
fat-free or low-fat mayonnaise
fat-free salad dressings
half and half
low-fat cream
non-fat or low-fat sour cream

Fruits

All fruits other than an avocado (dried, canned, frozen, fresh)

Other Proteins

Any peanut butter with added glucose, fructose, and/or sugar

Meats and Seafood

Any breaded or flour-covered meats
Beware of deli meats that have added sugar.

Miscellaneous Items

barbecue sauce
candy
cakes
caramel sauce
chocolate (both regular and dark)
ketchup
licorice
oatmeal
pies
sweet and sour sauce
sweet pickles

Vegetables

beans—navy, chickpeas, kidney, black beans, baked beans, refried beans
carrots
corn
peas
potatoes
pumpkin
squash
tomatoes

www.ingramcontent.com/pod-product-compliance
Lightning Source LLC
Chambersburg PA
CBHW051729260326
41914CB00040B/2027/J

* 9 7 8 0 9 8 1 5 8 2 7 5 7 *